C0-GAL-863

Immunobiology of Natural Killer Cells

Volume I

Editor

Eva Lotzová, Ph.D.
Department of General Surgery
University of Texas System Cancer Center
M.D. Anderson Hospital and Tumor Institute
Houston, Texas

Associate Editor

Ronald B. Herberman, M.D.
Pittsburgh Cancer Institute
Pittsburgh, Pennsylvania

RUTH SCARBOROUGH
LIBRARY
MAR 16 1987
0172308
SHEPHERD COLLEGE

CRC Press, Inc.
Boca Raton, Florida

Library of Congress Cataloging in Publication Data
Main entry under title:

Immunobiology of natural killer cells.

Includes bibliographies and index.
1. Killer cells. 2. Cell-mediated cytotoxicity.
I. Lotzová, Eva, 1936- . II. Herberman, Ronald B.,
1940- . [DNLM: 1. Immunity, Cellular. 2. Killer
Cells-immunology. QW 568 I317]
QR185.8.K54I46 1986 599′.029 85-12744
ISBN-0-8493-6542-2 (v.1)
ISBN-0-8493-6543-0 (v.2)

This book represents information obtained from authentic and highly regarded sources. Reprinted material is quoted with permission, and sources are indicated. A wide variety of references are listed. Every reasonable effort has been made to give reliable data and information, but the author and the publisher cannot assume responsibility for the validity of all materials or for the consequences of their use.

All rights reserved. This book, or any parts thereof, may not be reproduced in any form without written consent from the publisher.

Direct all inquiries to CRC Press, Inc., 2000 Corporate Blvd., N.W., Boca Raton, Florida, 33431.

© 1986 by CRC Press, Inc.

International Standard Book Number 0-8493-6542-2 (Volume I)
International Standard Book Number 0-8493-6543-0 (Volume II)

Library of Congress Card Number 85-12744
Printed in the United States

QR
185.8
.K54
I46
1986
v.1

PREFACE

It has become increasingly evident that natural killer (NK) cells may play an important role in defense against neoplasias and against exogenous intruders, such as viruses, bacteria, and parasites. More recent evidence also indicates involvement of NK cells in several other biological phenomena. For instance, NK cells were demonstrated to regulate growth and functions of lymphocytes, and to control proliferation and differentiation of myeloid and erythroid series of hemopoietic cells as well as pluripotential stem cells. Even though the mechanism of the effects of NK cells on hemopoiesis and lymphopoiesis has as yet not been elucidated, such regulation may be mediated by various soluble biological substances which are produced by NK cells. These are exemplified by different species of interferon, T cell and B cell growth factors, and colony-stimulating factor. It is quite plausible that NK cells, via their ability to regulate this wide array of biological functions, may represent a major component sustaining homeostasis of the organism. The early appearance of NK cells in phylogenetic development and their conservation through evolution to man, certainly supports this postulation.

Importantly, NK cells may have also a clinical relevance in cancer, nonmalignant diseases, and in the field of bone marrow transplantation. Available evidence indicates that the level of activity of these cells could be of prognostic value in relapse of leukemia or in assessing the severity of graft-vs.-host disease after allogeneic bone marrow transplantation, and perhaps these cells also may play a role in bone marrow graft rejection, benign hemopathies, and regulation of autoimmunity. There are also suggestions that NK cells may be therapeutically effective in cancer after their propagation in vitro.

The possible importance of NK cells in biology and medicine led us to review for the first time comprehensively various aspects of NK cells in a form of a book. This book will be composed of two volumes, and will include the techniques for NK cell quantification and characterization; the phylogeny and ontogeny of NK cells; the genetics of NK cell activity and the mechanisms of their functions; down- and up-regulation of NK cell activity; NK cell-suppressor cell relationships; and propagation and cloning of NK cells in vitro. We have also reviewed the cytotoxic profile of NK cells in cancer patients and its modulation by biological response modifying agents.

We hope that this book will contribute to the advancing knowledge of readers in the field of NK cells, and will be helpful as a teaching device. Furthermore, we trust that this publication will stimulate further research in this interesting and important field.

Eva Lotzová, Editor
Ronald B. Herberman, Associate Editor

THE EDITORS

Dr. Eva Lotzová is Professor of Immunology, Chief of the Division of Immunogenetics at the University of Texas System Cancer Center, M.D. Anderson Hospital and Tumor Institute, Houston. She is also Professor at the Graduate School of Biomedical Sciences, The University of Texas, Houston. Dr. Lotzová received her M.S. and Ph.D. degrees from Charles University, Prague, Czechoslovakia. She has been on the editorial boards of several scientific journals and is Editor-in-Chief of the journal *Natural Immunity and Cell Growth Regulation.* Furthermore, she is a contributing author to CRC Press and Academic Press Scientific Book Series. She has been a consultant to several governmental and private institutions in the area of biological response modification. Dr. Lotzová has been internationally recognized through her contributions to the fields of experimental bone marrow transplantation, natural cell-mediated immunity, and immunomodulation. She has contributed more than 150 publications to the scientific literature and is a member of several scientific organizations including the American Association of Immunologists, American Association for Cancer Research, Transplantation Society, and International Society for Experimental Hematology.

Dr. Ronald B. Herberman, formerly Chief of the Biological Therapeutics Branch, and Acting Associate Director for the Biological Response Modifiers Program, Division of Cancer Treatment, National Cancer Institute, Frederick, Maryland, has recently moved to Pittsburgh to become the first Director of the Pittsburgh Cancer Institute. Dr. Herberman received B.A. and M.D. degrees from New York University, graduating summa cum laude. After internship and residency in internal medicine at the Massachusetts General Hospital, Boston, Dr. Herberman joined the National Cancer Institute as a clinical associate in the Immunology Branch in 1966. He then held a series of positions at the National Cancer Institute, including Chief of the Laboratory of Immunodiagnosis. Dr. Herberman is a Diplomate of the American Board of Internal Medicine and is past president of the Reticuloendothelial Society. He has been or is currently on the editorial boards of a wide variety of oncology and immunology journals, including *Journal of Immunology, Cancer Research, Cellular Immunology, Journal of the National Cancer Institute,* and *Natural Immunity and Cell Growth Regulation.* He has published more than 600 papers in the fields of oncology and immunology and is the author of books on *Immunodiagnosis of Cancer, Natural Cell-Mediated Immunity Against Tumors,* and *NK Cells and Other Natural Effector Cells.*

CONTRIBUTORS

Paola Allavena
Visiting Fellow
Biological Therapeutics Branch
Biological Response Modifiers Program
National Cancer Institute
Frederick, Maryland
Istituto "Mario Negri"
Milan, Italy

Benjamin Bonavida
Professor
Department of Microbiology and Immunology
UCLA School of Medicine
Los Angeles, California

Robert C. Burton
Professor of Surgical Science
Faculty of Medicine
University of Newcastle
Newcastle, NSW, Australia

Denis M. Callewaert
Professor
Department of Chemistry
Oakland University
Rochester, Michigan

Edward A. Clark
Associate Professor
Department of Microbiology and Immunology
University of Washington School of Medicine
Seattle, Washington

Paula J. D'Amore
Departments of Surgery/Oncology and Pathology
UCLA School of Medicine
Los Angeles, California

Manlio Ferrarini
Associate Professor
Istituto Scientifico per lo Studio e la Cura dei Tumori
University of Genoa
Genoa, Italy

Sidney H. Golub
Professor
Department of Surgery/Oncology
UCLA School of Medicine
Los Angeles, California

Carlo E. Grossi
Department of Pathology
University of Alabama
Birmingham, Alabama

Tina Haliotis
Division of Molecular Immunology and Neurobiology
Mt. Sinai Hospital Research Institute
Toronto, Ontario, Canada

Tatsuo Kiyohara
Department of Urology
Nagasaki University School of Medicine
Nagasaki, Japan

Robert Lauzon
Division of Molecular Immunology and Neurobiology
Mt. Sinai Hospital Research Institute
Toronto, Ontario, Canada

Eva Lotzová
Professor of Immunology
Department of General Surgery and Graduate School of Biomedical Sciences
The University of Texas System Cancer Center
M.D. Anderson Hospital and Tumor Institute
Houston, Texas

John R. Ortaldo
Biological Therapeutics Branch
Biological Response Modifiers Program
National Cancer Institute
Frederick, Maryland

Sylvia B. Pollack
Research Professor
Department of Biological Structure
University of Washington School of Medicine
Seattle, Washington

Hugh F. Pross
Professor
Departments of Radiation Oncology and Microbiology and Immunology
Queen's University
Kingston, Ontario, Canada

Craig W. Reynolds
Senior Staff Fellow
Biological Response Modifiers Program
Division of Cancer Cause and Prevention
National Cancer Institute
Frederick, Maryland

John C. Roder
Division of Molecular Immunology and Neurobiology
Mt. Sinai Hospital Research Institute
Toronto, Ontario, Canada

Peter Rubin
Departments of Radiation Oncology and Microbiology and Immunology
Queen's University
Kingston, Ontario, Canada

Cherylyn A. Savary
Research Associate
Department of General Surgery
The University of Texas System Cancer Center
M.D. Anderson Hospital and Tumor Institute
Houston, Texas

Jerrold M. Ward
Laboratory of Comparative Carcinogenesis
Division of Cancer Cause and Prevention
National Cancer Institute
Frederick, Maryland

Susan C. Wright
Assistant Research Immunologist
Department of Microbiology and Immunology
UCLA School of Medicine
Los Angeles, California

IMMUNOBIOLOGY OF NATURAL KILLER CELLS

Volume I

Volume II

TABLE OF CONTENTS

Volume I

Chapter 1

ASSAYS FOR NK CELL CYTOTOXICITY — THEIR VALUES AND PITFALLS

Hugh F. Pross, Denis Callewaert, and Peter Rubin

TABLE OF CONTENTS

I. INTRODUCTION: A GENERAL OVERVIEW OF NK ASSAYS

It has been 10 years since the "background" cytotoxicity of normal human peripheral blood mononuclear cells against cultured tumor cell lines[1-4] was identified as being due to a subpopulation of lymphocytes,[5-10] now referred to as natural killer (NK) cells. Parallel observations were made simultaneously in murine systems,[11-13] and the ensuing exponential growth of the literature in this field attests to the interest that NK cells have generated in tumor biology, infectious disease, and hematopoietic regulation. It is obviously essential that in this morass of information we have some idea as to what we are talking about when we refer to NK cells and how we measure and quantitate their activity. In this chapter we will deal primarily with human systems and focus on aspects of NK assays which relate to quantification and the implications of using different techniques to measure NK function. The majority of information is applicable to murine systems as well.

The first question which must be assessed is "What is a natural killer cell?" Our original definition was "a lymphocyte found in the blood of normal individuals capable of lysing tumor cell lines in the apparent absence of disease, prior sensitization, or deliberate immunization". The definition is a functional one and has three components which restrict it in comparison with the definition of other cells which may be capable of tumor cell lysis — it is a lymphocyte, the donor is normal, and there is no sensitization. By this definition, the ability of macrophages (or any other nonlymphocytic cells) from normal donors to lyse NK-sensitive tumor targets does not make them NK cells and, similarly, cultured (i.e., in vitro activated) lymphocytes cannot be called NK cells simply because an NK sensitive target is lysed by them. Thus, although this definition was useful in defining the normal "fresh" NK cell and, conversely in categorizing tumor cells with respect to NK sensitivity, it fell short of what was needed in the analysis of patient populations or in studies of long-term cultured cells (greater than 48 hr). Considerable research has since been devoted to searching for markers which, alone or in combination, allow one to categorize a cell as being an NK cell with reasonable certainty and economy of effort. In this approach, the primary aim has been to find markers which identify virtually all NK cells, with regard for interesting but, in this context, nonuseful markers which are only on a proportion of the cells. Conversely, such markers must discriminate between NK and other cells, especially other cytotoxic cells. The remarks which follow reflect our own bias in this field, a bias which is best judged in the context of the other chapters in this book. At the onset, it should be pointed out that we are interested in identifying the majority population of NK cells, and believe that other cytotoxic lymphocytes which function differently should be identified, characterized, and named differently, as subpopulations of naturally occurring cytotoxic (NOC)[14] cells in general. Thus, while there may be heterogeneity in NOC cells, we define the NK cell fairly rigidly according to target (K562),[6,15] Fc gamma receptor status (positive),[5-9] and morphology (large granular lymphocyte [LGL]).[16,17] This definition applies to virtually all NK cells preexisting in peripheral blood and allows rapid identification of the nature of granulocyte-monocyte depleted lytic cells by (1) the elimination of lytic activity by depletion of Fc receptor (FcR)-positive cells, e.g., by EA rosette depletion, (2) the enrichment of cytotoxicity in the light density fractions of Percoll gradients, and (3) the demonstration of parallel effects of these procedures on the lysis of K562 by fresh peripheral blood lymphocytes (PBL). At present, we are reserving judgment on monoclonal antibodies (MoAbs) such as HNK-1,[18] N901,[19] and B73.1[20] for the exclusive identification of NK cells because of the high proportion of non-NK cells which are "marked" by them. A recently described MoAb B73.1 (Leull),[20] which is directed against the FcR, is more selective than HNK-1 and, like HNK-1, binds to virtually all NK cells. MoAb-defined markers on NK cells are discussed elsewhere in this volume and have proven to be extremely valuable in attempts to define the lineage of the NK cell. We feel, however, that it is not valid to describe the proportions of cells displaying currently available NK markers as being equivalent to either NK cells per se or NK function. This is a rapidly developing field, however, and the discovery of the elusive specific NK cell marker is only a matter of time.

Throughout this introduction we have referred to the erythroleukemia line K562 as the target of choice for the detection of NK cells. This cell line was developed by Lozzio and Lozzio[21] from the pleural effusion of a patient with chronic myelogenous leukemia in blast crisis. The line has many characteristics which make it unique and its selection by Jondal and Pross[6] from 19 other cell lines tested at the time was based on this fact. Its widespread use has resulted in a remarkable degree of consistency in the literature and has simplified the comparison of data from different laboratories. K562 was primarily selected for three reasons — its high NK sensitivity in short-term assays, the absence of Epstein-Barr nuclear antigen, and the fact that it is HLA-negative.[22] From the practical point of view, it is a suspension culture and therefore does not require trypsinization, a procedure which could affect NK target "antigens". Other T cell lines such as Molt-4[6] and HSB[23] are also highly sensitive but are not HLA-negative which, theoretically, could interfere with the interpretation of studies of mixed lymphocyte culture (MLC)-induced unrestricted cytotoxicity (see accompanying chaper in this volume) or of data obtained using lymphocytes from populations such as multiparous women or transplant recipients. The Chang cell line (hepatic carcinoma-derived) is also used by some investigators, but is comparatively insensitive. It has the advantage of being a good target in antibody-dependent cell-mediated cytotoxicity (ADCC) assays so that NK and K cells can be quantitated with one target.[24] The value of using K562 lies in the wealth of published experience with it. A pitfall in its sole use is that fine differences in effector lytic ability might not be detected and that interesting examples of heterogeneity in NOC cells could be overlooked.[26-28] Kimber and Moore[27] have reported on tonsillar lymphocytes which lyse K562, although weakly, and are not LGL although they possess low buoyant density and Masucci et al.[28] have described several populations of cytotoxic cells differing in Fc and E receptor status as well as the ability to lyse K562 and Daudi target cells. Another example of heterogeneity is the cell which mediates lysis of Herpes simplex virus (HSV)-infected fibroblasts, the so-called NK(HSV) cell.[26] This cell differs in function and surface markers (Ia+) from NK cells vs. K562 and unlike NK (K562) is unaffected by diseases such as severe combined immunodeficiency and certain leukemias.[26] Studies using USV-infected targets are also reported elsewhere in the book.

Many technical aspects of cytotoxicity assays were discussed in Bloom and David's text on in vitro cell-mediated immunity[29] and will not be dealt with in depth here since they still apply. However, there are four items relevant to NK assays that should be mentioned. They are mycoplasma infection, monocyte contamination, the time of assay, and the serum used in the assay. Mycoplasma contamination must be avoided since it enhances NK cytotoxicity,[30] especially when less-sensitive cell lines are used as targets. It has been postulated that NK activity itself is an artifact due to and dependent on mycoplasma contamination, but this is not so. The issue of monocyte contamination is less critical. Monocytes will apparently lyse K562 in short and long term (overnight) assays[31] but the monocyte-K562 ratio in iron plus magnetism, nylon wool passaged, or plastic-adhered cell preparations is ineffective in causing significant lysis. Although we believe that monocytes should be routinely removed from the mononuclear cells before doing NK assays, most investigators[5-9] have reported no effect or an increase in K562 lysis following monocyte depletion and do not usually remove them

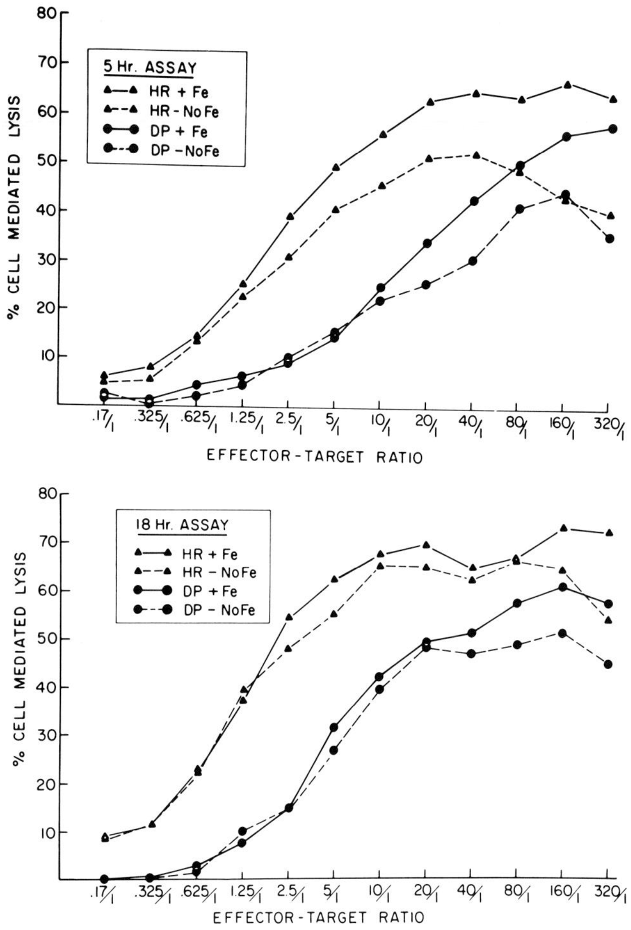

FIGURE 1. A comparison of NK assay results of a high NK donor (triangles) and low NK donor (circles) showing the effects of monocyte depletion (solid lines) vs. no depletion (dotted lines) in 5 hr vs. 18 hr assays. Monocytes were removed by iron plus magnetism (Fe) as described in the text. Both preparations contained approximately 5% phagocytic cells predepletion and approximately 0.5% postdepletion. Any cell containing one or more phagocytosed antibody-coated ox red blood cells was scored as positive; 400 cells were counted by two independent observers.

unless the cells are going to be further fractionated. Figure 1 shows the results of a set of NK assays done to demonstrate the effect of monocytes on NK activity against K562 in 5 and 18 hr assays. It can be seen that in the preparations which were not treated with iron plus magnetism (dotted lines), the NK activity was suppressed. This suppression was greater than would be expected simply on the basis of a dilution effect caused by the contaminating monocytes, which in this case made up only 5% of each of the total mononuclear cell populations (as judged by the phagocytosis of antibody-coated ox red blood cells). It is interesting that the effects were less marked in the overnight assay. We have also found that the proportion of monocytes recovered in routine Ficoll-Isopaque preparations varies markedly, especially in patient populations, and that this introduces an unnecessary variable. On the other hand, it may be said that the monocyte-containing mononuclear cell preparation more closely reflects in vivo reality because of possible cell-cell interactions and regulatory effects of monocytes. For this reason some investigators have routinely used the whole blood assay.[32,33] The whole blood assay combines the potential advantage of reflecting the in vivo situation with the disadvantage of containing a large proportion of granulocytes which may be inhibitory[34] per se or may inhibit simply because they are dying. Of course, the whole blood assay also incorporates autologous plasma. In our hands the effect of autologous serum on NK activity has varied markedly, even among normal donors. This is not related to the occasional presence of immune complexes.[34a] In an early study, the authors proved conclusively that the use of human AB positive, fetal calf, agamma newborn calf, or autologous serum, either in the assay itself or when used for long-term (>1 year) culture of the target cells had no effect on the presence or absence of NK-mediated lysis and made no difference to the rank order of cytotoxicity by NK cells from different donors.[35] The issue of the time of assay is perhaps more controversial. The short-term assay restricts the range of target cells judged as being NK-susceptible and, in some cases, differences between normal people and NK-deficient donors such as patients with Chediak-Higashi syndrome[36] appear to be more profound in short term assays.[37] It is possible that the induction of interferon (IFN) by the target cell may influence results in longer assays[38] but studies using anti-IFN to deplete in vitro IFN levels have shown little effect on NK activity vs. K562.[39] Assay results in which differences at 5 hr are apparently greater than at 18 hr are usually seen when the NK activity after 5 hr is below the threshold of detection of the assay for low NK donors, making comparisons with normal donors inaccurate. Theoretically, this may result in statistically significant differences in 5 hr assays becoming nonsignificant in 18 hr assays, but we have not observed this to happen in practice (e.g., in comparing Chediak-Higashi patients at 5 vs. 18 hr). The probability of this happening is lessened if the data are calculated accurately using equations such as the exponential fit equation (see below), which gives a more accurate expression of lytic units (LU) than does simple linear regression. In our laboratory, we usually do overnight assays and find that although absolute cytotoxicity is higher, the relative cytotoxicity of the individual donor to the group mean is usually the same as at 5 hr.[40] This is also illustrated in Figure 1. By comparing the effector-target ratios at similar levels of cell-mediated lysis (CML), it can be seen that there is approximately an eight fold difference between the high and low donors, and that this proportion is similar at both the 5 and 18 hr time points. This reflects our experience generally, although we have not done a large number of routine assays at both time points.

The concept of relative cytotoxicity or relative NK (RNK) is fundamental to NK assays because, whatever assay time, serum source, or cell line target is used, there is always day-to-day variability in the absolute level or cytotoxicity observed.[40-42] While some of this may be due to donor-related variables of which the investigator may be unaware, such as medications (e.g., prednisone,[43] aspirin,[44] dilantin[45]), smoking,[46] moderate exercise,[47] or "recreational" drug use (e.g., isobutyl nitrite[48]), it is mostly attributable to variability in the sensitivity of the target.[41] The problem is compounded by what we believe to be the greatest pitfall in assays of NK function — failure to express the data appropriately.

II. DATA EXPRESSION IN STANDARD CHROMIUM RELEASE ASSAYS

The most common method of assessing NK function is to use the chromium release assay in which fixed number of ^{51}Chromium(^{51}Cr)-labeled target cells are incubated with varying numbers of effector cells.[49] The percent CML is calculated from the following equation:

$$\% \text{ CML} = \frac{\text{CPM test} - \text{CPM spont}}{\text{CPM max} - \text{CPM spont}} \times 100\% \qquad (1)$$

where CPM test refers to the counts in supernatants from wells containing effector cells, CPM spont is the spontaneous release in medium only, and CPM max is the maximum incorporated counts obtained by lysis with detergent or by resuspension of the target cells. Usually four or more serial twofold dilutions are made of the effector cells, and each effector target ratio is plated in triplicate so that one lymphocyte preparation occupies 1 row of a 12-well, 8-row microtiter plate. Most investigators use microtiter plates instead of tubes, so that the assay can be "miniaturized" and many assays can be set up and harvested rapidly. In our studies, we use eight-prong multiple pipettors and deliver the supernatants symmetrically into 0.5 mℓ plastic tubes (LP2 tubes, Luckham Labs, Burgess Hill, U.K.) placed in flat-bottomed microtiter plates. The only advantage of the tube technique over the plate technique, aside from being necessary if large volumes have to be used, is that in the tube technique both supernatant and pellets are usually counted, which gives a more accurate expression of percent ^{51}Cr release and acts as a check that a similar number of labeled targets was added to each assay. It is also unnecessary to do separate tubes for the maximum counts. The assessment of maximum counts in microtiter plates can itself lead to some problems and pitfalls. We have found that the maximum ^{51}Cr release as defined by detergent lysis is never equal to the total incorporated label, usually being about 85 to 90% of the total.[40] On the other hand, resuspension of adherent targets is difficult and may give incorrectly low and very variable counts. In either case, the maximum Cr release as defined by the asymptote of CML is usually lower than values derived from either detergent-treated wells or resuspended wells. To avoid incorrect maximum counts with adherent targets, we use detergent in the wells to prevent adherence and then resuspend for total counts. To deal with the fact that the asymptote of the dose response curve is below 100% as defined by either detergent lysis or resuspension, the data must be mathematically reduced by nonlinear regression analysis.

III. THE ANALYSIS OF NK DATA

The methods and rationale for using nonlinear regression analysis for evaluating cytotoxicity data have been discussed at length by the authors and others in several previous publications.[25,40,50-56] Our own experience is with the "exponential fit" equation and the von Krogh equation.[40] The exponential fit equation may be written as follows:

$$y = A(1 - e^{-kx}) \qquad (2)$$

where y is the fractional Cr release, A is a constant equal to the asymptote of the curve, x is the E/T ratio, and k is a constant which, for curves having the same asymptote, is directly proportional to the NK activity. If the assay is plotted as a target survival curve, i.e., as $\ln(A-y)$ vs. x, the value k is the negative of the slope of resultant straight line. The exponential fit equation defines a sigmoid curve on a semilog plot (e.g., Figure 2) and, in our studies, this type of curve fit the data well. The von Krogh equation also defines a sigmoid curve, but contains a third variable which makes it possible to fit data in which there is a longer "lag phase" and a more abrupt rise in cytotoxicity in the exponential part of the curve.[54] To show the parallel with the exponential fit equation, the von Krogh equation can be written as follows:

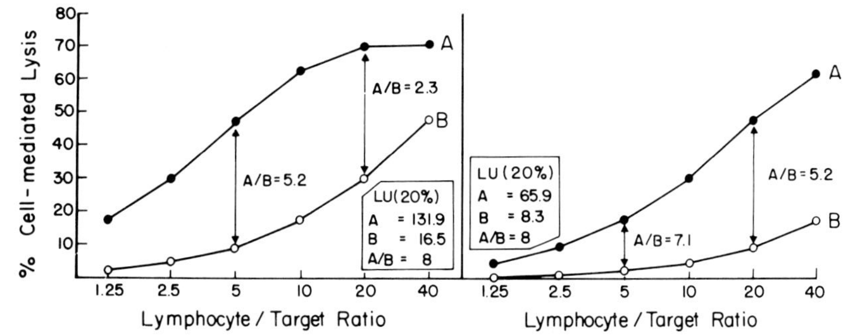

FIGURE 2. A diagram to illustrate the effect of expressing data as percent chromium release at an arbitrarily chosen E/T ratio on the expression of relative NK (RNK) of line A vs. line B. The lines were plotted using the exponential fit equation so that there is an eightfold difference between them in both cases. Because the curves are not linear, and because the absolute cytotoxicity may vary from time to time, comparing percent chromium release data can yield the rank order of two donors but not the proportion of one to the other. The diagram illustrates that the relative NK result as calculated by exponential fit equation is independent of assay variability [A/B = 8]. Right side: low K562 sensitivity; left side: high K562 sensitivity. This is not the case if percent lysis values are compared [A/B = 2.3, 5.2, or 7.1 depending on the reference point]. The von Krogh equation may be used similarly if "A" and "n" are constant.

$$y = \frac{A}{1 + (K/x)^n} \tag{3}$$

where y, x, and A are as in the exponential fit equation, n is a constant which defines the shape of the curve on the "standard" semilog plot, and K is a constant equal to x at y = 50% and is directly proportional to NK activity. (It is different from the k value of the exponential fit curve.) A family of curves with the same n and A will yield a series of parallel straight lines when plotted as $\ln(y/A-y)$ vs. ln x. We were unaware when describing these curves previously[40] that this form of data expression is known as the Hill transformation[55] and was used by Hill in 1910 to plot the binding of oxygen to hemoglobin,[58] 6 years before von Krogh described the equation named after him.[59] Fortran and Microsoft BASIC programs for the calculations described in this section are available on request.

The main reason for using such plots is to reduce a series of dose response data to a single number (with standard errors, etc.) which is based on all the data and whose value is directly proportional to NK lytic activity. This value is the k value of the exponential fit equation and the K value of the von Krogh equation; these values can be used to compare one dose response curve to another providing that the plateau (A) values are the same and, in the von Krogh equation, that n is the same for all the lines being compared. The plots are still valid if the constants are different but the k or K ratios between different lines are not an accurate expression of relative activity. These equations can also be used to calculate LU,[49] i.e., the value of x at a defined y, usually expressed as $LU/10^6$ effector cells, and the calculation of LU using these equations is more accurate than linear regression through the points on the exponential part of the curve.[40]

The point of these maneuvers is to obtain valid data which can be handled statistically and which yields meaningful numbers. This is illustrated in Figure 2. This figure shows 2 sets of curves plotted by the exponential fit equation to represent data obtained on different days in which the sensitivity of the target cells varied markedly. It can be seen from this figure that choosing an arbitrary E/T ratio to express percent cytotoxicity results in markedly different relative cytotoxicity both from day-to-day and depending on the E/T ratio chosen. The ratio of the k values or LU values is constant on both occasions because the curves were plotted with an eightfold difference in NK activity between them. The ratios of the LU values should (and do) give this result whatever the absolute cytotoxicity. The ratio of K values determined from the von Krogh equation can be used similarly, providing n and A are the same.

Because NK donors tend to be fairly constant in the rank order of their NK activity,[41] we routinely express our data as k (or LU) relative to the mean k value of a panel of normal fresh or cryopreserved controls done at the same time and corrected for their previously established NK activity relative to all normals.[42]

$$\text{RNK patient} = \frac{\text{k patient}}{\text{mean corrected control k}} \tag{4}$$

In this method, the k value from a particular contol donor who may be a "2 times normal" in terms of his NK activity (as defined over many previous assays) is corrected accordingly before the mean of all the controls is calculated. The application of these methods to patient populations has been discussed in depth recently.[42] The method has the advantage of relating to actual lytic activity, as discussed, as well as reducing intra-assay variation in data expression. It also makes the comparison of results between laboratories simpler since the average value for normal donors is by definition 1.0.

IV. KINETIC QUANTIFICATION OF NATURAL CYTOTOXICITY

An alternate approach to the quantification of cellular cytotoxicity reactions involves utilization of a kinetic model and equations that were originally derived for the study of simple enzyme-catalyzed reactions.[60] Kinetic analysis of cytotoxicity reactions was first applied to the study of cytotoxic T cells[61] followed by antibody-dependent cytotoxicity[62] and natural cytotoxicity.[63] While the use of these methods has been limited to date, recent advances in methods for data analysis and in the interpretation of the biological significance of the kinetic parameters obtained, to be discussed below, should have a significant impact on their use for the study of natural cytotoxicity.

A. A Kinetic Model for Natural Cytotoxicity

The proper application and interpretation of a kinetic method for cellular cytotoxicity reactions requires an understanding of the model on which it is based. A simple kinetic model for natural cytotoxicity, analogous to the one most frequently used for simple enzyme-catalyzed reactions, is presented in Figure 3. Here k_1 is the rate constant for the formation of an effector-target conjugate, k_{-1} is the rate constant for the nonlytic dissociation of a conjugate, and k_2 is the rate constant for target cell lysis. While the lysis of a target cell by an NK cell probably involves a number of additional steps, this simple model is still a valid representation of the rate-determining steps of the overall process.

For the model presented in Figure 3 one can derive the following equation:[64]

$$v = \frac{V_{max}[T]}{K_M^{app} + [T]} \tag{5}$$

where v is the rate of target cell lysis, [T] is the concentration of target cells tested, and V_{max} and K_M^{app} are defined by

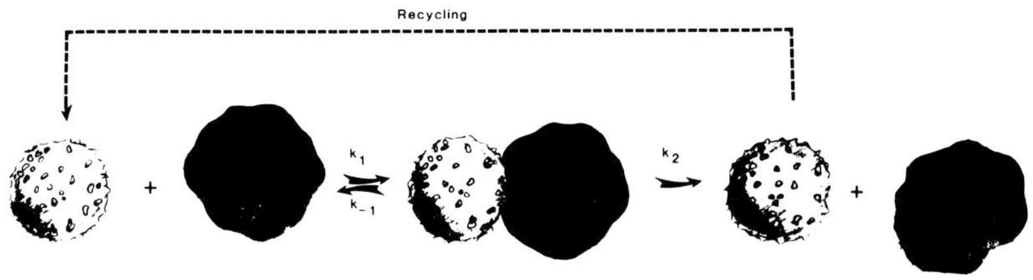

FIGURE 3. A kinetic model for natural cytotoxicity. The effector cell and the larger target cell combine to form an effector-target conjugate. The conjugate may then dissociate or lead to the destruction of the target cell with k_2 being the rate constant for the slow step in this process. The effector cell is then free to recycle, i.e., bind and lyse another target cell.

$$V_{max} = k_2[E] \tag{6}$$

$$K_M^{app} = K_M + [E] \tag{7}$$

for which [E] is the total concentration of NK effector cells in the assay that are capable of lysing the target cell employed and K_M, the standard Michaelis constant, is equal to $(k_{-1} + k_2)/k_1$.

Experimentally, the rate of lysis, v, is calculated using the equation:

$$v = \frac{\%CML[T]}{100t} \tag{8}$$

where t is the length of the assay in hours and %CML, the percentage of target cells lysed is determined by Equation 1.

Plots of v vs. [T] for natural cytotoxicity reactions yield a hyperbolic curve (Figure 4A) as predicted for the model presented in Figure 3. Furthermore, the values of K_M^{app} and V_{max} can be determined from a linear transformation of Equation 5, as shown in Figure 4B.

B. Interpretation of Experimentally Determined Kinetic Parameters

The maximal velocity, V_{max}, for a natural cytotoxicity reaction is a useful quantitative measure of the overall cytotoxic activity of the lymphocyte preparation against the target cell tested. As predicted (Equation 6), V_{max} increases linearly with increases in the concentration of lymphocytes in the assay. Thus V_{max} values are useful for the quantitative comparison of the relative cytotoxic activity of different lymphocyte preparations, as are appropriately calculated LU values.[40] Direct comparison of these two methods has demonstrated that they yield comparable estimates of relative cytotoxic activity.[56]

Interpretation of the physical significance of the apparent Michaelis constant, K_M^{app}, for natural cytotoxicity reactions has been more difficult. By analogy to simple enzyme-catalyzed reactions, early studies suggested that K_M^{app} was a measure of the dissociation constant for effector-target conjugates.[63,65,66] However, this interpretation requires the assumption that [E] is negligible compared to [T] and that $K_{-1} << k_2$ so that Equation 7 reduces to $K_M^{app} = k_{-1}/k_1$. While these assumptions are valid for many, but not all, enzyme-catalyzed reactions in vitro, they are not necessarily true for cytotoxicity reactions. In fact, K_M^{app} is not constant for cytotoxicity reactions but varies with the concentration of lymphocytes tested.[61-64] Recent experiments designed to determine the relative contribution of K_M and [E] to experimentally determined values

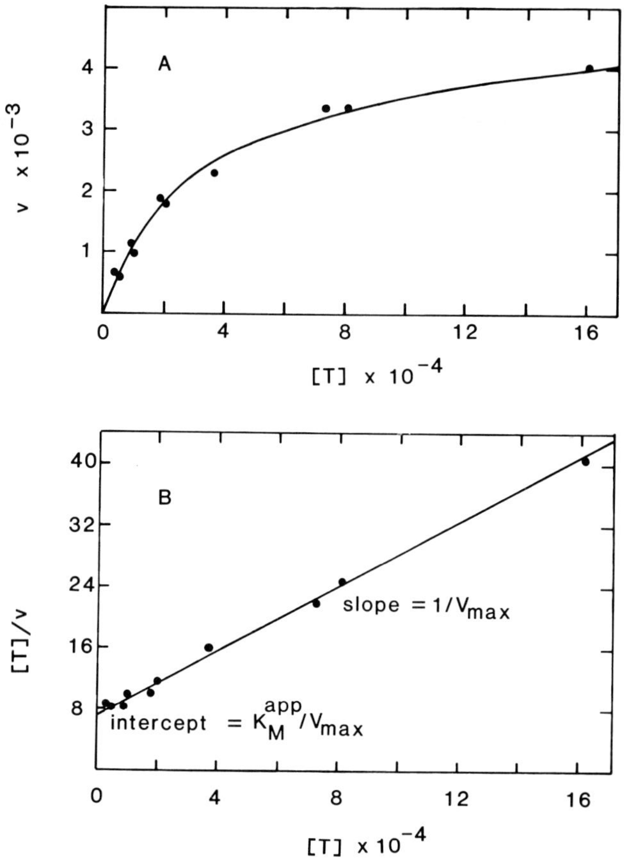

FIGURE 4. The fit of natural cytotoxicity data to the Michaelis-Menten equation. (A) A plot of v vs. [T] for natural cytotoxicity of HSB-2 target cells yields a hyperbolic curve typical of Michaelis-Menten kinetics. (B) The same data is plotted using the Hanes linear transformation of the Michaelis-Menten equation. Distribution-free statistical analysis of this data yields the following kinetic parameters (and 90% confidence intervals): $K^{app}{}_M = 3.49 \times 10^4$ ($3.13 - 3.56 \times 10^4$, $v_{max} = 4.72 \times 10^3$ ($4.59 - 4.85 \times 10^3$), and calculated values for %NK = 9.00 (8.07 − 9.18) and $k_2 = 0.135$ (0.133 − 0.138).

for K_M^{app} demonstrated that, for natural and antibody-dependent cellular cytotoxicity of various cell lines, $K_M << [E]$ so that K_M^{app} is approximately equal to [E].[64] This experimental situation does not allow for measurement of an effector-target dissociation constant. However, it is fortuitous in that is allows for the simultaneous determination of the frequency and activity of NK effector cells. The frequency of NK effector cells (%NK) in a given lymphocyte population can be estimated from the relationship:

$$\%NK = K_M^{app}/[L] \tag{9}$$

where [L] is the concentration of lymphocytes tested. The lytic activity per NK cell can also be evaluated in terms of k_2, the rate constant for the rate determining step of the reaction, using a rearrangement of Equation 6 and the fact that $K_M^{app} = [E]$:

$$k_2 = V_{max}/K_M^{app} \tag{10}$$

While K_M^{app} has been shown to be directly proportional to [E], one should use caution in the application of Equations 9 and 10 since the model on which they are based (Figure 3) is a simplification. For example, this model assumes one recognition site per NK cell, which is unlikely. Using this method, calculated values for %NK generally range from 3 to 20% of peripheral lymphocytes. These are probably overestimates. Likewise, calculated values for k_2 generally range from 0.02 to 0.2 target cells per hour per NK cell and are probably underestimates. Nevertheless, calculated values for %NK and k_2 are proportional to the NK cell frequency and lytic activity of a given lymphocyte preparation, and are therefore useful for quantitative comparisons between different donors, or for the study of effects of various drugs and metabolites on the frequency and activity of NK cells in a given lymphocyte preparation.

C. Statistical Methods for Determining Kinetic Parameters

Initial applications of kinetic methods to the study of natural cytotoxicity involved linear least-squares regression analysis of median v values using the Lineweaver-Burke (1/v vs. 1/[T]) transformation of the Michaelis-Menten equation.[63,65,66] The apparent precision of the kinetic parameters obtained by this approach was often unacceptable, partly because all of the data obtained at each [T] is reduced to a single mean value. In addition, the linear least-squares regression method is not intended for use with so few data points (4 to 10) and the Lineweaver-Burke transformation unequally weighs data obtained at low target cell concentrations.[67] Recently, the Hanes transformation ([T]/v vs. [T]) of the Michaelis-Menten equation and a powerful distribution-free statistical method have been adapted for use in the quantification of natural cytotoxicity reactions.[56] The median values for K_M^{app} and V_{max} obtained by this approach are not significantly different from the values obtained by previous methods, but the confidence intervals obtained are considerably narrower since all of the experimental data is included in the calculations. The distribution-free procedure requires rank-ordering of literally thousands of slope and intercept estimates, which is not practical without the aid of an appropriate computer program; however an available Fortran program[56] makes this a simple process.

D. Additional Considerations

The presence of nonviable cells in target cell cultures have recently been demonstrated to inhibit the lysis of the ^{51}Cr-labeled cells, thereby altering the experimentally determined kinetic parameters.[68] In addition to maintaining target cell cultures at high viability, one can correct for this inhibition by application of the following equations:

$$K_M^{app} = K_M^{observed}(1 + X) \tag{11}$$

$$V_{max} = V_{max}^{observed}(1 + X) \tag{12}$$

where X is the ratio of nonviable:viable cells in the target cell preparation.

The experimentally determined kinetic parameters for cytotoxicity reactions are also sensitive to inhibition by dead target cells that accumulate during the assay. Inhibition of this type is most likely to occur at low target cell concentrations for which a higher percentage of the target cells are lysed over a given time period. Product inhibition by lysed targets results in nonlinear Hanes plots and a simple correction factor cannot be employed. However, by using short-term assays, in which relatively few targets are lysed, this effect can be minimized. In addition, one can test for this type of inhibition by recalculating K_M^{app} and V_{max} after deleting data obtained at the lowest target cell concentration.[68] If this test results in a significant reduction in the observed value for K_M^{app}, then product inhibition at the low target cell concentrations is indicated.

Kinetic equations have also been derived for competitive inhibition of natural cytotoxicity by unlabeled viable cells homologous to the radiolabeled target cells.[68,69] The presence of homologous unlabeled inhibitor cells does not alter the observed value for V_{max}, but does result in an increase in the observed value for K_M^{app} compared to the value obtained in the absence of inhibitor cells. The magnitude of this increase can be predicted using the equation:

$$K_M^{observed} = K_M + [E] + [I] \tag{13}$$

where [I] is the concentration of inhibitor cells added to the assay.

Heterologous unlabeled inhibitor cells also exhibit a competitive inhibition pattern.[69] However, it has not yet been possible to derive suitable equations to predict or interpret the magnitude of inhibition in this case.

It is important to recognize that two of the situations discussed above, i.e., inhibition of natural cytotoxicity by nonviable or lysed target cells generated during the assay, should also influence LU values obtained in other assay systems.

V. THE SINGLE CELL NK ASSAY

In the study of human NK cells the overall cytotoxic activity of the effector cell population has been the primary source of information. In attempting to determine why individuals differ in their respective cytolytic capability it is important to bear in mind that the overall cytolytic activity is a function of two parameters: the frequency of the effector cell and its inherent recycling potential.

Various techniques have been used to assess effector cell frequency: limiting dilution analysis,[70] modified plaque assays,[71] kinetic analysis (see above), and recently, a single cell assay originally developed to determine cytotoxic T lymphocytes (CTL) frequency in murine spleen cell populations.[72,73] The development of the single cell assay in agarose was a major breakthrough in the field of cell-mediated cytotoxicity (CMC).[72-76] In this assay,[75] lymphocytes are conjugated with target cells, suspended in molten agarose, and incubated at 37°C on agarose-coated slides for varying lengths of time (usually 5 hr). The NK cell is prevented from recycling by the agar and the dead target cell can be identified by staining with trypan blue. The slides may then be fixed and the conjugates and lytic conjugates counted. The method has permitted investigators to directly determine the frequency of actively lytic cells, the kinetics of CML and the effect of drugs, biological response modifiers, and disease on NK frequency.[75,76] The original assay and modifications of it have also been used to define the phenotype of conjugate-forming cells (CFC) and lytic cells.[76-79]

Defining the phenotype of the CFC is essential to studies of NK specificity, NK binding kinetics, and the mechanism of action of NK modulating agents. We have consistently found that approximately 30 to 40% of lymphocytes bind to the tumor cell K562,[77] while other investigators have reported lower values of 10 to 20%.[74,80] This discrepancy may be partly due to our use of modified Cunningham chambers to enumerate conjugates.[79] The chambers have many advantages, one of which is the fact that the weight of the coverslip does not disrupt the conjugates. Whatever the frequency of conjugates observed is, the frequency of lytic NK cells is in the order of 1 to 5%. It is obvious from these figures that not all CFC can be NK cells. However, as Saksela et al.[81] and Opremack et al.[82] have demonstrated with conjugate depletion experiments, all NK cells are found within the conjugate pool.

The phenotype of the CFC has been ascertained using rosette and fluorescent monoclonal techniques.[77,78,83] The majority of conjugates were shown to be T cells, with the percentage of E rosette-forming conjugates being identical to the percentage of lymphocytes that formed E rosettes. While this might suggest that conjugate formation is a random event, we and others[77,78,83] have observed that the percentage of CFC that were stained with the NK "specific" markers OKM1, HNK-1 and Mac-1, was greater than the percentage of lymphocytes identified with these antibodies. Furthermore, Timonen et al.[16,84] have noted that the frequency of LGLs binding to K562 was four times higher than expected on the basis of their distribution in the lymphocyte pool. Thus, conjugates occur between NK targets and most lymphocyte subpopulations and, although binding parallels NK sensitivity to some extent,[79,85] by far the majority of CFC are neither NK nor pre-NK. It is interesting that variations in the technique which yield a high (30 to 40%) or low (10 to 15%) proportion of total conjugates by PBL have very little influence on the frequency of lytic cells expressed as a percent of lymphocytes as a whole.

The single cell assay itself has been used in both basic and clinical applications and has yielded much information concerning the mechanism of NK cytotoxicity. The examples which follow illustrate the value of this technique in the study of NK function. Ullberg and Jondal[80] have attempted to quantitate the recyclability of NK cells by applying Michaelis-Menten kinetics to an analysis of target cell lysis in conjunction with a single cell and ^{51}Cr release assay. By computing the V_{max} or maximum killing potential of the lytic process, a maximum recycling capacity value could be determined by dividing the V_{max} by the absolute number of killer cells. The methodology was applied to experiments designed to determine the mechanism of the effect of IFN on NK activity. It is well known that IFN can augment natural cytotoxicity. Experiments using the single cell assay indicate that IFN treatment of lymphocytes increases the frequency of lytic conjugates via recruitment of pre-NK cells and alters the kinetics of lysis.[86] Ullberg and Jondal[80] investigated the influence of IFN on three parameters contributing to NK cytotoxicity: V_{max}, the number of CFC, and effector cell frequency. Their data suggest a dual effect of IFN: first, effector cell recruitment and second, increased effector cell recycling.

In addition to measuring the frequency of NK cells, the single cell assay has been used to measure the frequency of K cells in peripheral blood. By using antibody-coated targets, Neville et al.[87] determined that K cells represent approximately 3% of the total lymphocyte population. Since this value is quite close to the frequency of NK cells, this would lend credence to the theory that both cytotoxic activities are mediated by the same cell. In fact Bradley and Bonavida[88] have documented, using a two-target conjugate assay, where a single effactor cell binds a fluorescent NK target and a nonfluorescent ADCC target, that a single effector cell can bind and kill both types of target cells. A similar approach has been used in the murine system to illustrate that a single CTL can mediate both specific as well as lectin-dependent cytotoxicity.[89]

NK activity is adversely affected in many disease states and the single cell assay can determine if the reduction in cytotoxic activity is due to a decrease in frequency of lytic CFC, the kinetics of lysis, or recycling of the effector cell. It is well established that normal individuals have a characteristic level of NK activity in peripheral blood[41] and Rubin et al.[77] have demonstrated that the difference between high and low donors is primarily attributable to the frequency of their NK cells. However, high frequency of NK cells does not necessarily result in augmented NK activity. We recently described[90] the first published case of a patient with "NK lymphocytosis", in which normal affinity E rosette-forming, FcR-positive NK cells were markedly increased in frequency, with only minimal augmentation of overall NK activity. This result suggested that the abnormal NK cells were deficient in recycling capacity, although it could not be ruled out that these cells represented a proliferation of a weakly lytic normal NK subpopulation.

Studies to define the marked NK abnormality in Chediak-Higashi syndrome[36] — an autosomal recessive defect in lysosomal enzyme production, revealed a normal binding capacity, a reduced percentage of active NK cells, but an apparently normal recycling ability.[91] This indicates that the active NK cell population which is present is capable of normal target cell lysis and recycling. Similarly, patients with systemic lupus erythematosus, who are often deficient in NK activity,[92-94] exhibit lower overall V_{max} values, with a reduced frequency of NK cells, indicating no abnormality in the ability to repeat the lytic sequence.[94]

This pattern of NK defect is markedly different from that observed by Steinhauer et al.[95] in a study of patients with malignant disease. These authors observed a decrease in overall cytotoxic activity with a concomitant reduction in V_{max}. The frequency of NK cells was normal, however, suggesting a defect in recycling. This inability to recycle may reflect a deficiency in cell motility or a physiological impairment in the functional recycling of the lytic moiety. Even within a single disease state one may observe NK defects at distinct steps in the lytic process. Merrill et al.[96] have shown that it is possible to distinguish different defects in NK activity in patients suffering from acute and chronic multiple sclerosis. Both groups demonstrated a reduction in cytotoxic activity, but the patients with acute disease had a decreased population of NK cells, whereas patients with chronic disease exhibited a normal frequency of NK cells which were less efficient killers.

In terms of pitfalls in this assay, it is tedious, extremely time consuming, and somewhat subjective. In studies of patients' PBL frequency, hundreds of conjugates must be counted if statistical comparisons are to be valid, because the frequency of NK cells in peripheral blood is so low. It is also essential to wash the trypan blue stained slides very thoroughly before fixation, since fixation kills all of the cells and, with time, the residual blue dye leaks out of the heavily stained originally dead cells to the agarose, on the one hand, and from inadequately washed agarose into the originally living cells on the other. As discussed above, another pitfall which must be avoided is the temptation to attach significance to lymphocyte-tumor binding per se.

In conclusion, it is apparent that the single cell assay, despite the problems involved in optimizing assay conditions, is a valuable means of studying different types of CMC directly and allows examination of many aspects of effector cell function and target specificity. This technique is an important addition to the armamentarium of the tumor immunologist.

VI. SUMMARY

The various methods currently employed for the experimental determination of natural cytotoxicity reactions are summarized in Table 1, along with the parameters obtained and brief comments about the utility of each method. All but one of these methods are based on determination of the relative ^{51}Cr-release from target cells compared to spontaneous and maximum release values. Of these, the simplest and most frequently used method — determination of the percentage of cytotoxicity at a single lymphocyte to target cell ratio — is the least quantitative. Values obtained by this method are not linearly related to actual cytotoxic activity. Its use is, therefore, not recommended unless one needs only a a qualitative measure of cytotoxicity, i.e., determination of whether or not a given cell line is killed by a given lymphocyte preparation.

Of the four methods involving determination of relative cytotoxic activity using a fixed concentration of target cells and several concentrations of lymphocytes, only two are suitable for quantitative work: linear regression analysis of Hill Plots and nonlinear least-squares analysis of semilog plots. The latter method has been used more extensively and demonstrated to yield meaningful quantitative estimates for the relative cytotoxic activity of different lymphocyte preparations.

Table 1
METHODS FOR DETERMINATION OF NATURAL CYTOTOXICITY

Experimental method	Calculation method	Parameter(s) obtained	Interpretation of parameters	Comments
Relative cytotoxicity at a single E:T ratio	% Cytotoxicity compared to sonicated or detergent lysed cells	% Cytotoxicity	Qualitative estimate of overall NK activity	%C is not a linear function of the E:T ratio; not useful for quantitative studies
Relative cytotoxicity determined using a single concentration of target cells and several concentrations of lymphocytes	None	Semilog plots of %CML vs. E:T ratio	Greater cytotoxicity causes a shift to lower E:T ratios	Qualitative; requires visual comparison of graphs
	Linear regression analysis of the "linear" portion of %C vs. E:T plots	LU	Proportional to the overall cytotoxic activity of the lymphocyte population tested	Semiquantitative; use of linear regression analysis for a few nonlinear data points is not recommended; can be misleading
	Transformation of data to linear Hill plots			Should prove to be useful for quantitative determinations
	Nonlinear regression analysis			Quantitative; an available computer program allows for determination of meaningful confidence intervals
Relative cytotoxicity determined using a single lymphocyte concentration and several concentrations of target cells	Linear transformation of the Michaelis-Menten equation	V_{max} K_M^{app}	Proportional to the overall cytotoxic activity of the lymphocyte population tested Proportional to the concentration of NK cells active against the target cell tested	Quantitative; an available computer program allows for simultaneous determination of both parameters and confidence intervals; the frequency of NK cells (%NK) in the lymphocyte preparation and K_2, the rate constant for lysis per NK cell, can also be estimated
Counting of lymphocytes, lymphocyte-target conjugates and lytic-conjugates	Conjugate to total lymphocyte ratio Lytic-conjugate to total lymphocyte ratio	Percentage of lymphocytes that form conjugates Percentage of lymphocytes that form lytic conjugates	Frequency of lymphocytes that bind to the target cell Proportional to the frequency of NK cells in the preparation tested	Since a rather large percent of lymphocytes bind to most target cells, this is probably not a valid estimate of NK binding; provides a semiquantitative estimate of the frequency of NK cells active against the target cell tested

The kinetic approach to the quantification of natural cytotoxicity is not extensively used at present. However, it has been shown to yield meaningful quantitative estimates for the relative cytotoxic activity of different lymphocyte preparations. The recent discovery that this method yields estimates for both the frequency and lytic activity of NK cells may lead to more widespread use.

Direct comparison of most methods involving ^{51}Cr-release[56] demonstrated that only nonlinear least-squares regression analysis of %C vs. log E:T ratio plots and V_{max} values obtained by a distribution-free statistical method were sufficiently precise for routine use in the quantification of natural cytotoxicity reactions.

The recently developed lytic-conjugate assay for natural cytotoxicity does not yield a quantitative estimate for the overall cytotoxic activity of a given lymphocyte preparation. However, the frequency of lytic conjugates does appear to be directly proportional to the frequency of NK cells in a lymphocyte preparation that are active against the target cell tested. Thus, while this method is relatively time-consuming and prone to subjectivity, it nonetheless provides a needed direct measure of lytic interactions. On the other hand, we caution against overinterpretation of the values for total (lytic plus nonlytic) conjugates measured in this assay. The relatively high frequency of lymphocyte-target cell conjugates frequently observed suggests that most do not involve NK cells. Thus, for example, the inability of a given compound to significantly reduce the total number of conjugates should not be interpreted as strong evidence that the compound does not block the binding step of natural cytotoxicity.

In conclusion, we believe that more rapid progress toward an understanding of the mechanism of natural cytotoxicity and its modulation by disease or drugs requires use of experimental methods that yield meaingful and precise estimates of cytotoxic activity. Suitable techniques have now been developed and should be more extensively employed.

ACKNOWLEDGMENTS

Supported by PHS Grants AI-12766 and CA-34112 from the National Institutes of Health; a Research Career Development Award (CA-00744) to D. M. Callewaert from the National Cancer Institute; and grants from the National Cancer Institute of Canada, the Medical Research Council of Canada, and the Ontario Cancer Treatment and Research Foundation to H. F. Pross. H. F. Pross is a Career Scientist of the O.C.T.R.F. We would like to thank Mrs. Christine Jackson and Ms. Joan Gibson for typing the manuscript.

REFERENCES

1. Takasugi, M., Mickey, M. R., and Terasaki, P. I., Reactivity of lymphocytes from normal persons on cultured tumor cells, *Cancer Res.*, 33, 2898, 1973.
2. Rosenberg, E. B., McCoy, J. L., Green, S. S., Donelly, F. C., Siwarski, D. F., Levine, P. H., and Herberman, R. B., Destruction of human lymphoid tissue-culture cell lines by human peripheral lymphocytes in ^{51}Cr-release cellular cytotoxic assays, *J. Natl. Cancer Inst.*, 52, 345, 1974.
3. De Vries, J. E., Cornain, S., and Rumke, P., Cytotoxicity of non-T-versus T-lymphocytes from melanoma patients and healthy donors on short- and long-term cultured melanoma cells, *Int. J. Cancer*, 14, 427, 1974.
4. Pavie-Fischer, J., Kourilsky, F. M., Picard, F., Banzet, P., and Puissant, A., Cytotoxicity of lymphocytes from healthy subjects and from melanoma patients against cultured melanoma cells, *Clin. Exp. Immunol.*, 21, 430, 1975.

5. Pross, H. F. and Jondal, M., Cytotoxic lymphocytes from normal donors. A functional marker of human non-T-lymphocytes, *Clin. Exp. Immunol.,* 21, 226, 1975.
6. Jondal, M. and Pross, H. F., Surface markers on human B- and T-lymphocytes. VI. Cytotoxicity against cell lines as functional markers for lymphocyte subpopulations, *Int. J. Cancer,* 15, 596, 1975.
7. Hersey, P., Edwards, A., Edwards, J., Adams, E., Milton, G. W., and Nelson, D. S., Specificity of cell-mediated cytotoxicity against human melanoma lines: evidence for "non-specific" killing by activated T-cells, *Int. J. Cancer,* 16, 173, 1975.
8. Peter, H. H., Pavie-Fischer, J., Fridman, W. H., Aubert, C., Cesarini, J. P., Rougin, R., and Kourilsky, K. M., Cell-mediated cytotoxicity in vitro of human lymphocytes against a tissue culture melanoma cell line (IGR3), *J. Immunol.,* 115, 539, 1975.
9. Matthews, N. and MacLaurin, P. B., Spontaneous cytotoxic activity as a test of human lymphocyte function, *Lancet,* 1, 581, 1975.
10. De Vries, J. E., Meyering, M., Van Dongen, A., and Rumke, P., The influence of different isolation procedures and the use of target cells from melanoma cell lines and short-term cultures of the non-specific cytotoxic effects of lymphocytes from healthy donors, *Int. J. Cancer,* 15, 391, 1975.
11. Kiessling, R., Klein, E., and Wigzell, H., Natural killer cells in the mouse. I. Cytotoxic cells with specificity for mouse Moloney leukemia cells. Specificity and distribution according to genotype, *Eur. J. Immunol.,* 5, 112, 1975.
12. Kiessling, R., Klein, E., Pross, H., and Wigzell, H., "Natural" killer cells in the mouse. II. Cytotoxic cells with specificity for mouse Moloney leukemia cells. Characteristics of the killer cell, *Eur. J. Immunol,* 5, 117, 1975.
13. Herberman, R. B., Nunn, M. E., and Lavrin, D. H., Natural cytotoxic reactivity of mouse lymphoid cells against syngeneic and allogeneic tumors. II. Characterization of effector cells, *Int. J. Cancer,* 16, 230, 1975.
14. Behelak, U., Banerjee, D., and Richter, M., Immunocompetent cells in patients with malignant disease. I. The lack of naturally occurring killer cell activity in the unfractionated circulating lymphocytes from patients with chronic lymphocytic leukemia (CLL), *Cancer,* 38, 2274, 1976.
15. West, W. H., Cannon, G. B., Kay, H. K., Bonnard, G. D., and Herberman, R. B., Natural cytotoxic reactivity of human lymphocytes against a myeloid cell line: Characterization of effector cells, *J. Immunol.,* 118, 355, 1977.
16. Timonen, T., Ranki, A., Saksela, E., and Hayry, P., Fractionation, morphological and functional characterization of effector cells responsible for human natural killer activity against cell-line targets, *Cell. Immunol.,* 48, 121, 1979.
17. Timonen, T., Ortaldo, J. R., and Herberman, R. B., Characteristics of human large granular lymphocytes and relationship to natural killer and K cells, *J. Exp. Med.,* 153, 569, 1981.
18. Abo, T. and Balch, C. M., A differentiation antigen of human NK and K cells identified by a monoclonal antibody (HNK-1), *J. Immunol.,* 127, 1024, 1981.
19. Griffin, J. D., Hercend, T., Beveridge, R., and Schlossman, S. F., Characterization of an antigen expressed by human natural killer cells, *J. Immunol.,* 130, 2947, 1983.
20. Perussia, B., Starr, S., Abraham, S., Fanning, V., and Trinchieri, G., Human natural killer cells analyzed by B73.1, a monoclonal antibody blocking Fc receptor functions. I. Characterization of the lymphocyte subset reactive with B73.1, *J. Immunol.,* 130, 2133, 1983.
21. Lozzio, C. B. and Lozzio, B. B., Cytotoxicity of a factor isolated from human spleen, *J. Natl. Cancer Inst.,* 50, 535, 1973.
22. Klein, E., Ben-Bassat, H., Newman, H., Ralph, P., Zeuthen, J., Polliack, A., and Vanky, F., Properties of the K562 cell line derived from a patient with chronic myeloid leukemia, *Int. J. Cancer,* 18, 421, 1976.
23. Jondal, M., Spina, C., and Targan, S., Human spontaneous killer cells selective for tumor derived target cells, *Nature (London),* 272, 62, 1978.
24. Blomgren, H., Baral, E., Edsmyr, F., Strender, L. E., Petrini, B., and Wasserman, J., Natural killer activity in peripheral lymphocyte population following local radiation therapy, *Acta Radiol. Oncol.,* 19, 139, 1980.
25. MacLennan, I. C. M., Campbell, A. C., and Gale, D. G. L., Quantitation of K cells, in *In Vitro Methods in Cell-Mediated and Tumor Immunity,* Bloom, B. R. and David, J. R., Eds, Academic Press, New York, 1976, 511.
26. Lopez, C., Kirkpatrick, D., Sorell, M., O'Reilly, R. J., and Ching, C., Association between pre-transplant natural kill and graft-versus-host disease after stem-cell transplantation, *Lancet,* 2, 1103, 1979.
27. Kimber, I. and Moore, M., Naturally cytotoxic tonsillar lymphocytes: a manifestation of heterogeneity among human NK cells, *Scand. J. Immunol.,* 17, 29, 1983.
28. Masucci, G., Masucci, J. G., Bejarano, M. T., and Klein, E., Comparison of highly NK active human lymphocyte subsets separated by various procedures involving E, EA rosetting, density gradients and adherence to immune complexes, *J. Immunol. Methods,* 63, 57, 1983.

29. Bloom, B. R. and David, J. R., Eds., *In Vitro Methods in Cell-Mediated and Tumor Immunity*, Academic Press, New York, 1976.
30. Brooks, C. G., Rees, R. C., and Leach, R. H., High nonspecific reactivity of normal lymphocytes against mycoplasma-infected targets in cytotoxicity assays, *Eur. J. Immunol.*, 9, 159, 1979.
31. Fischer, D. G., Hubbard, W. J., and Koren, H. S., Tumor cell killing by freshly isolated peripheral blood monocytes, *Cell. Immunol.*, 58, 426, 1981.
32. Ottenhof, P. C., Morales, A., and Baines, M. G., Quantitation of a whole blood assay for human natural killer cell activity, *J. Immunol. Methods*, 42, 305, 1981.
33. Rees, R. C. and Platts, A. A., A modified short-term cytotoxicity test: assessment of natural cell-mediated cytotoxicity in whole blood, *J. Immunol. Methods*, 62, 79, 1983.
34. Kay, H. D. and Smith, D. L., Regulation of human lymphocyte-mediated natural killer (NK) cell activity. I. Inhibition in vitro by peripheral blood granulocytes, *J. Immunol.*, 130, 475, 1983.
34a. Dorval, G., Pross, H. F., and Baines, M. G., unpublished.
35. Pross, H. F., Luk, S., and Baines, M. G., Spontaneous human lymphocyte-mediated cytoxicity against tumor target cells. V. The role of serum-derived heterologous membrane antigens, *Int. J. Cancer*, 21, 291, 1978.
36. Roder, J. C., Haliotis, T., Klein, M., Korec, S., Jett, J., Ortaldo, J., Herberman, R. B., Katz, P., and Fauci, A. S., A new immunodeficiency disorder in humans involving NK cells, *Nature*, 284, 553, 1980.
37. Targan, S. R. and Oseas, R., The "Lazy" NK cells of Chediak-Higashi Syndrome, *J. Immunol.*, 130, 2671, 1983.
38. Timonen, T., Saksela, E., Virtanen, I., and Cantell, K., Natural killer cells are responsible for the interferon production induced in human lymphocytes by tumor cell contact, *Eur. J. Immunol.*, 10, 422, 1980.
39. Copeland, C. S., Koren, H. S., and Jensen, P. J., Natural killing can be independent of interferon generated in vitro, *Cell Immunol.*, 62, 220, 1981.
40. Pross, H. F., Baines, M. G., Rubin, P., Shragge, P., and Patterson, M., Spontaneous human lymphocyte-mediated cytotoxicity against tumor target cells. IX. Quantitation of natural killer (NK) cell activity, *J. Clin. Immunol.* 1, 51, 1981.
41. Pross, H. F. and Baines, M. G., Studies of human natural killer cells. I. In vivo parameters affecting normal cytotoxic function, *Int. J. Cancer*, 29, 383, 1982.
42. Pross, H. F. and Maroun, J. A., The standardization of NK cell assays for use in studies of biological response modifiers, *J. Immunol. Methods*, in press.
43. Onsrud, M. and Thorsby, E., Influence of in vivo hydrocortisone on some human blood lymphocyte populations, *Scand. J. Immunol.*, 13, 573, 1981.
44. Porzolst, F. and Wolf, W., Modulation of natural killer activity by aspirin. I. In vitro effect of aspirin, *J. Interferon Res.*, 3, 11, 1983.
45. Thatcher, N., Wan, H. H., Swindell, R., Wilkinson, P. M., and Crowther, D., Effects of diphylhydantoin on killer cell activity and other immunological functions, *Int. J. Immunopharmacol.*, 4, 167, 1982.
46. Ferson, F., Edwards, A., Lind, A., Milton, G. W., and Hersey, P., Low natural killer-cell activity and immunoglobulin levels associated with smoking in human subjects, *Int. J. Cancer*, 23, 603, 1983.
47. Targan, S., Britvan, L., and Dorey, F., Activation of human NKCC by moderate exercise: increased frequency of NK cells with enhanced capability of effector-target lytic interactions, *Clin. Exp. Immunol.*, 45, 352, 1981.
48. Hersh, E. M., Reuben, J. M., Bogard, H., Rosenblum, M., Bielski, M., Mansell, P. W., Rios, A., Newell, G. R., and Sonnenfeld, G., Effect of the recreational agent isobutyl nitrite on human peripheral blood leukocytes and in vitro interferon production, *Cancer Res.*, 43, 1365, 1983.
49. Brunner, K. T., Manuel, J., Cerottini, J. C., and Chapuis, B., Quantitative assay of the lytic action of immune lymphoid cells on ^{51}Cr-labelled allogeneic target cells in vitro: inhibition by isoantibody and drugs, *Immunology*, 14, 181, 1968.
50. Miller, R. G. and Dunkley, M., Quantitative analysis of the ^{51}Cr release cytotoxic assay for cytotoxic lymphocytes, *Cell Immunol.*, 14, 284, 1974.
51. Clark, D. A., Phillips, R. A., and Miller, R. G., Characterization of cells that suppress the cytotoxic activity of T lymphocytes. I. Quantitative measurement of inhibitor cells, *J. Immunol.*, 116, 1020, 1976.
52. Trinchieri, G., De Marchi, M., Mayr, W., Sari, M., and Ceppellini, R., Lymphocyte antibody lymphocyte interaction (LALI) with special emphasis on HLA, *Transplant Proc.*, 5, 1631, 1973.
53. Kabat, E. A. and Mayer, M. M., *Experimental Immunochemistry*, 2nd ed., Charles C Thomas, Springfield, Ill., 1967.
54. Bloom, E. T. and Korn, E. L., Quantification of natural cytotoxicity by human lymphocyte subpopulations isolated by density: heterogeneity of the effector cells, *J. Immunol. Methods*, 58, 323, 1983.

55. Krebs, H. J. and Norrild, B., Quantitation and estimation of cooperation between target-binding sites in natural and antibody-dependent cell-mediated cytotoxicity by use of a mathematical transformation, *Scand. J. Immunol.*, 17, 123, 1983.
56. Callewaert, D. M., Smeekens, S. P., and Mahle, N. H., Improved quantification of cellular cytotoxicity reactions: determination of kinetic parameters for natural cytotoxicity by a distribution-free procedure, *J. Immunol. Methods*, 49, 25, 1982.
57. Thatcher, N., Swindell, R., and Crowther, D., Effects of Corynbacterium parvum and BCG therapy on immune parameters in patients with disseminated melanoma. A sequential study over 28 days, *Clin. Exp. Immunol.*, 35, 171, 1979.
58. Hill, A. V., The possible effect of the aggregation of the molecules of hemoglobin on its dissociation curves, *J. Physiol.*, (London) 4, 40, 1910.
59. Von Krogh, M., Colloidal chemistry and immunology, *J. Infect. Dis.*, 19, 452, 1916.
60. Michaelis, L. and Menten, M. L., Kinetics of invertase action, *Biochemistry*, 49, 333, 1913.
61. Thorn, R. M. and Henney, C. S., Kinetic analysis of target cell destruction by effector T cells. I. Delineation of parameters related to the frequency and lytic efficiency of killer cells, *J. Immunol.*, 117, 2213, 1976.
62. Zeijlemaker, W. P., Van Oers, R. H. J., DeGoede, R. E. Y., and Schellekens, P. T. H., Cytotoxic activity of human lymphocytes: quantitative analysis of T cell and K cell cytotoxicity, revealed by enzyme-like kinetics, *J. Immunol.*, 119, 1507, 1977.
63. Callewaert, D. M., Johnson, D. F., and Kearney, J., Spontaneous cytotoxicity of cultured human cell lines mediated by normal peripheral blood lymphocytes. III. Kinetic parameters, *J. Immunol.*, 121, 710, 1978.
64. Callewaert, D.M., Genyea, J., Mahle, N. H., Dayner, S., Korzeniewski, C., and Schult, S., Simultaneous determination of the concentration and lytic activity of effector cells that mediate natural and antibody-dependent cytotoxicity, *Scand. J. Immunol.*, 17, 479, 1983.
65. Pollack, S. B and Emmons, S. L., Kinetic analysis of human spontaneous cell-mediated cytotoxicity, *J. Immunol.*, 123, 160, 1979.
66. Forbes, J. T. and Oldham, R. K., Kinetic analysis of specificity in human natural cell-mediated cytotoxicity, in *Natural Cell-Mediated Immunity Against Tumors*, Herberman, R. B., Ed., Academic Press, New York, 1982, 819.
67. Atkins, G. L. and Nimmo, I. A., Current Trends in the estimation of Michaelis-Menten parameters, *Anal. Biochem.*, 104, 1, 1980.
68. Callewaert, D. M., Genya, J., Mahle, N. H., Korzeniewski, C., and Schult, S., Simultaneous determination of the concentration and lytic activity of effector cells that mediate natural and antibody-dependent cytotoxicity, *J. Immunol. Methods*, in press.
69. Callewaert, D. M., Mahle, N. H., Dayner, S., Earnshaw, B., Bowman, S., and O'Connor, M., Kinetic analysis of the specificity of human natural cytotoxicity, *Scand. J. Immunol.*, in press.
70. Pross, H. F., Wilberforce, K., Dean, D., Kennedy, J. C., and Baines, M. G., Spontaneous human lymphocyte-mediated cytoxicity against tumor target cells. VIII. Characteristics of normal lymphocytes showing consistently high or low natural killer (NK) cell activity, in *The Molecular Basis of Immune Cell Function*, J. Gordin Kaplan, Ed., Elsevier, Amsterdam, 1979, 580.
71. Bonavida, B., Ikerjiri, B., and Kedar, E., Direct estimation of frequency of cytotoxic T lymphocytes by a modified plaque assay, *Nature*, 263, 769, 1976.
72. Grimm, E. A. and Bonavida, B., Studies on the induction and expression of T cell mediated immunity. VI. Heterogeneity of lytic efficiency exhibited by isolated cytotoxic T lymphocytes prepared from highly enriched populations of effector-target conjugates, *J. Immunol.*, 119, 1041, 1977.
73. Grimm, E. and Bonavida, B., Mechanism of cell-mediated cytotoxicity at the single cell level. I. Estimation of cytotoxic T lymphocyte frequency and relative lytic efficiency, *J. Immunol.* 123, 2861, 1979.
74. Targan, S., A single cell marker of active NK cytotoxicity: only a fraction of target binding lymphocytes are killer cells, *J. Clin. Lab. Immunol.*, 4, 165, 1980.
75. Bonavida, B., Bradley, T. P., and Grimm, E. A., The single-cell assay in cell-mediated cytotoxicity, *Immunol. Today*, 4, 196, 1983.
76. Bonavida, B., Bradley, T., and Grimm, E. A., Frequency determination of killer cells by a single-cell cytotoxic assay, *Methods Enzymol.*, 93, 270, 1983.
77. Rubin, P., Pross, H. F., and Roder, J. C., Studies of human natural killer cells, II. Analysis at the single cell level, *J. Immunol.*, 128, 2553, 1982.
78. Vargas-Cortes, V., Hellstrom, U., and Perlmann, P., Surface markers of human natural killer cells as analyzed in a modified single cell cytotoxicity assay on poly-L-lysine coated cover slips, *J. Immunol. Methods*, 62, 87, 1983.
79. Pross, H. F., Gallinger, L. A., Rubin, P., and Baines, M. G., The use of modified Cunningham chambers for the enumeration of H rosettes, E. rosettes, and lymphocyte-tumor cell conjugates, *Int. Arch. Allergy Appl. Immunol.*, 66, 365, 1981.

80. Ullberg, M. and Jondal, M., Recycling and target binding capacity of human natural killer cells, *J. Exp. Med.,* 153, 615, 1983.
81. Saksela, E., Timonen, T., Ranki, A., and Hayry, P., Morphological and functional characterization of isolated effector cells responsible for human natural killer activity to fetal fibroblasts and to cultured cell lines, *Immunol. Rev.,* 44, 71, 1979.
82. Opremack, E. M., Bakenhaster, K., and Whisler, R. L., NK and K cell characteristics of human lymphocytes enriched for subpopulations isolated from NK tumor cell conjugates, *Cell. Immunol.,* 58, 415, 1981.
83. Salata, R. A., Schaeter, B. Z., and Ellner, J. J., Recruitment of OKM1 staining lymphocytes with selective binding of K562 tumour targets by interferon, *Clin. Exp. Immunol.,* 52, 185, 1983.
84. Timonen, T., Ortaldo, J. R., and Herberman, R. B., Analysis by a single cell cytotoxicity assay of natural killer (NK) cell frequencies among human large granular lymphocytes and of the effects of interferon on their activity, *J. Immunol.,* 128, 2514, 1982.
85. Stewart, L. D. and Ades, E. W., Human natural killer cells: correlation of a lytic assay with a visual binding assay, *J. Clin. Lab. Immunol.,* 10, 203, 1983.
86. Targan, S. and Dorey, F., Interferon activation of "pre-SK" cells and alterations in kinetics of lysis of both pre-SK and active SK cells, *J. Immunol.,* 124, 2157, 1980.
87. Neville, M. E., Grimm, E. A., and Bonavida, B., Frequency determination of K cells by a single cell cytotoxic assay, *J. Immunol. Methods,* 36, 255, 1980.
88. Bradley, T. P. and Bonavida, B., Mechanisms of cell-mediated cytotoxicity at the single cell level. IV. Natural killing and antibody-dependent cellular cytotoxicity can be mediated by the same human effector cell as determined by the two-target conjugate assay, *J. Immunol.,* 129, 2260, 1983.
89. Bradley, T. P. and Bonavida, B., Mechanisms of cell-mediated cytotoxicity at the single cell level. III. Evidence that cytotoxic T lymphocytes lyse both antigen-specific and -nonspecific targets pretreated with lectins or periodate, *J. Immunol.,* 128, 208, 1981.
90. Pross, H. F., Pater, J., Dwosh, I., Giles, A., Gallinger, L. A., Rubin, P., Corbett, W. E. N., Galbraith, P., and Baines, M. G., Studies of human natural killer cells. III. Neutropenia associated with unusual characteristics of antibody-dependent and natural killer cell-mediated cytotoxicity, *J. Clin. Immunol.,* 2, 126, 1982.
91. Katz, P., Zaytoun, A., and Fauci, A. S., Deficiency of active natural killer cells in the Chediak-Higashi syndrome, *J. Clin. Invest.,* 69, 1231, 1982.
92. Sibbitt, W. L., Mathews, P. M., and Bankhurst, A. D., Natural killer cell in systemic lupus erythematosus defects, in effector lytic activity and response to interferon and interferon inducers, *J. Clin. Invest.,* 71, 1230, 1983.
93. Karsh, J., Dorval, G., and Osterland, C. K., Natural cytotoxicity in rheumatoid arthritis and systemic lupus erythematosus, *Clin. Immunol. Immunopathol.,* 19, 437, 1981.
94. Katz, P., Zaytoun, A. M., Lee, J. H., Panush, R. S., and Longley, S., Abnormal natural killer cell activity in systemic lupus erythematosus: an intrinsic defect in the lytic event, *J. Immunol.,* 129, 1966, 1982.
95. Steinhauer, E. H., Doyle, A. T., Reed, J., and Kadish, A. S., Defective natural cytotoxicity in patients with cancer: normal number of effector cells but decreased recycling capacity in patients with advanced disease, *J. Immunol.,* 129, 2255, 1982.
96. Merrill, J., Jondal, M., Seely, J. Vilberg, M., and Siden, A., Decreased NK killing in patients with multiple sclerosis: an analysis on the level of the single effector cell in peripheral blood and cerebrospinal fluid in relation to the activity of the disease, *Clin. Exp. Immunol.,* 47, 419, 1982.

Chapter 2

SEPARATION AND CHARACTERIZATION OF PHENOTYPICALLY DISTINCT SUBSETS OF NK CELLS

Paola Allavena and John R. Ortaldo

TABLE OF CONTENTS

I. INTRODUCTION

Investigations on natural killer (NK) activity[1] considerably advanced when the fractionation of nonadherent blood lymphocytes on Percoll density gradient led to the enrichment of large granular lymphocytes (LGL) with high NK activity.[2,3] Functionally, in a single-cell assay, the majority, up to about 80% of LGL, are active NK cells.[4] Their surface phenotype[5] and their pattern of specificity[6] against tumor and nontumor targets have been extensively studied and revealed that in spite of their homogeneous morphology, the population of LGL clearly presents heterogeneous characteristics and probably consists of different antigenic and functional subsets.

This hypothesis of heterogeneity of NK cells has been recently confirmed at the clonal level[7-9] by studying, in detail, clones derived from NK cells and expanded in the presence of interleukin 2 (IL-2). With such evidence in mind, we have tried to further separate the LGL population. The approach we have used is to separate phenotypically distinguishable subsets of LGL, each one having or lacking a surface marker recognized by monoclonal antibodies (MoAb). The question we addressed was, "Do antigenically different subsets of LGL differ also in their functional activities?"

Some of the surface characteristics of NK cells that have been studied for the identification and isolation of different subpopulations are listed in Table 1. When peripheral blood lymphocytes (PBL) were separated on the basis of the sheep erthrocyte receptor into E^+ and E^- subsets, only a portion of NK cells (∼50%) were found to have a low affinity for sheep red blood cells (SRBC), and E^- lymphocytes were more active in NK activity than the E^+ cells.[10,11] On the contrary, all the EA^+ lymphocytes expressing the Fc_γ receptor have NK activity, while the EA^- cells are poorly cytotoxic.[10-13]

In addition, some MoAb selective for human NK cells have recently been produced. Among them, B73.1 recognizes the Fc_γ receptor on NK cells.[14] In agreement with previous results, B73.1$^+$ cells sorted by flow cytometry were found to have high NK activity, while B73.1$^-$ cells lacking the Fc receptor (FcR) were not cytotoxic.

The association between phenotypic markers on NK cells and cytotoxic activity was initially approached by the complement-lysis technique, which only indicates the extent of activity by antigen-negative cells, but do not reveal the reactivity of antigen-positive cells. Zarling et al.[15] showed that elimination of OKM1$^+$ and OKT11$^+$ cells from PBL dramatically decreased the NK activity. Ortaldo et al.[5] showed that elimination of OKT10,$^+$ OKT11$^+$ and OKM1$^+$ LGL on antimouse Ig-coated plastic dishes decreased the NK activity of the remaining lymphocytes, suggesting that the NK effectors are bearing these markers.

In the present study we have used a different technique: a Sepharose 4B immunoadsorbent gel coupled with an $F(ab')_2$ goat antimouse Ig, for separating MoAb-treated cells. This technique has the following advantages over complement-mediated lysis: (1) it allows the recovery of both positive and negative reactivity with the MoAb, (2) the purity of the negative and positive fractions are very high, and (3) it allows the recovery of a high proportion of cells (>77 ± 5%). When highly purified populations of LGL were fractionated into different subsets according to reactivity with various MoAb NK activity was shown to be mainly restricted to the B73-1$^+$, OKM1$^+$, OKT11$^+$, OKT10$^+$, OKT3$^-$ subsets of cells. The subsets B73.1$^-$, OKM1$^-$, were completely devoid of NK activity; some reactivity was occasionally found in the OKT11$^-$ and OKT10$^-$ LGL and in both the positive and negative fractions for OKT8 and anti-Ia markers.

Early in vivo studies in mice demonstrated a bone marrow origin of NK cells.[16] We were interested in further studying the characteristics of the progenitors of NK cells, which might be present in peripheral blood. As peripheral blood LGL can grow in vitro in the presence of IL-2,[17] we have utilized a limiting dilution analysis[18] to examine the frequency of proliferative and cytotoxic (NK) progenitors among the subsets of

Table 1
SURFACE CHARACTERISTICS USED FOR THE IDENTIFICATION OF SUBPOPULATIONS OF HUMAN NK CELLS

Characteristics	Ref.
Low affinity receptor for SRBC (E^+)	10, 11
Receptor for Fc-IgG (EA^+)	10, 12
Plastic nonadherent E^-EA^+	13
Reactivity with MoAb	
OKM1	26, 27
OKM1/OKT11	15
OKM1/OKT8/OKT10/OKT11	5
αIa	28
HNK-1	29
VEP 13	30
B73.1	14
H25, H366	31
N901	32

peripheral blood LGL.[19] The results demonstrated that the frequency of cytotoxic progenitors was higher (i.e., more precursors) in the $OKM1^+$, $OKT11^+$, and $B73.1^-$ subsets of LGL. On the other hand, the highest frequency of progenitors proliferative cells was found in the $OKM1^-$, $B73.1^-$, but $OKT11^+$ subsets.

II. EXPERIMENTAL PROCEDURES

A. Isolation of LGL

LGL were isolated from normal donors' blood on Percoll density gradients, as described elsewhere[2,3] and purified by rosetting at 29°C with SRBC for 1 hr.[3] By morphology, on Giemsa-stained cytopreps, 80 to 90% of the cells were LGL. The above LGL population was subsequently separated into different subsets and will be referred to hereafter as the "whole" LGL population.

B. Separation of LGL Subsets

The pattern of specificity for each of the MoAb used and the percentage of LGL reacting with them can be found in Table 2. MoAb BRL αMϕ was purchased from Bethesda Research Laboratories, Gaithersburg, Md., OKT3, OKT8, OKT10, OKT11, OKM1 from Ortho Pharmaceutical Corp., Raritan, N.J., B73.1 was kindly provided by Dr. G. Trinchieri, Wistar Institute, Philadelphia, Pa., HNK-1 was kindly provided by Dr. Toru Abo, University of Alabama, Birmingham, and αIa was purchased from Becton Dickinson, Mountain View, Calif.

LGL subsets were separated on antimouse immunoadsorbent gel following a modified method of Schlossman[20] and Nelson.[21] The immunoadsorbent gel was a CnBr-activated Sepharose 4B (Pharmacia) and was coupled with an affinity-purified $F(ab')_2$ goat antimouse IgG (Cappel Labs, Cochranville, Pa.) as previously described.[21] Whole LGL preparations were treated with appropriate dilutions of MoAb[5] and loaded on top of a column of packed immunoadsorbent gel. Negative cells were eluted immediately at a very slow flow rate (12 drops/min). Positive cells were subsequently recovered by mechanical agitation with a Pasteur pipette followed by extensive washing at faster flowrate.

In other experiments, whole LGL were separated into antigen-positive and negative cells by flow cytometry using a Cytofluorograf® cell sorter (Ortho).

Table 2
PATTERN OF SPECIFICITY OF MoAb

MoAb	Positive LGL %	Other specificities	Structure recognized
OKT3	<3	Mature T lymphocytes	Unknown T cell receptor related protein
OKT8	25—35	Suppressor/cytotoxic T Lymphocytes	Unknown
OKT10	50—60	Thymocytes, activated T lymphocytes	Unknown
OKT11	55—65	E^+ T lymphocytes	Receptor for sheep erythrocyte
OKM1	60—70	Monocytes-granulocytes	Unknown C3bi
αIa	20—30	Monocytes, B lymphocytes, Activated T lymphocytes	Unknown class II antigen, MHC product
B73.1	60—75	Few granulocytes	Fc_γ receptor
HNK-1	45—55	Some T lymphocytes	Unknown

C. Cytotoxic Assay

NK activity was measured by a standard ^{51}chromium(^{51}Cr)-release assay of 4 hr.[3] The following targets were used: K562 (derived from a patient with chronic myelogeneous leukemia in blast crisis); MOLT-4 (a T cell line derived from a patient with acute lymphocytic leukemia); Daudi (a B cell line derived from a patient with Burkitt's lymphoma); and Alab (derived from a patient with breast carcinoma). The target for ADCC was RL♂1 (a murine T lymphoma), coated with 1:100 dilution of a rabbit antimouse brain serum (Flow Labs, Rockville, Md.).

D. Limiting Dilution Analysis (LDA)

The LDA for the determination of the frequency of proliferative progenitors and of cytotoxic NK progenitors was performed as previously described.[19] Briefly, different concentrations of whole or separated LGL populations (10,000 to 10 cells per well) were cultured in RPMI 1640 medium + 10% human AB serum + 10% partially purified human IL-2 (Associate Biomedic Systems, Buffalo, N.Y.), or 50% crude supernatant of the gibbon lymphosarcoma cell line MLA 144 constitutively producing IL-2[22] (kindly provided by Dr. H. Rabin, Frederick, Md.). A small amount of phytohaemagglutinin (PHA) (Wellcome, England), 0.1 μg/mℓ, was added to initiate proliferation. In other experiments, it was determined that using the cells from the same donor, the human IL-2 and gibbon IL-2 gave similar frequencies of progenitors.

Proliferation was assessed by uptake of ^{3}H-thymidine after culture of 7 days. Cytotoxicity was measured as described above after 8 days. Results were calculated by linear regression analysis as previously described.[18]

III. RESULTS

A. Validity of the Method

In some experimental systems, e.g., with the cytotoxic T lymphocytes, lysis can be blocked by the addition of MoAb. Therefore, preliminary experiments were designed to investigate whether MoAb treatment or simple passage through immunoadsorbent columns would affect the NK activity of LGL. Cells were incubated with MoAb (OKT3, OKM1, OKT11) or with heterologous antiserum (mouse Thy 1), or were passed through an $F(ab')_2$ immunoadsorbent column without any MoAb pretreatment and immediately tested in the 4-hr cytotoxicity assay. In both cases, NK activity was comparable to control values (Table 3), indicating that neither treatment was affecting the cytotoxic activity of LGL.

Table 3
EFFECT OF PRETREATMENTS ON NK ACTIVITY OF HUMAN LGL

Pretreatment[a]	% Specific lysis[b] ± S. D. (E:T 20:1)
None	33.7 ± 1.5
S4B column alone	34.4 ± 0.9
Thy 1 alone	32.0 ± 1.3
OKM1 alone	33.9 ± 1.1
OKT11 alone	35.0 ± 1.9
OKT3 alone	32.3 ± 0.8

[a] Effector cells were tested with MoAb (OKT3, OKM1, OKT11) or with heterologous serum (anti-Thy 1), or were passed through a $F(ab')_2$ column, without any pretreatment, and immediately tested for cytotoxicity.

[b] Cytotoxic activity was measured in a standard 4-hr ^{51}Cr-release assay against K562. Specific lysis was calculated as follows:

$$\% \text{ specific lysis} = \frac{\text{cpm in experimental wells} - \text{cpm in wells with target cells alone}}{\text{cpm incorporated in target cells}} \times 100$$

When MoAb-treated LGL were separated into positive and negative fractions on immunoadsorbent columns, the total recovery of the cells was 77 ± 5% as assessed in four independent experiments with a panel of eight different MoAb (data not shown). Although the viability of positive cells recovered from the gel was greater than 90%, their functional activity was inhibited when immediately tested, but it was fully recovered after 12 hr; therefore, after the fractionation procedures the cells were incubated overnight at 37°C in medium RPMI 1640 + 10% FCS and tested for cytotoxicity the following day. Reanalysis of the isolated populations by flow cytometry revealed that contamination with "inappropriate" cells was less than 5% in the negative fraction, while the positive fraction contained 70 to 83% of fluorescent-stained cells. This percentage of positive cells was probably an underestimate, however, since by morphological criterion >97% of B73.1$^+$ cells were LGL. This discrepancy between morphology and fluorescence analysis may be explained by the fact that during the physical detachment of the positive cells from the columns some antibody/antigen complexes may have been removed. These cells could not be relabeled with the same MoAb and fluorescent secondary antibody.

As fractionation with the Cytofluorograf® cell sorter has been, up to now, the method providing cell subsets with the smallest contamination of "inappropriate" cells, it was important to compare the NK activity of subsets separated with the Sepharose 4B columns and with the cell sorter. These data, presented in Table 4, show that the results from both methods are fully comparable. One important advantage of the immunoadsorbent columns is that the total recovery of cells is appreciably higher than with the cell sorter.

B. NK Activity of Different LGL Subsets

In subsequent experiments we tested the NK activity of different MoAb positive and negative fraction of LGL. Table 5 shows a representative experiment in which most NK activity was recovered in the fractions OKT3$^-$, OKM1$^+$, B73.1$^+$, OKT11$^+$, OKT10$^+$, and αIa$^-$ LGL. OKM1$^+$ and OKT3$^-$ LGL were four and three times more active, respectively, than untreated LGL. NK activity was found in both the OKT8$^-$ and OKT8$^+$

Table 4
COMPARISON OF CYTOTOXIC ACTIVITY OF LGL SUBSETS SEPARATED BY TWO DIFFERENT METHODS

	Flow cytometry		Sepharose 4B columns	
LGL subset[a]	LU[b]	Control (%)	LU	Control (%)
LGL	150	100	270	100
B73.1⁻	23	15	7	2
B73.1⁺	211	140	444	164
OKM1⁻	3	2	7	2
OKM1⁺	181	120	948	350
OKT10⁻	20	13	74	27
OKT10⁺	135	90	265	98

[a] LGL were pretreated with MoAb and then separated on Sepharose 4B columns, or were sorted by flow cytometry into negative and positive fractions. Control LGL were passed through the Sepharose 4B column without any pretreatment.

[b] LU were calculated at 30% specific lysis per 10^7 effector cells.

Table 5
CYTOXOCITY OF HUMAN LGL SUBSETS

LGL subset[b]		Cytotoxicity to K562[a]: $LU^{30}/10^7$ cells[c]	Cytotoxicity to K562[a]: % Compared to control	% Recovery of input cells
LGL		406	100	100
BRL-Mϕ	−	558	137	60
	+	134	33	23
OKT3	−	1187	293	50
	+	164	40	27
OKT8	−	716	176	39
	+	368	90	35
OKT10	−	112	27	37
	+	398	98	44
OKT11	−	64	16	24
	+	719	177	53
OKM1	−	10	2	32
	+	1632	402	52
αIa	−	474	117	52
	+	129	32	28
B73.1	−	11	2	30
	+	667	164	55

[a] Cytotoxicity assay was a standard 4-hr ^{51}Cr-release assay.

[b] LGL were pretreated with MoAb and then separated on Sepharose 4B columns (see Section II) into negative and positive fractions. Control LGL were passed through the Sepharose 4B column without any pretreatment.

[c] LU were calculated at 30% specific lysis per 10^7 effector cells.

Table 6
CYTOTOXIC ACTIVITY OF DIFFERENT LGL SUBSETS AGAINST NK-SUSCEPTIBLE TARGETS

LGL subset[a]		(%) Specific lysis[b]			
		K562	ADCC	Daudi	Alab
LGL		42	22	32	26
BRL Mϕ	−	46	10	39	19
BRL Mϕ	+	12	11	22	24
OKT3	−	40	10	32	22
OKT3	+	16	10	14	22
OKT10	−	31	7	24	4
OKT10	+	47	13	34	33
OKM1	−	3	2	9	8
OKM1	+	46	23	40	28
OKT11	−	10	8	6	4
OKT11	+	45	13	43	25
OKT8	−	41	16	28	13
OKT8	+	36	14	36	21
αIa	−	35	13	29	16
αIa	+	22	13	11	28
B73.1	−	5	1	8	7
B73.1	+	51	32	29	20

[a] LGL were treated with MoAb and separated on Sepharose 4B columns into positive and negative fractions. Control LGL were passed through the Sepharose 4B column without any pretreatment.

[b] Effector cells were tested against the various targets in a standard 4-hr ^{51}Cr-rlease assay at 20:1 E:T ratio.

fractions, with the OKT8⁻ population having higher activity. Similar results were consistently obtained in four independent experiments. In the experiment shown in Table 5, αIa⁻ LGL were very active while the αIa⁺ LGL were poorly cytotoxic. In other assays this difference was not as great, with NK activity usually recovered in both fractions. In addition, OKT11⁻ LGL occasionally had appreciable reactivity in the NK assay, though always less than the OKT11⁺ LGL.

C. Cytotoxic Activity of the LGL Subsets Against a Panel of NK-Susceptible Target Cells

As the K562 cell line is generally the most susceptible and widely used target for human NK activity, it is possible that differences among the LGL subsets might occur in the inability to kill other NK-susceptible targets. When the various subsets were tested against a wider panel of NK-susceptible targets (Table 6), with few exceptions, similar results as against the K562 were obtained. For instance, Alab, which is derived from a human breast carcinoma and is an anchorage-dependent cell line, was lysed not only by OKM1⁺ T11⁺ cells that are highly enriched in LGL, but also by OKT3⁺ and BRL Mϕ⁺ cells. The same effector cells that killed the NK targets were also active in antibody-dependent cell-mediated cytotoxicity (ADCC), with the B73.1⁺ cells, bearing the FcR, being the most efficient subset.

D. Analysis of NK Cell Progenitors

Previous studies have been performed with cells selected on the basis of their surface antigens and tested for NK activity. In order to characterize the progenitors of NK cells, we conducted a series of experiments to determine the frequency of both proliferative and NK-like cytotoxic progenitors following lectin stimulation and culture in

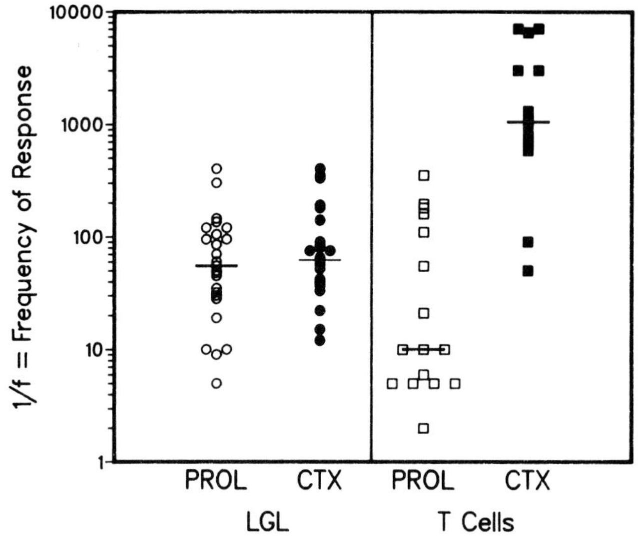

FIGURE 1. Scatter graph of the frequencies of proliferative (prol) and cytotoxic (ctx) progenitors from highly purified preparations of LGL and T lymphocytes. Each dot is a separate experiment. Responder cells were plated at different concentrations and cultured in IL-2-containing medium. Horizontal lines indicate median of frequencies. The determination of the proliferative progenitor frequency was assessed by uptake of ^{3}H-thymidine after 7 days and that of the cytotoxic progenitors with a ^{51}Cr-release assay after 8 days. Assessment of results was performed by the linear regression analysis as described in Taswell, C., *J. Immunol.*, 126, 1614, 1981.

the presence of IL-2. Experiments were performed with both antigen/antibody-selected and unseparated LGL populations.

Figure 1 shows that the unfractionated LGL from 25 different normal donors had a median frequency of proliferative progenitors of 1/55 and of cytotoxic progenitors of 1/62. In contrast, purified T lymphocytes (95% E$^+$, from the high density fraction of the Percoll gradient) from 16 donors, studied in parallel, had a much higher rate of proliferation (1/10) but generated very few killers (1/950).

The same parameters were calculated for subsets of LGL separated either by flow cytometry or affinity chromatography. Table 7 shows the frequencies of cytotoxic and proliferative progenitors of various phenotypically distinct subsets of LGL.

The cytotoxic precursors among the LGL population were found predominantly in the OKT11$^+$ (Experiment 2); cells that were OKT11$^-$ had low frequencies for both the proliferative and the cytotoxic percursors. OKT11$^+$ and OKM1$^-$ subsets had similar cytotoxic frequencies, but within the OKM1$^-$ only a small percentage of proliferating cells were cytotoxic. On the other hand, OKM1$^-$ cells contained a high number of proliferative progenitors and, among them, those cells which formed rosettes with sheep erythrocytes (E$^+$) accounted for most of the proliferation (Experiment 4).

Cytotoxic progenitors were also contained in the subsets OKT10$^+$ and OKT8$^-$; however, the OKT10$^-$ and OKT8$^+$ cells had also NK progenitors at a frequency comparable to the whole LGL population.

Cells that were B73.1$^-$ had a high frequency of proliferative progenitors and a somewhat lower frequency of cytotoxic progenitors than the control unseparated LGL population. However, compared to the B73.1$^+$ cells, which have low frequencies for both progenitors, it appears that B73.1$^-$ cells account for most of the generation of the cytotoxic cells.

IV. CONCLUDING REMARKS

In the last few years, MoAbs have been extensively used for the characterization of the surface phenotype of NK cells. The results of these studies extended the previous indications for heterogeneity among NK cells. In the context of such diversity, it is of interest to determine whether subpopulations isolated on the basis of their surface markers as detected by MoAb, also varied in their ability to indicate NK activity against a panel of NK-susceptible target cells.

To perform these experiments, we have mainly used a Sepharose 4B immunoabsorbent gel, coupled with an $F(ab')_2$ goat antimouse Ig, to separate MoAb-treated LGL into different subsets, each one expressing or lacking the marker recognized by MoAb; in some experiments cells were similarly sorted into positive and negative subsets by flow cytometry. Each subset has been tested for NK activity against the K562 cell line and other NK-susceptible targets and for ADCC activity. Previous studies by Ortaldo et al.[5] and Zarling et al.[15] have demonstrated that depletion of $OKM1^+$, $OKT11^+$ and $OKT10^+$ cells dramatically decreased NK activity. However, direct evidence on the levels of reactivity of the antigen-positive subsets can be obtained only by testing the cells bearing these markers. With the above techniques we demonstrated that, indeed, $OKM1^+$, $OKT10^+$, $OKT11^+$, and $B73.1^+$ LGL were considerably more cytotoxic against all of the NK targets tested than were the cells lacking these markers. $OKT11^-$ and $OKT10^-$ cells occasionally contained some cytotoxicity, while $OKM1^-$ and $B73.1^-$ cells had little or no NK activity. When LGL were separated with the MoAb OKT8 and αIa, NK activity was found in both positive and negative fractions, indicating that these two markers do not discriminate from functional NK activity. Recently, Perussia et al.[24] reported similar results to what we have presented here, showing that $OKT8^+$ nonadherent lymphocytes sorted by flow cytometry mediate the same level of cytotoxicity as $OKT8^-$ cells.

We also characterized the progenitors of proliferative and cytotoxic cells which are generated in vitro in the presence of IL-2. Using a limiting dilution assay we were able to estimate the frequency of these progenitors among various subsets of LGL. Most of the progenitors of cytotoxic cells were $OKT11^+$ and $OKM1^+$. In contrast, cytotoxic cells did not originate from $OKM1^-$ and $OKT11^-$ subsets. Such results were not surprising since these markers are on most NK cells from peripheral blood.

It was initially reported by Zarling et al.[15] and confirmed in our experiments that about half of the $OKM1^+$ LGL also express the receptor for SRBC. As shown in Table 7 (Experiment 4), the $OKM1^+$ E^+ subpopulation of LGL, which is equivalent to the $OKM1^+$ subset, had a high frequency of cytotoxic NK progenitors. The frequency of proliferative progenitors of $OKT11^-$ cells (Experiment 2) was very low; similarly, $OKM1^+$ E^- subset (Experiment 4) had a lower frequency than $OKM1^+$ E^+ cells. It is worth noting that $OKM1^-$ E^+ and $OKM1^+$ E^+ subsets had the same frequency of proliferative precursors, but only the cells bearing the OKM1 marker generated in vitro an appreciable number of cytotoxic progenitors.

$B73.1^+$ cells, that account for most of the activity in the NK assay, contained very few cytotoxic and proliferative progenitors; on the other hand, $B73.1^-$ cells had a high frequency of proliferative progenitors. It is of interest that the majority of cytotoxic NK progenitors were found in the $B73.1^-$ subset. We cannot exclude, however, that $B73.1^+$ cells can also generate in vitro cytotoxic cells, in fact, the cytotoxic frequency from $B73.1^+$ cells was even higher than the frequency of proliferative progenitors. This divergency has been rarely seen, but with the MOAb B73.1, it has been somewhat consistent in three repeated experiments with the cells of three different donors. It may be possible that the ^{51}Cr release cytotoxicity assay is a more sensitive method than the ^{3}H-thymidine uptake assay. Another possibility is that the $B73.1^+$ effectors are very

Table 7
FREQUENCY OF PROLIFERATIVE AND CYTOTOXIC PROGENITORS FROM HUMAN LGL SUBSETS

LGL subset[a]	Proliferative progenitor frequency[b]	Cytotoxic progenitor frequency[c]
Expt 1[d]		
LGL	1/30	1/82
LGL OKM1$^-$	1/13	1/259
LGL OKM1$^+$	1/118	1/187
LGL OKT10$^-$	1/10	1/67
LGL OKT10$^+$	1/20	1/40
Expt 2[d]		
LGL	1/46	1/83
LGL B73.1$^-$	1/32	1/162
LGL B73.1$^+$	1/6231	1/861
LGL OKT11$^-$	1/387	1/425
LGL OKT11$^+$	1/24	1/50
Expt 3[d]		
LGL	1/148	1/197
LGL OKT8$^-$	1/114	1/126
LGL OKT8$^+$	1/285	1/177
Expt 4[e]		
LGL	1/163	1/152
LGL OKM1$^-$ E$^-$	1/921	1/1978
LGL OKM1$^-$ E$^+$	1/67	1/440
LGL OKM1$^+$ E$^-$	1/137	1/130
LGL OKM1$^+$ E$^+$	1/62	1/184
Expt 5[d]		
LGL	1/44	1/55
LGL HNK-1$^-$	1/77	1/64
LGL HNK-1$^+$	1/62	1/120

[a] See Footnote b, Table 5.
[b] Determination of the proliferative progenitor frequency was assessed by uptake of ^{3}H-thymidine after 7 days in a LDA.
[c] Determination of the cytotoxic progenitor frequency was assessed by ^{51}Cr-release from labeled targets after 8 days in a LDA.
[d] Experiments performed with cells sorted by flow cytometry.
[e] Experiment performed with cells separated into OKM1$^-$ and OKM1$^+$ by immunoadsorbent columns. Each subset was subsequently rosetted with sheep erythrocytes for 1 hr at 4°C and divided into E$^+$ and E$^-$ fractions by centrifugation on Ficoll-Hypaque gradient.

active NK cells and have a high recycling capability, so that the same effector cell can lyse multiple tumor targets.

Previous studies by Ortaldo et al.[25] on the in vitro generation of NK cells, have shown that cells with NK activity are generated after 7 days culture from FcR-depleted lymphocytes, which correspond to the B73.1$^-$ cells. This and our experiments demonstrated that NK cells can originate from B73.1$^-$ cells, suggesting that some progenitors in the PBL are distinct from the mature NK population, but rather are a small population of less differentiated preNK cells.

In conclusion, the results of this study indicate that NK cells are generated in vitro from progenitors bearing the phenotype: OKM1$^+$, OKT11$^+$, both B73.1$^+$ and B73.1$^-$, the last ones being more immature cells with a higher proliferative rate than the B73.1$^+$ cells. These data provide new and useful information regarding the characteristics and heterogeneity of NK cells and their progenitors.

REFERENCES

1. Herberman, R. B. and Ortaldo, J. R., Natural killer cells: their role in defense against disease, *Science,* 214, 24, 1981.
2. Timonen, T. and Saksela, E., Isolation of human natural killer cells by density gradrient centrifugation, *J. Immunol. Methods,* 36, 285, 1980.
3. Timonen, T., Ortaldo, J. R., and Herberman, R. B., Characteristics of human large granular lymphocytes and relationship to natural killer and K cells, *J. Exp. Med.,* 153, 569, 1981.
4. Timonen, T., Ortaldo, J. R., and Herberman, R. B., Analysis by a single cell cytotoxicity assay of natural killer (NK) cell frequencies among human large granular lymphocytes and of the effects of interferon on their activity, *J. Immunol.,* 128, 2514, 1982.
5. Ortaldo, J. R., Sharrow, S. O., Timonen, T., and Herberman, R. B., Determination of surface antigens on highly purified human NK cells by flow cytometry with monoclonal antibodies, *J. Immunol.,* 127, 2401, 1982.
6. Ortaldo, J. R. and Herberman, R. B., Specificity of NK cells, in *Natural Killer Cells,* Vol. 4, Serrou, B., Rosenfeld, C., and Herberman, R. B., Eds., Elsevier/North-Holland, Amsterdam, 1982, 17.
7. Pawelec, G. P., Hadam, M. R., Schneider, E. M., and Wernet, P., Clonally restricted natural killer-like cytotoxicity displayed by cloned human T cell lines., *J. Immunol.,* 128, 2271, 1982.
8. Hercend, T., Reinherz, E. L., Meuer, S., Schlossman, S. F., and Ritz, J., Phenotypic and functional heterogeneity of human cloned natural killer cell lines, *Nature,* 301, 5896, 1983.
9. Allavena, P. and Ortaldo, J. R., Specificity and phenotype of IL-2 expanded clones of human large granular lymphocyte clones, *J. Immunol.,* 132, 2363, 1984.
10. Kay, H. D., Bonnard, G. D., West, W. H., and Herberman, R. B., A functional comparison of human Fc-receptor-bearing lymphocytes active in natural cytotoxicity and antibody-dependent cellular cytotoxicity, *J. Immunol.,* 118, 2058, 1977.
11. West, W. H., Cannon, G. B., Kay, H. D., Bonnard, G. D., and Herberman, R. B., Natural cytotoxic reactivity of human lymphocytes against myeloid cell line: characterization of the effector cells, *J. Immunol.,* 118, 355, 1977.
12. Eremin, O., Ashby, J., and Plumb, D., Antibody-dependent cellular cytotoxicity and natural cytotoxicity: effect of pretreatment of human lymphocytes with deionised water and ammonium chloride. *J. Immunol. Methods,* 24, 257, 1978.
13. Masucci, G., Masucci, M. G., and Klein, E., Human blood lymphocyte subset separated on the basis of nylon adherence, SRBC and EA rosetting: natural cytotoxicity and characterization with monoclonal reagents, *Cell. Immunol.,* 69, 166, 1982.
14. Perussia, B., Starr, S., Abraham, S., Fanning, V., and Trinchieri, G., Human natural killer cells analyzed by B.73.1, a monoclonal antibody blocking Fc receptor functions. I. Characterization of the lymphocyte subset reactive with B.73.1, *J. Immunol.,* 130, 2133, 1983.
15. Zarling, J. M., Clouse, K. A., Biddison, W. E., and Kung, P. C., Phenotypes of human natural killer cell populations detected with monoclonal antibodies, *J. Immunol.,* 127, 2575, 1981.
16. Häller, O., Kiessling, R., Örn, A., and Wigzell, H., Generation of natural killer cells: an autonomous function of the bone marrow, *J. Exp. Med.,* 145, 1411, 1977.
17. Timonen, T., Ortaldo, J. R., Stadler, B. M., Bonnard, G. D., Sharrow, S., and Herberman, R. B., Cultures of purified human natural killer cells. Growth in the presence of IL-2, *Cell. Immunol.,* 72, 198, 1982.
18. Taswell, C., Limiting dilution assasys for the determination of immunocompetent cell frequencies. I. Data analysis, *J. Immunol.,* 126, 1614, 1981.
19. Vose, B. M. and Bonnard, G. D., Limiting dilution analysis of the frequency of human T and large granular lymphocytes proliferating in response to interleukin 2, *J. Immunol.,* 130, 687, 1983.
20. Schlossman, S. F. and Hudson, L., Specific purification of lymphocyte populations on a digestible immunoabsorbent, *J. Immunol.,* 110, 313, 1973.
21. Nelson, D. L., Bundy, B. M., Pitchon, H. E., Blaese, R. M., and Strober, W., The effector cells in human peripheral blood mediating mitogen-induced cellular cytotoxicity and antibody-dependent cellular cytotoxicity, *J. Immunol.,* 117, 1472, 1976.
22. Rabin, H., Hopkins, R. F., Ruscetti, F. W., Neubauer, R. H., Brown, R. L., and Kawakaui, T. G., Spontaneous release of a fraction of properties of T cell growth factor from a continuous line of primate tumor T cells, *J. Immunol.,* 127, 1852, 1981.
23. Nakayama, E., Shiku, H., Stockert, E., Oettgen, H. F., and Old, L. J., Cytotoxic T cells: lyt phenotype and blocking of killing activity by Lyt antisera, *Proc. Natl. Acad. Sci. U.S.A.,* 76, 1977, 1979.
24. Perussia, B., Fanning, V., and Trinchieri, G., A human NK and K cell subset shares with cytotoxic T cells expression of the antigen recognized by antibody OKT8, *J. Immunol.,* 131, 223, 1983.
25. Ortaldo, J. R., Bonnard, G. D., and Herberman, R. B., Cytotoxic reactivity of human lymphocytes cultured *in vitro, J. Immunol.,* 119, 1351, 1977.

26. Breard, J., Reinherz, E. L., Kung, P. C., Goldstein, G., and Schlossman, S. F., A monoclonal antibody reactive with human peripheral blood monocytes. *J. Immunol.*, 124, 1943, 1980.
27. Kay, H. D. and Horwitz, D. A., Evidence by reactivity with hybridoma antibodies for a probable myeloid origin of antibody-dependent cell-mediated cytotoxicity, *J. Clin. Invest.*, 66, 847, 1980.
28. Ng, A.-K., Indiveri, F., Pellegrino, M. A., Molinaro, G. A., Quaranta, V., and Ferrone, S., Natural cytotoxicity and antibody-dependent cellular cytotoxicity of human lymphocytes depleted of HLA-DR bearing cells with monoclonal HLA-DR antibodies, *J. Immunol.*, 124, 2336, 1980.
29. Abo, T. and Balch, C. M., A differentiation antigen of human NK and K cells identified by a monoclonal antibody (HNK-1), *J. Immunol.*, 127, 1024, 1981.
30. Rumpold, H., Kraft, D., Obexer, G., Böck, G., and Gebhart, W., A monoclonal antibody against a surface antigen shared by human large granular lymphocytes and granulocytes, *J. Immunol.*, 129, 1458, 1982.
31. Bai, Y., Beverley, P. C. L., Knowles, R. W., and Bodmer, W. F., Two monoclonal antibodies identifying a subset of human peripheral mononuclear cells with natural killer cell activity. *Eur. J. Immunol.*, 13, 521, 1983.
32. Griffin, J. D., Hercend, T., Beveridge, R., and Schlossman, S. F., Characterization of an antigen expressed by human natural killer cells, *J. Immunol.*, 130, 2947, 1983.

Chapter 3

ULTRASTRUCTURE AND CYTOCHEMISTRY OF THE HUMAN LARGE GRANULAR LYMPHOCYTES

Manlio Ferrarini and Carlo E. Grossi

TABLE OF CONTENTS

I. INTRODUCTION

Large granular lymphocytes (LGL) are operationally defined as lymphoid cells with an extended cytoplasm containing numerous azurophilic granules.[1,2] Cytoplasmic granules staining metachromatically red with the Azur B component of the panoptic stains (Wright's, Giemsa) are found in other leukocytes and are particularly numerous in monocytes. However, LGL are distinguishable from monocytes since they are nonadherent, nonphagocytic, peroxidase-negative cells.[3]

LGL have been show to constitute the bulk of the so-called Tγ cells (i.e., lymphocytes forming E rosettes with sheep erythrocytes and expressing receptors for the Fc portion of IgG, Fc receptor [FcR]) and of the third population cells (TPC) (i.e., non-T, non-B cells with FcR).[4] In addition to LGL with avid FcR there are also granular lymphocytes which lack this marker.[5-7] Since the early studies with classical, i.e., nonmonoclonal markers, it was evident that there was some heterogeneity among LGL. This heterogeneity, on one hand, made it more difficult to obtain highly purified LGL populations and, on the other hand, raised the problem of whether or not LGL could be considered as a single, homogeneous population. Additional data such as differences in surface phenotype determined by monoclonal reagents and two or three-color fluorescence analysis,[8-13] and disparate functional activities (cytotoxicity, suppression, regulation of cell proliferation),[6,14-19] reinforced the possibility that LGL were heterogeneous.

In this article, we shall review the basic morphological and cytochemical features of LGL as well as their variances. Moreover, the problem of the relationship between differences in morphology and function of LGL will be discussed.

II. THE METHODOLOGICAL APPROACH TO THE STUDY OF LGL MORPHOLOGY AND CYTOCHEMISTRY

Before describing the basic morphological features of LGL, it seems appropriate to examine briefly the techniques used for LGL separation.

The early studies reported observations on Tγ or TPC which, although enriched for LGL, also contain other cell types.[4] Lately, separation on Percoll density gradients[2] or sorting for cells expressing LGL-specific surface antigens[12,13,20] have been employed. All of these methods have drawbacks which should be considered when trying to assess the typical LGL morphology. For example, none of the above techniques is suitable for the purification of the entire LGL population and different methods select for different cell fractions. Moreover, in most cases, a variable degree of contamination with other cell types may create problems regarding cell identification. Finally, with each method, cells undergo some manipulation that can cause artifacts, particularly at the ultrastructural level. For instance, cells separated as rosettes may be damaged by treatment with lysing media whereas cells fractionated by Percoll gradients or cell sorting may exhibit the results of physical injury.[21] Figure 1 shows a characteristic membrane artifact observed on a LGL from a Chediak-Higashi patient separated on Percoll gradients.

Immunohistochemical methods on sections have recently allowed the identification of LGL in tissues.[22-25] Although these techniques seem very promising and have revealed some ultrastructural differences between cells examined in suspension or in sections,[26] owing to the scarce number of observations it is premature to draw any firm conclusion. Therefore, our review will be centered on work on cell suspensions obtained mainly from normal peripheral blood.

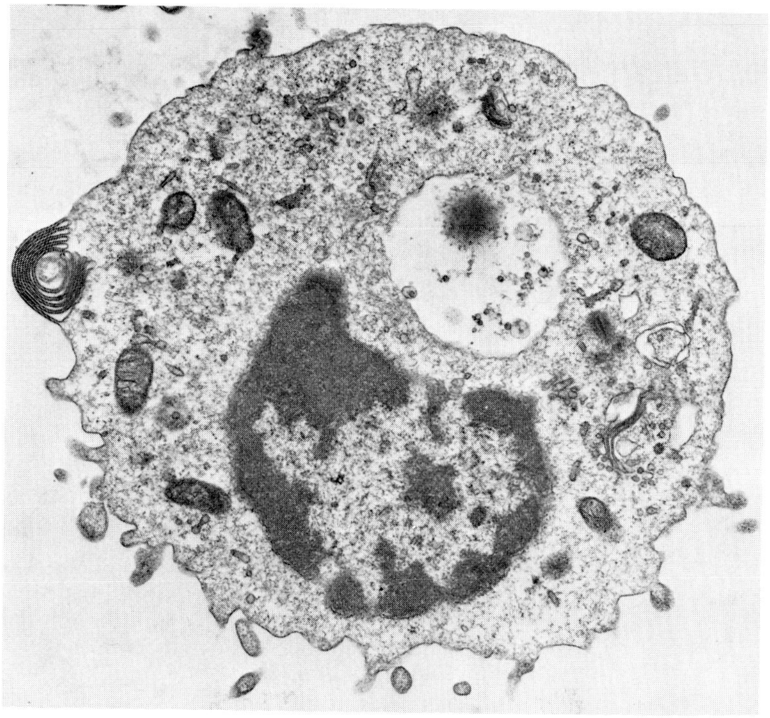

FIGURE 1. Ultrastructure of a LGL fractionated on Percoll density gradient from peripheral blood of a Chediak-Higashi patient. The large cytoplasmic inclusion is of note. The surface membrane displays a myelin figure. This is a fixation artifact due to a focal damage of the cell surface which occurred presumably during cell fractionation. (Magnification × 8500.)

III. ULTRASTRUCTURE OF LGL

The fine structure of a typical LGL is illustrated in Figure 2. It should be noted preliminarily that there are variations among the cells as for some of the features described below, particularly for the number and the characteristics of the granules.

LGL have a relatively low nuclear to cytoplasmic ratio. Nuclei are usually indented with dispersed chromatin and sometimes display prominent nucleoli. The cytoplasm is extended and contains a variety of organelles. The Golgi apparatus is located in the nuclear notch and consists of single or multiple stacks of cisternae. Smooth vesicles (round or cup-shaped) are seen at the concave aspect of the Golgi apparatus. Other vesicles that are smaller in size and bear an external coat (coated vesicles), are observed mainly in the proximity of the Golgi area, but are also scattered in the cytoplasm. Centrioles, sparse mitochondria and single strands of rough endoplasmic reticulum (RER) are also detected.

A number of round granules of variable size are found in the LGL cytoplasm. They are bound by unit membranes and contain a matrix of uniform electron opacity. These granules are more numerous in the nuclear notch, close to the Golgi apparatus, but are also found dispersely in the cytoplasm. The electron-opaque granules most likely correspond to the azurophilic granules seen by light microscopy in Giemsa-stained preparations. However, other organelles have been related to the azurophilic granules and namely the so-called parallel tubular arrays (PTA) which are found sporadically in LGL,[27-29] and also in other cell types such as malignant B cells or T-ALL lymphoblasts.[30] At the ultrastructural level, PTA appear as stacks of parallel tubules which

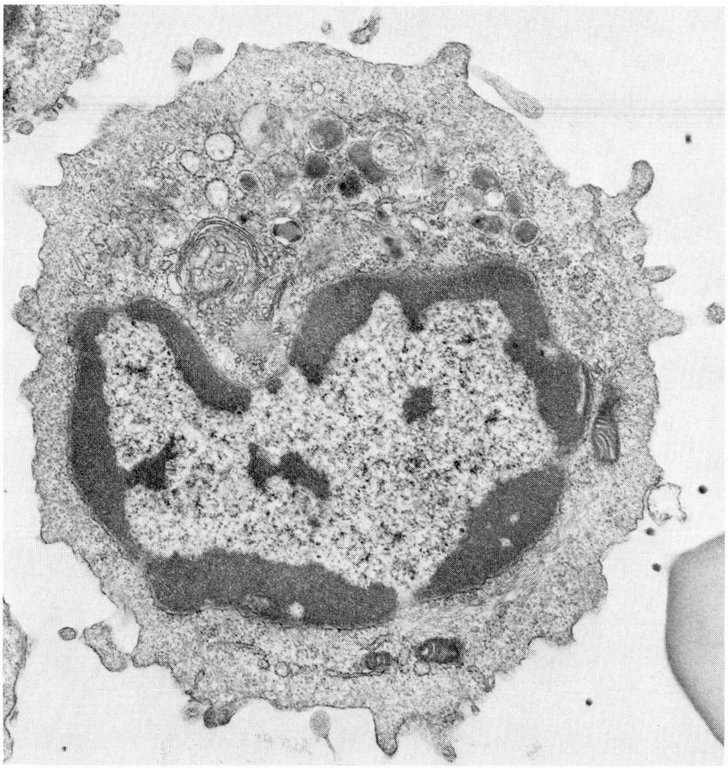

FIGURE 2. Ultrastructure of a peripheral blood LGL. An extended Golgi apparatus is found in the proximity of the nuclear notch. The cytoplasm contains numerous electron-dense granules. (Magnification × 8500.)

may be free in the cytoplasmic matrix or delimited by a unit membrane (Figure 3). Since the number of PTA varies considerably according to the different laboratories and to the different procedures used,[21,31] it seems unlikely that they account for all of the azurophilic granules. Also, the variations reported raise the possibility that PTA may at least in part be the result of technical artifacts.

Morphological variants of the electron-dense granules described above and shown in Figure 4, are represented by vesicles containing a flocculent, moderately electron-dense matrix which is separated from the limiting membrane by an electron-translucent, apparently empty, space. Membranes, sometimes arranged in parallel arrays, and residual vesicles are also found within the matrix (Figure 5). These organelles could represent maturing granules and are frequently detected in LGL from patients with lymphoproliferative disorders (and increased LGL numbers) or from normal peripheral blood subsets of LGL expressing T-cell markers.[32,33]

In a small proportion of complement receptor positive ($C3R^+$) normal peripheral blood LGL and in the cells from some patients with abnormally expanded LGL populations, there are additional cytoplasmic organelles, that are not generally seen in LGL.[32,33] These are multivesicular bodies (MVB) consisting of clusters of small vesicles (some of which are of the coated type) which are surrounded by a limiting membrane. Some MVB have a central core of electron-dense matrix. Together with MVB, these LGL also contain electron-dense granules which display residual vesicles in their peripheral matrix. All the above features suggest, although do not definitively prove, that MVB transform into electron-dense granules.

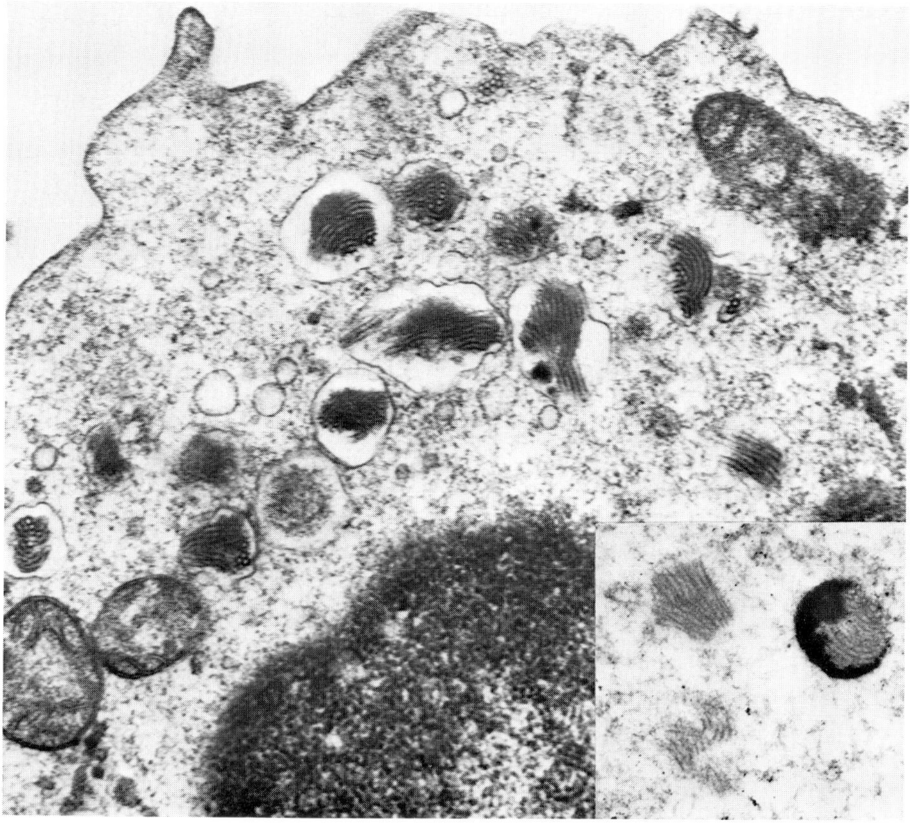

FIGURE 3. Ultrastructure of a peripheral blood LGL. The majority of the cytoplasmic inclusions are parallel tubular arrays (PTA), commonly surrounded by unit membranes. The inset shows the AP localization in a similar cell. The reaction product is detected in the space between the PTA and the limiting membrane. PTA which are free in the cytoplasmic matrix are AP-negative. (Magnification × 12,500.)

IV. CYTOCHEMISTRY AND ULTRASTRUCTURAL CYTOCHEMISTRY OF LGL

The extension of the Golgi apparatus, the high number of Golgi-related vesicles and the presence of azurophilic (electron-dense) granules suggests that the Golgi-lysosomal system is particularly well developed in LGL.[1,4,34] This hypothesis was confirmed by cytochemical studies showing that lysosome markers such as acid hydrolases are expressed in LGL. At the light microscopy level, acid phosphatase (AP), beta glucuronidase (BG) and alpha naphthyl acid esterase (ANAE) have been used most commonly to stain and identify LGL (Figure 6). Most, if not all, LGL are positive for AP or BG with scattered granular pattern of cytochemical staining.[4,35] The number of granules detected by these cytochemical techniques is higher than that of the azurophilic granules, suggesting that cytoplasmic organelles other than granules and yet related to the lysosomal system react for AP and BG; 50% or less of the LGL are positive for ANAE with a scattered granular or a diffuse paranuclear pattern of staining.[33] AP^{+}-BG^{+}-$ANAE^{-}$ cells are detected in both E rosette-positive and -negative fractions of peripheral blood mononuclear cells[4] and are particularly numerous in $C3R^{+}$ LGL[31] or among the cells from some patients with expanded LGL populations of possible malignant origin.[32] In some studies, $ANAE^{-}$LGL have been shown to have some phenotypic and functional natural killer (NK) features of immaturity and it has been suggested that, as

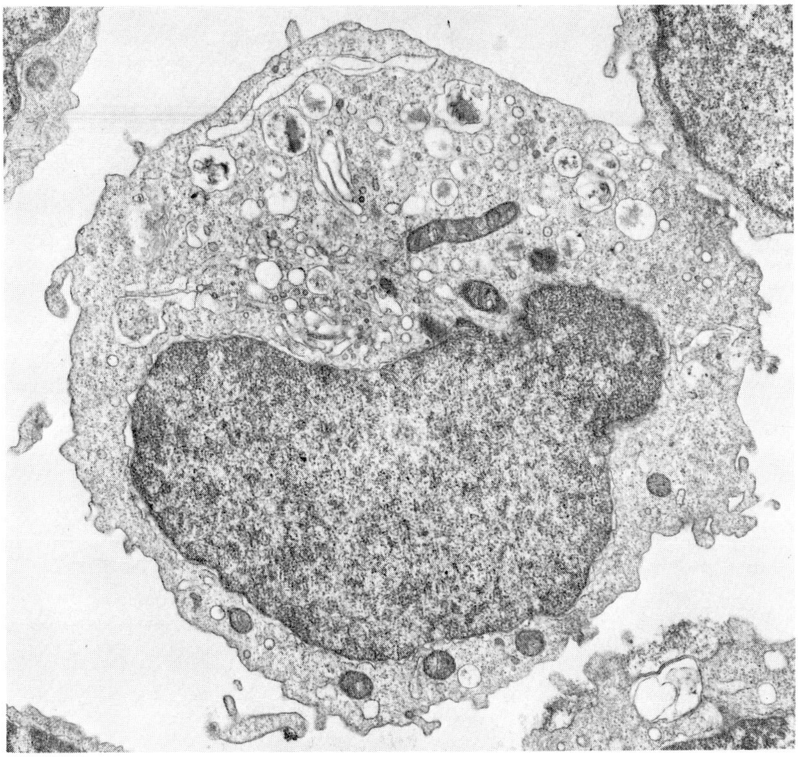

FIGURE 4. Ultrastructure of a peripheral blood LGL. As compared to the cell shown in Figure 2, the granules of this LGL show different ultrastructural characteristics (see text). (Magnification × 9200.)

for other lymphocyte populations (i.e., T or B cells), acid hydrolases could be expressed sequentially during maturation.[32] In other studies, however, a correlation between the presence or absence of ANAE and LGL subsets with distinct surface phenotype and function was detected (Table 1). Thus, E rosette$^+$-T8$^+$-M1$^+$ LGL stain strongly for ANAE, considerably suppress T cell proliferation and have no NK activity.[7] In contrast, Leu 11$^+$-Leu7$^-$ LGL comprise cells with high NK activity[12] that are consistently ANAE$^-$ (Table 1).

Recently, it has been reported that LGL also express napthol-AS-D-chloroacetate esterase (NASDCA), with a scattered granular pattern of cytochemical staining.[36] Interestingly this enzyme marker has been regarded as specific for the granulocytic lineage.

Cytochemical studies at the ultrastructural level have shown that AP is localized in the electron-dense granules (Figure 7) thus confirming their lysosomal nature.[3] Additional sites where the AP reaction product has been detected comprise PTA,[37] a variety of smooth vesicles, coated vesicles, and MVB.[3,32] In a small proportion of normal, circulating LGL and in expanded LGL populations with features of immaturity, AP activity has also been detected in the perinuclear cisterna and in some strands of the RER. The variety of AP-positive organelles detected in LGL by electron microscopy provides an explanation for the discrepancy in the number of granules detected by Giemsa staining as compared to that found by light microscopy cytochemistry.

Another enzyme detected in LGL by ultrastructural cytochemistry is thiamine pyrophosphatase (TPP), a marker of the transmost cisternae of the Golgi apparatus.[3,32] TPP activity has been shown in the perinuclear cisterna, in strands of RER, and in

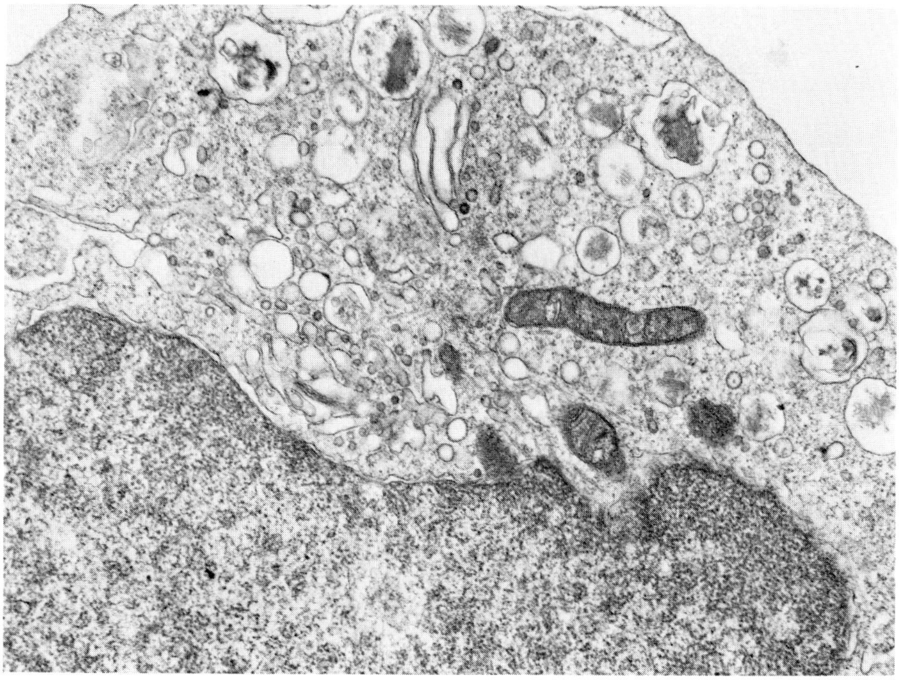

FIGURE 5. A higher magnification of the cell shown in Figure 4, to illustrate the ultrastructural heterogeneity of the granules. The numerous smooth and coated vesicles are also of note. (Magnification × 14,800.)

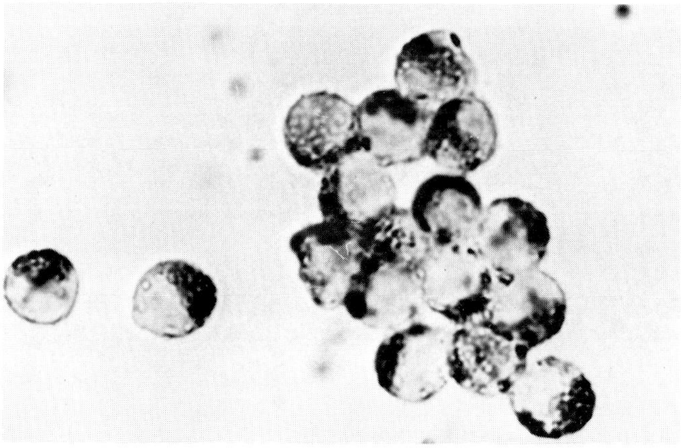

FIGURE 6. Cytochemical localization of phosphatase in a preparation enriched for LGL. Virtually all of the cells show a scattered granular pattern of staining. (Magnification × 650.)

stacks of cisternae at the concave aspect of the Golgi apparatus, but not in the granules. Furthermore, some cup-shaped vesicles and the limiting membrane of some MVB are TPP-positive. Since cup-shaped vesicles and MVB are found in LGL involved in active granulogenesis, it has been suggested that the limiting membrane of the granules is Golgi-derived whereas the matrix could originate from AP-positive smooth and coated vesicles.[38,39]

Table 1
EXPRESSION OF LYSOSOMAL ACID HYDROLASES IN GRANULAR LYMPHOCYTE SUBSETS

	Acid hydrolases			
Surface phenotype	AP	BG	ANAE	NK function
$T11^+$-$T3^+$-$T8^+$-$M1^+$-$Leu11^-$	+	+	+	−
$T11^+$-$T3^+$-$T8^+$-$M1^-$-$Leu11^-$	+	+	−	±
$T11^+$-$T3^-$-$T8^-$-$M1^+$-$Leu11^+$	+	+	−	+
$Leu7^+$-$Leu11^-$	+	+	+	±
$Leu7^-$-$Leu11^+$	+	+	−	+

Data shown in this table are derived from Refs. 6, 7, 9, and 12 and from unpublished experiments by A. Tilden, C. M. Balch, and C. E. Grossi.

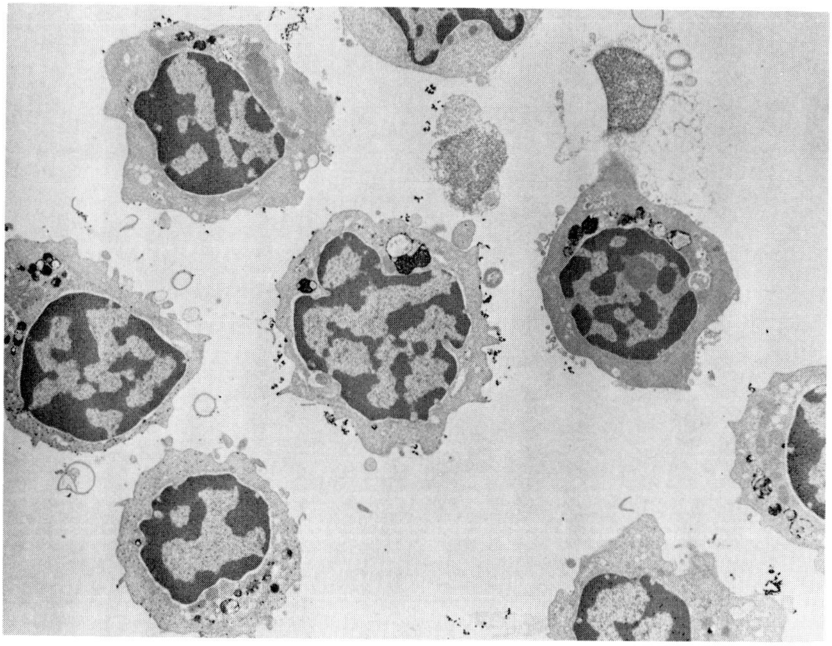

FIGURE 7. Ultrastructural localization of acid phosphatase in a LGL-enriched cell population. The electron-dense reaction product is detected primarily within the matrix of the granules. (Magnification × 2200.)

V. THE PROBLEM OF LGL HETEROGENEITY

The data presented above indicate that LGL are heterogeneous as for the expression of acid hydrolases and for some ultrastructural features such as the type and number of granules and vesicles, the extension of the Golgi apparatus, and the presence or absence of other organelles such as MVB or PTA. These differences may indicate that there are various LGL subsets specialized for different functions. Alternatively, these "subsets" may simply represent maturational stages of a single cell type. Comparative analysis of surface marker phenotype and morphological features leads to the delineation of distinct LGL subpopulations. For example, $T3^+$-$T8^+$-$Leu7^+$-$M1^-$ LGL have scarce granules.[9] The same morphology and phenotype have been reported for the cells from patients with granulocytopenia and expanded populations of LGL.[32] Since these cells are relatively inefficient in NK activity and are engaged in active granulogenesis, it has been proposed that they might correspond to immature LGL. It is of note, in this connection, that LGL expanded in continuous cell lines, seem to change their predominant surface phenotype from $T8^-$-$M1^+$ to $T8^+$-$M1^-$.[39a] These data would indicate that actively proliferating LGL express the T8 marker. A switch from one to the other phenotype has been reported in other types of cytotoxic cells following activation. This is, for example, the case of lymphokine-activated killers that originate from $M1^+$ cells and express the T3-T8 markers.[40,41]

Another example of correlation between surface phenotype and morphology is provided by the observation that besides being poor NK effectors,[3] LGL with C3R have fewer granules and lack ANAE activity.

A third case of defined LGL surface phenotype with particular morphological features is represented by the $T8^+$-$M1^+$-$Leu7^+$ cells which do not express FcR. These cells, that have been found both in normal peripheral blood and in a case of LGL lymphoproliferative disorder, have suppressor but not cytotoxic activity, stain strongly for ANAE and contain numerous granules.[6,7]

A final example along this line is offered by a special LGL subset of cells with high NK activity, which display a FcR^+-Leu 11^+-$Leu7^{+/-}$ phenotype and are negative for ANAE (see Table 1).

Clearly, some of the data so far obtained appear sometimes to confuse, rather than to clarify the issue. A better classification of the LGL subsets, together with the stages of maturation, will be probably reached by using a combination of cytochemical and ultrastructural observations in conjunction with surface marker analysis and functional studies.

REFERENCES

1. Grossi, C. E. Webb, S. R., Zicca, A., Lydyard, P. M., Moretta, L., Mingari, M. C., and Cooper, M. D., Morphological and histochemical analyses of two human T-cell subpopulations bearing receptors for IgM or IgG, *J. Exp. Med.*, 147, 1495, 1978.
2. Timonen, T., Ortaldo, J. R., and Herberman, R. B., Characterization of human large granular lymphocytes and relationship to natural killer and K cells, *J. Exp. Med.*, 153, 569, 1981.
3. Grossi, C. E., Cadoni, A., Zicca, A., Leprini, A., and Ferrarini, M., Large granular lymphocytes in human peripheral blood. Ultrastructural and cytochemical characterization of the granules, *Blood*, 59, 277, 1982.
4. Ferrarini, M., Cadoni, A., Franzi, A. T., Ghigliotti, C. Leprini, A., Zicca, A., and Grossi, C. E., Ultrastructure and cytochemistry of human peripheral blood lymphocytes. Similarities between the cells of the third population and T_G lymphocytes, *Eur. J. Immunol.*, 10, 562, 1980.
5. Zicca, A., Leprini, A., Cadoni, A., Franzi, A. T., Ferrarini, M., and Grossi, C. E., Ultrastructural localization of alpha-naphthyl acid esterase in human T_M lymphocytes, *Am. J. Pathol.*, 105, 40, 1981.
6. Landay, A., Gartland, G. L., and Clement, L. T., Characterization of a phenotypically distinct subpopulation of $Leu2^+$ cells that suppress T-cell proliferative responses, *J. Immunol.*, 1983, 131, 2757, 1983.
7. Landay, A., Clement, L. T., and Grossi, C. E., Phenotypically and functionally distinct subpopulations of human lymphocytes with T-cell markers also exhibit different cytochemical patterns of staining for lysosomal enzymes, *Blood*, in press.
8. Ortaldo, J. R., Sharrow, S. O., Timonen, T., and Herberman, R. B., Determination of surface antigens on highly purified human NK cells by flow cytometry with monoclonal antibodies, *J. Immunol.*, 127, 2041, 1981.
9. Abo, T., Cooper, M. D., and Balch, C. M., Characterization of HNK-$1/^+$(Leu7) human lymphocytes. I. Two distinct phenotypes of human NK cells with different cytotoxic capability, *J. Immunol.*, 129, 1752, 1982.

10. Rumpold, H., Kraft, D., Obexer, G., Bock, G., and Gebhart, W., A monoclonal antibody against a surface antigen shared by human large granular lymphocytes, *J. Immunol.*, 129, 1458, 1982.
11. Perussia, B., Starr, S., Abraham, S., Fanning, V., and Trinchieri, G., Human natural killer cells analyzed by B73.1, a monoclonal antibody blocking Fc receptor functions. I. Characterization of the lymphocyte subset reactive with B73.1, *J. Immunol.*, 130, 2133, 1983.
12. Lanier, L. L., Le, A. M., Phillips, J. H., Warner, N. L., and Babcock, G. F., Subpopulations of human natural killer cells defined by expression of the Leu 7 (HNK-1) and Leu 11 (NK-15) antigens, *J. Immunol.*, 131, 1789, 1983.
13. Lanier, L. L. and Loken, M. R., Human lymphocyte subpopulations identified by using three color immunofluorescence and flow cytometry analysis: correlation of Leu2, Leu3, Leu7, Leu8 and Leu11 cell surface antigen expression, *J. Immunol.*, 132, 151, 1984.
14. Herberman, R. B., Djeu, J. Y., Kay, D., Ortaldo, J. R., Riccardi, C., Bonnard, G. D., Holden, K. T., Fagnani, R., Santoni, A., and Puccetti, P., Natural killer cells: characteristics and regulation of activity, *Immunol. Rev.*, 44, 43, 1979.
15. Tilden, A., Abo, T., and Balch, C. M., Suppressor cell function of human granular lymphocytes identified by the HNK-1 (Leu 7) monoclonal antibody, *J. Immunol.*, 130, 1171, 1983.
16. Arai, S., Yamamoto, H., Itoh, K., and Kumagai, K., Suppressive effect of human natural killer cells on pokeweed-mitogen induced B-cell differentiation, *J. Immunol.*, 131, 651, 1983.
17. Hansson, M., Bevan, M., Anderson, B., and Kiessling, R., Inhibition of in vitro granulopoiesis by autologous and allogeneic human NK cells, *J. Immunol.*, 129, 126, 1982.
18. Pistoia, V., Nocera, A., Ghio, R., Leprini, A., Perata, A., Pistone, M., and Ferrarini, M., PHA-induced human T-cell colony formation: enhancing effect of large granular lymphocytes, *Exp. Hematol.*, 11, 251, 1983.
19. Pistoia, V., Nocera, A., Perata, A., Leprini, A., Ghio, R., and Ferrarini, M., Large granular lymphocytes have a regulatory role on the growth of human peripheral blood T cell and erythroid colonies, *Surv. Synth. Pathol. Res.*, 2, 47, 1983.
20. Abo, T. and Balch, C. M., A differentiation antigen of human NK and K cells identified by a monoclonal antibody (HNK-1), *J. Immunol.*, 127, 1024, 1981.
21. Payne, C. M., Glasser, L., Fiederlein, R., and Lindberg, R., New ultrastructural observations: parallel tubular arrays in human Tγ lymphoid cells, *J. Immunol. Methods*, 65, 307, 1983.
22. Ritchie, A. W. S., James, K., and Micklem, H. S., The distribution and possible significance of cells identified in human lymphoid tissue by the monoclonal antibody HNK-1, *Clin. Exp. Immunol.*, 51, 439, 1983.
23. Si, L. and Whiteside, T., Tissue distribution of human NK cells studied with an anti-Leu7 monoclonal antibody, *J. Immunol.*, 130, 2149, 1983.
24. Banerjee, D. and Thibert, R. F., Natural Killer-like cells found in B-cell compartments of human lymphoid tissues, *Nature*, 304, 270, 1983.
25. Mori, S., Mohri, N., Morita, H., Yamaguchi, K., and Shimamine, T., The distribution of cells expressing a natural killer cell marker (HNK-1) in normal human lymphoid organs and malignant lymphomas, *Virchows Arch. Cell Pathol.*, 43, 253, 1983.
26. Cerf-Bensusson, N., Schneeberger, E. E., and Ghan, A. K., Immunohistologic and immunoelectron microscopic characterization of the mucosal lymphocytes of human small intestine by the use of monoclonal antibodies, *J. Immunol.*, 130, 2615, 1983.
27. Payne, C. M., Jones, J., F., Sieber, O. F., Jr., and Fulginiti, V. A., Parallel tubular arrays in severe combined immunodeficiency disease. An ultrastructural study of peripheral blood lymphocytes, *Blood*, 50, 55, 1977.
28. Payne, C. M. and Glaser, L., Evaluation of surface markers on normal human lymphocytes containing parallel tubular arrays: a quantitative ultrastructural study, *Blood*, 57, 567, 1981.
29. Smit, J. W., Blom, N. R., Van Luyn, M., and Halie, M. R., Lymphocytes with parallel tubular structures: morphologically a distinctive subpopulation, *Blut*, 46, 311, 1983.
30. Greaves, M. F., Habeshaw, J. A., and Stansfeld, A. G., Lymphoproliferative disorders, in *Atlas of Blood Cells, Function and Pathology*, Zucker-Franklin, D. Greaves, M. F., Grossi, C. E., and Marmont, A. M., Eds., Lea & Febiger, Philadelphia, 1981.
31. Smit, J. W., Blom, N. R., Van Luyn, M. J. A., and Halie, M. R., Susceptibility of the expression of parallel tubular structures in lymphocytes to the exposure to ammonium chloride buffer, *J. Immunol. Methods*, 61, 49, 1983.
32. Ferrarini, M., Romagnani, S., Montesoro, E., Zicca, A., Del Prete, G. F., Nocera, A., Maggi, E., Leprini A., and Grossi, C. E., A lymphoproliferative disorder of the large granular lymphocytes with natural killer activity, *J. Clin. Immunol.*, 3, 30, 1983.
33. Nocera, A., Montesoro, E., Balbo, P., Ferrarini, M., Leprini, A., Zicca, A., and Grossi, C. E., Complement receptor distinguishes two subsets of large granular lymphocytes with different NK activity and cytochemical and ultrastructural features, *Scand. J. Immunol.*, 18, 345, 1983.

34. Saksela, E., Timonen, T., Ranki, A., and Hayry, P., Morphological and functional characterization of isolated effector cells responsible for human natural killer activity to fetal fibroblasts and to cultured cell line targets, *Immunol. Rev.*, 44, 71, 1979.
35. Crockard, A. D., MacFarlane, E., Jess, H., and Catovsky, D., Correlation of lymphocyte β-glucuronidase and N-acetyl-β-glucosaminidase with E-rosette formation, *Histochem. J.*, 15, 179, 1983.
36. Heumann, D., Colombatti, M., and Mach, J. P., Human large granular lymphocytes contain an esterase activity usually considered as specific for the myeloid series, *Eur. J. Immunol.*, 13, 154, 1983.
37. Costello, C., Catovsky, D., O'Brien, M., Morilla, R., and Varardi, S., Chronic T-cell leukemias. I. Morphology, cytochemistry and ultrastructure, *Leukemia Res.*, 4, 463, 1980.
38. Grossi, C. E. and Ferrarini, M., Morphology and cytochemistry of human large granular lymphocytes, in, *NK Cells and Other Natural Effector Cells*, R. B. Herberman, Ed., Academic Press, New York, 1982, 1.
39. Grossi, C. E., Zicca, A., Leprini, A., Cadoni, A., Pandolfi, F., Burgio, V. L., Romagnani, S., Guglielmi, C., and Ferrarini, M., Granule formation in large granular lymphocytes (LGL). Ultrastructural and cytochemical studies in patients with abnormally expanded LGL population, *J. Submicrosc. Cytol.*, 16, 759, 1984.
39a. Nocera, A., unpublished.
40. Grimm, E. A., Mazumder, A., Zhang, H. Z., and Rosenberg, S. A., Lymphokine-activated killer cell phenomenon. I. Lysis of natural killer-resistant fresh solid tumor cells by interleukin 2-activated autologous human peripheral blood lymphocytes, *J. Exp. Med.*, 155, 1823, 1982.
41. Grimm, E. A., Ramsey, K. M., Mazumder, A., Wilson, D. J., Djeu, J. Y., and Rosenberg, S. A., Lymphokine-activated killer cell phenomenon. II. Precursor phenotype is serologically distinct from peripheral T lymphocytes, memory cytotoxic thymus-derived lymphocytes and natural killer cells, *J. Exp. Med.*, 157, 884, 1983.

Chapter 4

PHYLOGENY AND ONTOGENY OF NK CELLS

Cherylyn A. Savary and Eva Lotzová

TABLE OF CONTENTS

I. INTRODUCTION

As discussed in other chapters in this book, natural killer (NK) cells, although initially recognized for their anticancer activity, appear to be involved in a multitude of biological processes, including defense against bacterial and viral infections,[1] resistance to parasites,[2] rejection of hemopoietic transplants,[3-7] and regulation of the growth and/or differentiation of erythroid, myeloid, and lymphoid cell types.[8-12] Thus, NK cells may represent a population whose complex functional activities arise from a basic responsibility of maintenance of homeostasis within the biological system. Such a functional unit would be expected, therefore, to be well preserved throughout phylogenetic development, since it is a basic premise of the theory of evolution that characteristics or adaptations which are favorable to the survival of an organism will be highly conserved. Analysis of the origin and development of NK cell activity within the evolutionary scale could therefore provide insight into the adaptive advantage created by the NK cell system and could contribute to an understanding of its precise biological role(s) in man.

The characteristics of NK cells, their functional properties, and their mechanism of action have been, and are currently, under intensive investigation. However, the phylogeny and ontogeny of this important effector cell population have not been so thoroughly explored. In this chapter, we will summarize the available data regarding the presence of NK or NK-like cells in various invertebrate and vertebrate species, and discuss the current knowledge pertaining to the ontogenetic development of NK cell activity.

II. PHYLOGENY OF NK CELLS

A. Invertebrates

While NK cell activity was first detected in vertebrates, there is now evidence to suggest that naturally cytotoxic cells bearing some resemblance to mammalian NK cells are also present in invertebrates (Table 1).[13-17] For instance, in unsegmented worm, *Sipunculus nudus,* cells within the coelomic cavity (coelomocytes) resembling vertebrate leukocytes, exert rapid spontaneous cytolysis of allogeneic and xenogeneic erythrocytes in vitro.[14] Natural cytotoxic reactivity directed against erythrocytes is also displayed by other invertebrate species, including annelids, echinoderms, and mollusks.[14,15] In echinoderms and mollusks the cytolytic activity is also directed against normal mononuclear cells.[15] In addition to spontaneous cytotoxicity against normal tissues, invertebrates also mediate cytotoxic reactivity against malignant cells.[13,15,17] Among the echinoderms, coelomocytes of *Pisaster gigantus* were found to effectively lyse murine P815 mastocytoma tumor, as well as a human B cell line,[15] and cells from the axial organ of *Asterias rubens* are cytolytically active against various types of murine tumor cells.[17] Antitumor activity was also detected in annelids, as exampled by the bloodworm *Glycera Sp-C,*[15] and in arthropods, including crayfish *Parachaeraps bicarinatus* and lobster *Homarus americanus.*[13,16]

The effector cells in invertebrates were not conclusively characterized; however, they are functionally and morphologically similar to mammalian NK cells. For instance, the coelomocytes of annelids mediating lysis of allogeneic leukocytes are nylon wool-nonadherent,[14] the spontaneously active effector cells of echinoderms and mollusks are nonspecific esterase-negative, and their cytotoxic function is inhibited by monosaccharides.[15] Moreover, coelomocytes of the earthworm, *Lumbricus terrestris,* which are involved in the rejection of xenogeneic skin grafts, display large granular lymphocyte (LGL) morphology,[18,19] the morphology displayed by NK cells of most vertebrates.

Table 1
SPONTANEOUS CYTOTOXICITY IN VARIOUS INVERTEBRATE SPECIES

Phylum	Species	Type of target cells killed: Normal	Type of target cells killed: Malignant
Sipunculids	*Sipunculus nudus* (unsegmented worms)	Allogeneic and xenogeneic erythrocytes	—
Annelids	*Eisenia fetida* (earthworm)	Allogeneic leukocytes	—
	Lumbricus terrestris (earthworm)	Xenogeneic skin grafts	—
	Glycera Sp-C (bloodworm)	Xenogeneic erythrocytes	Xenogeneic mastocytoma
Echinoderms	*Pisaster gigantus* (starfish)	Xenogeneic erythrocytes and mononuclear cells	Xenogeneic mastocytoma and B cell line
	Asterias rubens (starfish)	—	Xenogeneic cell lines
Mollusks	*Megathura crenulata* (keyhole limpet)	Xenogeneic erythrocytes and mononuclear cells	—
Arthropods	*Parachaeraps bicarinatus* (crayfish)	—	Xenogeneic ascites
	Homarus americanus (lobster)	No reactivity to sheep erythrocytes or autologous cells	Xenogeneic mastocytoma

Note: — = not tested.

B. Vertebrates

1. Fish and Amphibians

Primitive vertebrates, as represented by fish and amphibians, also possess NK-like cytotoxic activity (Table 2). Fresh water fish, including *Cyprinus carpio* (carp), *Carassius cuvieri* (crucian carp), *Ctenopharyngodon idella* (grass carp), *Misgrunus anguillicandatus* (oriental weather fish), and *Channa argus* (northern snakehead), display spontaneous in vitro cytotoxicity to established mammalian cell lines of both normal and malignant derivation.[20] In these species, highest cytotoxicity was found in the kidney (a hemopoietic organ in fish), and lower and variable reactivity in peripheral blood and spleen. The cytotoxic activity resembled that of mammalian NK cells by the rapid lysis (occurring within 6 hr of contact with target cells) and no species restriction.

Natural cytotoxic cells were also detected in the nurse shark *(Ginglymostoma cirratum)*[21] and in amphibian *Xenopus laevis*.[16] In the amphibia, the splenocytes were the main source of effector cells, whereas bone marrow and thymus exhibited only negligible levels of cytotoxicity (Table 3).[16]

2. Avians

In avian species, chicken and quail exhibited spontaneous lytic activity against normal and malignant targets of allogeneic and xenogeneic origin.[22-25] The cells mediating cytotoxicity in both species were found in spleen and peripheral blood, but not in thymus and bursa of Fabricius (tested in chickens only, Table 3).[22-25] Splenic effector cells of quail were characterized as nonadherent to plastic, and not expressing specific T- or B-cell antigens. One group of investigators reported, however, that peripheral blood effector cells in both of the species were removed by adherence to plastic or nylon wool and were decreased after carbonyl iron treatment.[25] The latter observation suggests that some of the spontaneously cytotoxic cells may be of possible macrophage nature. Nevertheless, the cells with typical LGL characteristics are present in chicken peripheral blood,[26] even though their cytotoxic potential has not yet been explored (Table 4).

Table 2
SPONTANEOUS CYTOTOXICITY IN VARIOUS VERTEBRATE SPECIES

Species	Type of target cells killed: Normal	Malignant
Fish	Xenogeneic amnion, kidney, and fibroblast cells	Xenogeneic carcinoma and lymphomas
Amphibians	—	Xenogeneic lymphoma
Avians	Allogeneic embryonic cells	Xenogeneic and allogenic lymphoma; xenogeneic plasmocytoma, thymoma, mastocytoma, melanoma, and leukemia
Mice	Syngeneic and allogeneic bone marrow, thymocytes and macrophages; allogeneic fibroblasts	Syngeneic, allogeneic, and xenogeneic leukemia, lymphoma and solid tumors
Rat	Allogeneic kidney cells and embryonic cells	Syngeneic, allogeneic, and xenogeneic, lymphoma and leukemia; syngeneic and allogeneic solid tumors
Hamster	Allogeneic and xenogeneic kidney cells; xenogeneic fibroblasts	Syngeneic, allogeneic and xenogeneic lymphoma; xenogeneic lymphoma; xenogeneic leukemia
Guinea pig	Syngeneic and xenogeneic fibroblasts and liver cells	Syngeneic and allogeneic solid tumors; xenogeneic leukemia
Felines	Allogeneic and xenogeneic kidney cells	Xenogeneic lymphoma
Canine	Allogeneic testicular cells, thymus cells	Allogeneic solid tumors; xenogeneic leukemia
Swine	—	Xenogeneic lymphoma and leukemia
Nonhuman primates	No reactivity to murine bone marrow cells or thymocytes	Allogeneic, B cell lines; xenogeneic lymphomas and leukemia
Humans	Autologous and allogeneic bone marrow; allogeneic thymocytes; xenogeneic splenocytes	Autologous, allogeneic, and xenogeneic lymphoma, leukemia, and solid tumors

Note: — = not tested.

3. *Rodents*

NK cells were first described in mice,[27,28] and with the possible exception of humans, natural cytotoxicity has been most thoroughly analyzed in the murine system. The spontaneous cytotoxic tumor-directed cells were subsequently detected in other rodents, including rats, hamsters, and guinea pigs (Table 2).[29-40] In addition to antitumor activity, NK cells in these species were also found to display cytotoxicity against normal tissues.[38-42] NK cells in all rodents were characterized as rapidly reactive, nonphagocytic, and relatively nonadherent, without any species-specific or histocompatibility restriction for function.[27,43]

In rodents, highest NK cell activity is present in the spleen and peripheral blood; furthermore, high levels of NK activity were detected in the lamina propria and intestinal epithelium of mice (Table 3).[44] Lower NK cell reactivity is present in lymph nodes, bone marrow, lungs, and liver of all rodents tested.[30-40,45] In peritoneal exudate of most rodents, NK cell activity is very low or nonexistent, with the exception of some strains of rats in which a high degree of cytotoxicity has been observed.[32,34,35] Thymus is virtually devoid of NK cell activity. However, it must be pointed out that most of the studies on tissue distribution of NK cells have been done with unpurified cell preparations and thus the presence of NK cells may have been obscured by the other cell populations or the presence of suppressor cells. In fact, a subpopulation of murine thymocytes obtained by separation on Percoll density gradients has been shown to exert significant levels of NK cell cytotoxicity.[46]

Table 3
TISSUE DISTRIBUTION OF NK CELL ACTIVITY IN VARIOUS SPECIES OF VERTEBRATES

Species	Tissue and the levels of NK cell reactivity
Fish	Kidney (H); peripheral blood (V); spleen (V)
Amphibians	Spleen (H); bone marrow (L); thymus (L)
Avians	Peripheral blood (H); spleen (H); thymus (N); bursa of Fabricius (N)
Mice	Peripheral blood (H); spleen (H); intestinal epithelium (H); lamina propria (M); bone marrow (L); lymph node (V); thymus (N); peritoneal exudate (L); lungs (L); liver (L)
Rats	Peripheral blood (H); spleen (H); bone marrow (N); lymph node (L); thymus (N); peritoneal exudate (V); lungs (L); liver (L)
Hamsters	Peripheral blood (H); spleen (H); bone marrow (L); lymph node (L); thymus (N); peritoneal exudate (L)
Guinea pigs	Peripheral blood (H); spleen (H); bone marrow (L); lymph node (L); thymus (N); peritoneal exudate (L)
Felines	Peripheral blood (H)
Canines	Peripheral blood (H); spleen (V)
Swine	Peripheral blood (H); spleen (L); bone marrow (N); lymph node (N); thymus (N); tonsils (N)
Nonhuman primates	Peripheral blood (H); spleen (H); thymus (N)
Humans	Peripheral blood (H); spleen (H); bone marrow (L); lymph node (L); thymus (N); peritoneal exudate (N); lungs (L); tonsils (V)

Note: H=high; M=medium; L=low; V=variable; N=none.

NK cell activity in rats has been associated with cells displaying LGL morphology, as represented by relatively large size, large cytoplasm-to-nucleus ratio, and azurophilic granules in the cytoplasm (Plate 1*).[33] In mice, these cells are of medium rather than large size, and may not be responsible for all cytotoxic activity in this species.[26,47] As indicated in other chapters in this book, LGL of rats and mice are distributed among various lymphoid tissues, including the spleen, peripheral blood, lungs, lamina propria, and intestinal epithelium; negligible or lower numbers of LGL have been detected in bone marrow, lymph nodes, and peritoneal exudate in these two species (Table 4).[33-35,48] LGL have also been detected in hamster peripheral blood.[26,38] In contrast to LGL of other species which are of low density, LGL of hamsters were found to be of higher density as determined by separation on discontinous Percoll gradients.[38]

A suggestion has been made that spontaneous reactivity of guinea pigs may be mediated by an unusual mononuclear cell population designated as Kurloff cells.[49] These cells are easily distinguished morphologically by their characteristic intracytoplasmic inclusion body, which resembles, by its staining properties, azurophilic granules of LGL described in mammals.[50,51] While these structures in guinea pigs predominantly contain proteoglycans, similar to human LGL, they were also found to contain acid phosphatase.[50] In parallel with the tissue distribution of NK cell activity, Kurloff cells were found predominantly in the spleen, and to a lesser extent in peripheral blood and lymph nodes,[49] and were not detected in thymus tissue. Like NK cells of other species, Kurloff cells are nonphagocytic, lack nonspecific esterase activity, and express Fc receptors (FcR).[49,50] Additionally, 50 to 75% of these cells form spontaneous rosettes with rabbit erythrocytes, the characteristic of guinea pig T cells.[49]

* Plate 1 appears after page 54.

Table 4
TISSUE DISTRIBUTION OF LGL IN VARIOUS SPECIES OF VERTEBRATES

Species	Tissue (% LGL)
Avians	Peripheral blood (6)
Mice	Peripheral blood (6—11), spleen (0.4—3), bone marrow (1), lymph node (0.5), thymus (0), peritoneal exudate (<0.5), lungs (4), lamina propria (13), intestinal epithelium (38)
Rats	Peripheral blood (4—14), spleen (2—6), bone marrow (<0.5), lymph node (0.5—1), thymus (<0.5), peritoneal exudate (2—4), lungs (3—10)
Hamsters	Peripheral blood (5—10)[a]
Guinea pigs	Peripheral blood (9)
Felines	Peripheral blood (1)
Canines	Peripheral blood (1—13)
Swine	Peripheral blood (3)
Nonhuman primates	Peripheral blood (6—26)
Humans	Peripheral blood (5—17), spleen (5), bone marrow (1)

[a] Percoll density gradient enriched cell fraction.

4. Felines

Very early investigations in felines failed to demonstrate spontaneous antitumor effector cells in these animals.[52] More exploratory studies, using a larger panel of tumor cell lines, however, demonstrated substantial levels of peripheral blood cytotoxicity directed against xenogeneic targets in domestic cats (Table 2).[53] Reactivity to allogeneic targets (both normal and virus-transformed) was found to be absent or low, unless the targets were previously infected with a Herpes simplex virus (HSV). Similar to other vertebrates, cat NK cells are nonadherent to plastic, and some, but not all, possess high affinity FcR.[53] Approximately 1% of feline peripheral blood mononuclear cells display LGL morphology (Table 4).[26] Spontaneous cell-mediated cytotoxicity (CMC) was also observed in Sumatran tigers; in these studies, ^{75}Se-selenomethionine-labeled xenogeneic lymphoma cells were found to be sensitive to lysis by tiger peripheral blood mononuclear cells.[24]

5. Canines

Spontaneous cytolytic activity against allogeneic and xenogeneic target cells of both normal and malignant derivation was detected in peripheral blood of canines (Table 2).[54-56] However, a great degree of variability in NK cell cytotoxic potential was observed among individual mongrel dogs.[54] In our laboratory, we investigated NK cell cytotoxic potential of mongrel dogs against K-562 and canine thyroid adenocarcinoma (CTAC) cell lines. We found low levels of NK cell cytotoxicity against K-562 target, but significant levels against CTAC target in peripheral blood of most mongrel dogs after longer time of incubation (Table 5). Characterization studies have shown that the effector cells are nonadherent to nylon wool and of a low density, as determined by separation on Percoll density gradients.[56a] As can be seen from Figure 1, the parallelism between levels of NK cell cytotoxicity and LGL content was observed in various fractions after Percoll separation. These data, along with our observation that canine LGL bind to susceptible tumor target, suggest that these cells may be responsible for NK cell-mediated reactions in dogs.

In other studies on NK cell cytotoxicity in dogs, carbonyl-iron ingesting and B cell-depleted peripheral blood mononuclear cells of specific pathogen-free beagles were found to exert significant cytolytic activity to canine distemper virus-infected, but not to uninfected normal testicular cells.[55] Such findings, along with the observation that

Table 5
NK CELL CYTOTOXICITY OF CANINE PERIPHERAL BLOOD MONONUCLEAR CELLS

Time of incubation (hr)	Target	$LU_{10}/10^7$ mononuclear cells[a] Unseparated	Nylon wool-filtered
4	CTAC	<1	<1
	K-562	<1	<1
7	CTAC	3.1 ± 1.5	1.1 ± 0.3
	K-562	<1	<1
16	CTAC	22.8 ± 1.9	19.0 ± 1.4
	K-562	2.7 ± 0.8	—

Note: — = not tested.

[a] Lytic units were determined by linear regression analysis of cytotoxicity values obtained at various target-to-effector cell ratios (1:25, 1:50, 1:100).

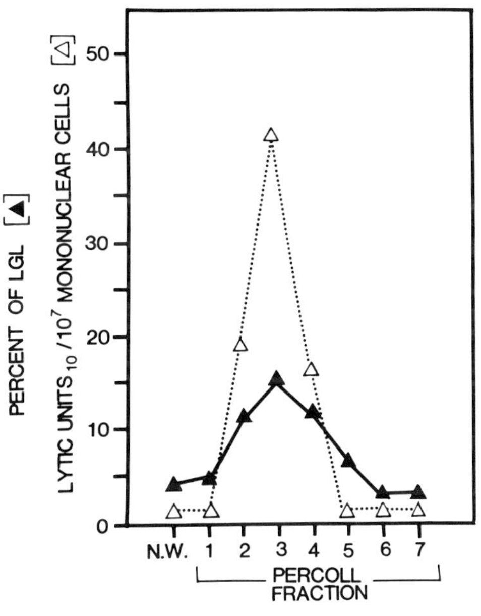

FIGURE 1. Enrichment of canine peripheral blood NK cell cytotoxicity and LGL following Percoll density gradient fractionation. Cytotoxicity to CTAC tumor cells was tested in a 16 hr ^{51}Cr release assay. Lytic units were calculated by linear regression analysis of cytotoxicity values obtained at various target-to-effector cell ratios (1:3, 1:6, 1:12, 1:25). N.W. = nylon wool-filtered (input) cells.

NK cell reactivity to distemper virus-infected targets is increased following immunization of dogs with this virus, suggest that NK cells may play a role in in vivo resistance to canine distemper virus-mediated disease.

6. Swine

Studies in specific pathogen- or germ-free Minnesota miniature swine,[57,58] as well as in conventionally raised pigs,[24] demonstrated natural cytotoxic reactivity in peripheral blood of these species which was directed against various xenogeneic lymphomas and leukemias (Table 2).[57,58] Splenic NK activity was either absent or was quite low, and bone marrow, lymph nodes, tonsils, and thymus appeared to be devoid of NK cell cytolytic capacity.[58] Characterization studies indicated that the effector cells were non-adherent to plastic, and unlike T cells, most of them lacked detectable receptors for sheep red blood cells (SRBC).[57] No attempt, however, was made to evaluate the possible presence of low-affinity SRBC receptors (found to be characteristic of human NK cells) on porcine NK cells. LGL were detected in peripheral blood of pigs (Table 4), suggesting that these cells may be responsible for NK cell reactivity observed in this tissue.[26] However, the involvement of LGL in spontaneous cytotoxicity of pigs remains to be determined.

7. Human and Nonhuman Primates

Both Old and New World monkeys demonstrate significant peripheral blood and splenic NK cell cytotoxic activity against various types of allogeneic and xenogeneic tumor cell lines in vitro (Table 2).[59,60] Recently, we have shown in our laboratory that NK cell reactivity of Rhesus monkeys is associated with nylon wool-filtered peripheral blood mononuclear cells displaying LGL morphology (Plate 1, Table 4). Percoll density gradient separation of monkey LGL demonstrated that these cells display relatively low density (Figure 2). These results suggest that NK cells of nonhuman primates have many similarities in common with the NK cells of the phylogenetically close human species and indicate that monkeys may prove to be a useful animal model for extrapolation of experimental results to the human situation.

Cells with NK cell reactivity have been conserved in the phylogenetically highest species, man. A detailed discussion of the characteristics and functional properties of this effector cell population in humans is beyond the scope of this chapter, and is covered in other chapters of this book. However, for comparison with other vertebrate species, the target specificity, tissue distribution, and NK cell morphological characteristics in man are summarized in Tables 2, 3, and 4, and Plate 1.

8. Other Vertebrate Species

Besides the above discussed species, there is one report describing spontaneously cytolytic cells in peripheral blood of horses, cattle, and mink.[24] Although the reactivity of individual animals was quite variable, significant NK cell reactivity to xenogeneic targets was observed in all three species. In cattle, NK cells were characterized as plastic nonadherent and nonphagocytic. LGL have also been detected in peripheral blood of cattle;[26] however, their relation to cytotoxic reaction was not explored in these animals.

III. ONTOGENY OF NK CELLS

A. Avians

Quail and chickens less than 3 weeks old lack significant levels of splenic natural cytolytic activity.[22,23] The cytotoxic potential is fully developed 4 weeks after birth in quail[23] and by at least 8 weeks in chickens.[22] Even though the endogenous NK cell activity is not present or is very low in young chickens, it could be induced following immunization with the Marek's disease virus.[61] These findings, along with the observation that such treatment prevents Marek's virus-induced neoplasia, suggests a possible role for NK cells in the control of this syndrome. This is further supported by the observation that adoptive transfer of adult spleen cells, depleted of macrophages and

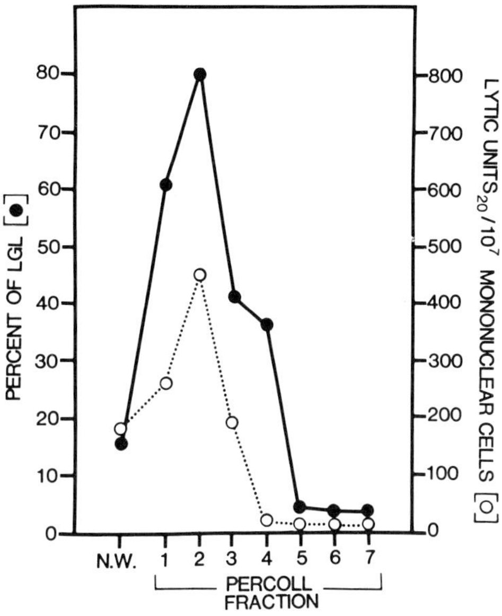

FIGURE 2. Enrichment of rhesus monkey peripheral blood NK cell cytotoxicity and LGL following Percoll density gradient fractionation. Cytotoxicity to K-562 tumor cells was tested in a 3 hr ^{51}Cr release assay. Lytic units were calculated by linear regression analysis of cytotoxicity values obtained at various target-to-effector cell ratios (1:3, 1:6, 1:12). N.W. = nylon wool-filtered (input) cells.

T cells, or obtained from bursectomized chickens, protected newly hatched chickens from Marek's disease infection.[62]

B. Swine

Miniature swine display negligible levels of NK cell activity at birth.[63] Cytotoxicity is first detected in specific pathogen-free piglets within 2 to 3 weeks after birth. In contrast, NK cell reactivity develops slightly later (3 to 4 weeks) in hysterectomy-derived colostrum-deprived, germ-free piglets of the same strain. Evidence suggests that the accelerated maturation of NK cell reactivity in the specific pathogen-free piglets may be due to the exposure to microfloral bacteria which are absent in the latter group of animals. These results, therefore, allude to a possible contribution of the environment in development of NK cytolytic potential. However, the fact that the piglets maintained in germ-free environments acquire NK cell activity within a month after birth indicates that maturation of NK cell reactivity is not totally dependent on environmental stimulation.[63] This is supported by observations in rodents, including detection of high levels of cytotoxicity in gnotobiotic mice and rats and comparable levels of NK activity in germ-free and conventionally maintained animals.[64,65]

C. Rodents

In rodents, fetal development of the NK cell system has been studied only in mice. Effector cells obtained from the yolk sac of 10-day-old mouse embryos of Balb/c strain exert significant spontaneous cytotoxic reactivity to allogeneic YAC-1 lymphoma in vitro.[66] Analysis of effector cells in yolk sac have indicated that these cells share some characteristics with NK cells of adult mice. They are, for instance, nonadherent to plastic and resistant to trypsin treatment;[67] there are, however, differences in embry-

Table 6
PRESENCE OF NK-1.1 POSITIVE CELLS IN FETAL TISSUES OF C57BL/6 MICE

Age of fetus (days)	NK-1.1-positive cells (%)		
	Liver	Thymus	Spleen
14	15	18	0
16	30	5	32
18	38	3	33
20	5	2	35

Extrapolated from Koo, G. C., Peppard, J. R., and Hatzfeld, A., *J. Immunol.*, 129, 867, 1982.

onic and mature NK cells with regard to expression of cell surface antigens, such as Ly-5, Thy-1, NK-1, Qa-5, and asialo GM1, which are expressed only on the latter category of cells.

Significant levels of NK-1.1-positive cells (NK-1.1 antigen is considered to be primarily expressed on NK cells) have been detected also in fetal liver, thymus, and spleen of C57BL/6 mice (Table 6).[68] In the liver at 14 days of gestation, approximately 15% of cells express NK-1.1 antigen. This population increases to 30 to 38% between 16 to 18 days of fetal life, but negligible levels of NK-1.1 positive cells are detected in this tissue at the time of birth. A relatively high proportion (18%) of NK-1.1-positive cells is present in thymus of 14-day-old fetuses of the same strain; these cells rapidly decrease to approximately 5% by 16 days of gestation.[68] However, a small percentage (<5%) of thymocytes continue to express NK-1.1 antigen throughout adulthood. Asialo GM1 positive cells display a parallel occurrence with NK-1.1 cells in fetal thymus.[69] No attempt, however, has been made to determine if asialo GM1 and NK-1.1 antigens are coexpressed or if they represent a separate thymocyte population. Although these findings suggest that at least a subpopulation of NK cells home to the thymus during ontogenetic development, the presence of fully functional NK cells in congenitally athymic animals[34,70] indicates a thymic independent maturation pathway. Nevertheless, there is suggestive evidence for regulation of NK cell functions by mature thymocytes.[71] In contrast to studies on NK cell surface phenotype, neither liver nor thymic neonatal tissue was tested for NK cell cytotoxic potential.

Cells expressing NK-1.1 antigen are first detected in spleens of C57BL/6 mice at 16 days of gestation and comprise approximately 32% of the splenic compartment.[68] Approximately the same percentage of splenic NK-1.1 positive cells is present in infant mice until 3 weeks of age. In mature mice of the same strain (>3 weeks of age), the proportion of NK-1.1-positive cells in the spleen decreases to 5 to 10% and remains at this level through adulthood. In contrast to the high proportion of splenic NK-1.1-positive cells present in infant mice, NK cell reactivity of these animals has consistently been found to be low or nonexistent.[3,68,72,73] These results suggest that NK cells may be inactive in these young animals, or negatively influenced by suppressor cells. In fact, we have demonstrated significant suppression of adult splenic NK cell cytotoxicity by splenocytes of infant mice in coculture experiments[72] and such suppression was confirmed by other groups of investigators.[73] The fact that NK-1.1-positive cells of infant mice can bind in normal frequency to YAC-1 tumor cells, indicates that the regulation of cytotoxicity is manifested on the lytic level.[68] However, we have observed that the lack of cytotoxic potential of infant mice could be reversed following treatment with

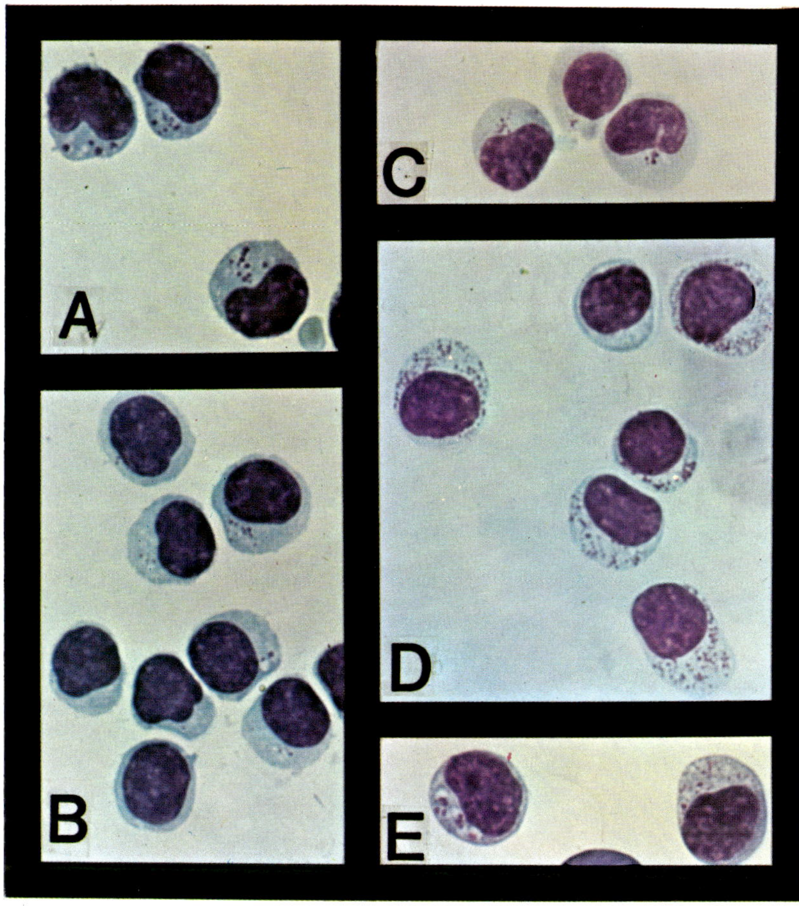

PLATE 1. Large granular lymphocytes of various mammalian species. (A) Human, (B) monkey, (C) canine, (D) rat, (E) mice. Percoll-separated (A, C, D) and nylon wool-filtered (B, E) cells were prepared by May-Grünwald-Giemsa staining of cytocentrifuge slides. Data from our laboratory.

interferon (IFN) inducers of the pyrimidinone group.[74] Splenic NK cell cytotoxic reactivity reaches a peak in 5 to 8-week-old mice of most strains and declines with advanced age. In contrast, levels of NK-1.1-positive cells are similar in young adult and aged C57BL/6 mice,[68] despite the differences in these mice in cytotoxic potential. The age-related change in splenic NK cell activity correlated with levels of LGL detected in this tissue. For example, LGL (enumerated after Percoll separation) were shown to be present in higher proportions (20 to 30%) in the spleen of young C3H mice and declined to lower levels (approximately 2%) in aged animals of the same strain.[48]

Although only low levels of NK cell activity have been found in murine bone marrow, a large percentage of NK-1.1-positive cells has been detected in this tissue of C57BL/6 mouse strain.[75] Since the NK-1.1-positive cells bind, but do not lyse, YAC-1 tumor target, they appear to represent a less mature step of NK cell differentiation. Cells with LGL morphology were also found in low frequency (1.0%) in bone marrow of adult C3H/HeN mice.[76] Even though bone marrow is not a tissue with high NK cell cytotoxic potential, it appears to be important for NK cell origin and, most likely, also for NK cell differentiation. The dependence of NK cells on an intact bone marrow microenvironment is supported by the following observations: first, mice irradiated by bone marrow seeking isotope ^{89}Sr remain deficient in NK cell activity in spite of the renewal of T cell, B cell, and macrophage functions, mediated via splenic hemopoietic stem cell activities;[77-79] second, such animals cannot be restored by reconstitution with bone marrow cells from fully NK cell reactive syngeneic mice.[80] Influence of the bone marrow on NK cell development was further demonstrated by studies in which the NK cell reactivity of congenitally or experimentally NK-deficient mice could be restored by adoptive transfer of bone marrow cells from highly NK cell responsive strains.[81]

The ontogeny of NK cell activity in other rodent species has not been as well analyzed. Low or no NK cell activity was detected in spleen and peripheral blood of various strains of newborn hamsters.[36-38] In the latter species, as well as in guinea pigs, cytotoxic activity was observed in animals >3 weeks of age.[36-39] No definable age-related peak of NK activity could be identified in these two species, due to the variability between individuals in all age groups tested. Neither hamsters nor guinea pigs displayed decline in NK cell antitumor reactivity with advanced age (1 $^1/_2$ to 3 years).

In rats, the development of NK cell reactivity is also an age-dependent phenomenon. We have recently shown that in both congenitally athymic and euthymic rats of N:NIH and Rowett strains, NK cell antitumor activity was not detected before 4 weeks of age in any tissue tested, including spleen, bone marrow, peritoneal exudate, and peripheral blood, when unseparated effector cells were tested.[35,82] However, we found significant levels of NK cell activity in the nylon wool-filtered fraction of the spleens of young rats, indicating that they are not absolutely devoid of NK cells;[35] thus, the lack of NK cell activity could be due to lower number of NK cells present in this tissue or by suppressor cells. Significant NK CMC was observed in spleen and peritoneal exudate of N:NIH rats >4 weeks of age; NK cell cytolytic potential of peripheral blood cells was first detected at 6 to 7 weeks in this strain. Significant cytotoxicity in all three tissues was not observed until 7 weeks in athymic Rowett rats, suggesting that maturation of NK cell activity may be, to some extent, strain-dependent. Peak levels of NK cell cytotoxicity occurred in all tissues of both strains of rats at 8 to 10 weeks of age.[35,82] The bone marrow was the only exception, since in this tissue NK cell activity was not detected in any of the age groups.[35,82] We have not observed in either athymic or euthymic rats of NIH and Rowett strains, any abrupt decline of NK cell reactivity with age; in fact, rats >20 weeks of age displayed significant levels of NK cell reactivity. A slight decrease in NK cell antitumor reactivity has been reported by some investigators in old rats of a W/Fu strain, indicating that reduced NK cell activity in older rats may

Table 7
DISTRIBUTION OF NK CELL CYTOTOXICITY AND HNK-1-POSITIVE CELLS IN FETAL TISSUES OF HUMANS

		%					
Tissue	Parameter tested	9[a]	11	13	15	16	19
Liver	Cytotoxicity	25.3	10.5	—	7.0	—	13.0
	HNK-1 positive cells				0.2		
Thymus	Cytotoxicity	—	—	—	—	—	−0.7
	HNK-1 positive cells				<0.05		
Bone marrow	Cytotoxicity	—	—	3.9	—	3.5	−0.5
	HNK-1 positive cells			0.06		0.1	
Spleen	Cytotoxicity	—	—	—	—	—	13.0
	HNK-1 positive cells				0.2		

[a] Age of fetus in weeks.

Extrapolated from Uksila, J., Lassilo, O., Hirvonen, T., and Toivanen, P., *J. Immunol.*, 130, 153, 1983, and Abo, T., Miller, C. A., Gartland, G. L., and Balch, C. M., *J. Exp. Med.*, 157, 273, 1983.

be strain-dependent.[33] Moreover, since decreased splenic, but not peripheral blood NK cell cytolytic activity was reported in the latter strain of rats,[33] the age-related decline in NK cell cytotoxic potential may also be tissue-dependent.

D. Humans

In humans, NK cell cytotoxic activity against K-562 tumor was detected in fetal liver at 9 to 19 weeks of gestation (Table 7).[83] Although significant, this activity was generally lower than that observed in peripheral blood of most normal adults. In line with these studies is the observation that 13 to 17-week-old fetal liver cells contain a small percentage (0.2%) of HNK-1-positive cells,[84,85] the antigen expressed on the majority of NK cells. Cytotoxic activity against K-562 is not detected in unseparated bone marrow of human fetuses, where HNK-1-positive cells represent 0.06 to 0.1% of the cell population.[85] NK cell lytic activity was demonstrated, however, in bone marrow of fetuses after enrichment for HNK-1-positive cells.[85] Low levels of HNK-1-positive cells (0.1 to 0.8%) are maintained in the bone marrow after birth and throughout adulthood. In contrast to fetal bone marrow, the majority of HNK-1-positive cells in the adult bone marrow coexpress T3 and T8 (T-cell associated) surface antigens. Morphologically, these cells resemble LGL, but contain only a few cytoplasmic granules, suggesting that they could represent an immature stage in NK cell development.[85]

The data concerning the presence of splenic NK cells in human fetuses are limited. Significant NK cell reactivity was found in this tissue in 19-week-old fetuses.[83] Independently, levels (0.2%) of HNK-1-positive cells were detected in fetal spleen.[85] There are relatively little data concerning splenic NK cells in adult humans; we and others have found substantial levels of NK cell cytotoxicity in spleens of adult individuals.[43,86] Approximately 5% of adult splenocytes display LGL morphology (Table 4), and 10% express HNK-1 antigen.[85]

In the fetal thymus, <0.05% of thymocytes bear the HNK-1 antigen; this population remains at negligible levels in thymus of neonates and adults. Similar to bone marrow, the majority of HNK-1-positive thymocytes express T3 and T8 surface antigens.[85]

The time of appearance of NK cell activity in human peripheral blood is still a controversial issue. High levels of cytotoxic reactivity to K-562 tumor cell line (often of the order observed in adults) were detected in cord blood of some, while no or very low NK cell cytotoxicity was demonstrable in the same tissue of other infants.[86-88] This variation in NK cell activity may be due, in part, to the methods of collection of cord blood samples. In fact, the main problem associated with this technique, which may contribute to the discrepant results, is the possibility of contamination of the cord blood sample with maternal peripheral blood lymphocytes. Therefore, studies on cord blood NK cell cytotoxicity must be interpreted with caution. Moreover, the demonstration of NK cell reactivity in cord blood may also be dependent on the type of target cell used; some investigators detected low cytotoxicity levels against K-562 tumor, but cytotoxicity comparable to adults against Molt-4 cells.[88] The frequency of lymphocytes expressing HNK-1 antigen is very low in cord blood (0.3%) in comparison to adult peripheral blood (14%); the majority of cord blood HNK-1-positive lymphocytes also express T3 antigen.[85] Morphologically, the majority of HNK-1-positive cord blood cells appear to resemble those of bone marrow LGL, with regard to their sparsely granulated cytoplasm.[85] A small percentage of cord blood HNK-1-positive cells display highly granulated cytoplasm, the characteristic of LGL in adult peripheral blood.[85] In fact, a differentiation pathway of NK cells from small agranular HNK-1-positive, T3-negative, M1-negative cells in the fetus, to the sparsely granulated, HNK-1-positive, T3-positive, M1-negative cell type within the bone marrow, with final differentiation into the highly granular HNK-1-positive, T3-negative, M1-positive cell population, found in peripheral lymphoid tissues, has been proposed.[85] This model, however, awaits further confirmation.

We and others have found no difference in the cytolytic potential of young or old individuals within the normal donor population (ranging in age from 20 to 70 years).[89-91] The great degree of variability in NK cell activity amond normal individuals complicates determination of the effect of age on human NK cell antitumor-directed cytotoxicity. This is not due to day-to-day variability in NK assay, since we and others have observed minor fluctuations of NK cell cytotoxicity of normal donors tested repeatedly during a period of months, and in some cases, years.[89,90] In fact, this stability in reactivity has allowed for recognition of high, medium, and low NK cell responders within the normal adult population.[89] Analysis of these responder classes in various age groups may aid in further determination of the effect of age on human NK cell reactivity. Such studies, however, will require a larger panel of normal individuals.

IV. CONCLUSIONS

Even though naturally cytotoxic cells are present in the phylogenetically highest species, man, they appear to represent an evolutionary very old lymphocyte population as evidenced by their occurrence also in primitive invertebrates. The finding of spontaneously cytotoxic cells in unsegmented worms suggests that this effector cell population may precede development of primordial T and B cells, since these invertebrates lack an anamnestic response and recognizable antibody production. The simultaneous presence of these cytotoxic cells with phagocytic and granulocytic coelomocytes, however, does not allow for determination of their exact time of origin with respect to that of granulocytes or macrophages.

Although naturally cytolytic cells in invertebrates display reactivity to tumor targets, malignant transformation is not a common occurrence in these lower life forms. Instead, this activity may represent an early manifestation of cellular defense against microbial infection, thus explaining the adaptive advantage created by acquisition of NK-like effector function. The involvement of LGL-like effector cells in the graft rejection phenomenon of earthworms also illustrates the possible early functional capacity of such cells to recognize "nonself" (or absence of "self") antigens. The implication of NK cells in resistance to viral infections in dogs, cats, rodents, and humans, as well as their proposed involvement in resistance to viral, bacterial, parasitic, and fungal infections, indicates the stability of such functions throughout time. Therefore, while their first recognized functional activity in vertebrates suggested involvement of NK cells in antitumor resistance, this may be a consequence (or specialization) of a more primary functional role.

Another NK cell function, i.e., reactivity to normal tissue targets, is also manifested in invertebrates, inferring that regulation of proliferation of other cell types (a functional activity attributed to NK cells in the human species) may also be a fundamental property of this cell population. The reactivity of NK cells against tumors therefore, could stem from an ability to recognize and regulate rapidly dividing cell populations. This would explain the sensitivity of bone marrow cells and thymocytes to NK cell-mediated lysis (CML). In fact, increased susceptibility of less-differentiated vs. well-differentiated tumor cell variants to NK cell cytotoxic activity, and the rather generalized immaturity of cells composing the thymic and bone marrow compartments, have led to the postulation that NK cells may be preferentially targeted toward less mature cell populations. Thus, NK cells could represent a line of defense against both externally and internally originating disturbances in the biological integrity of the organism.

ACKNOWLEDGMENT

The authors would like to acknowledge Abbas Khan for his technical assistance in experiments performed in our laboratory and for his help in the preparation of illustrations used in this chapter. We also wish to acknowledge Ann Childers for her secretarial assistance in the preparation of this manuscript. The work from this laboratory was supported by Grant CA 31394 from the National Cancer Institute.

REFERENCES

1. Lopez, C., Genetic resistance to herpes virus infections: role of natural killer cells, in *Genetic Control of Natural Resistance to Infection and Malignancy,* Skamene, S., Kongshavn, P. A. L., and Landy, M., Eds., Academic Press, New York, 1980, 253.
2. Eugui, E. M. and Allison, A. C., Natural cell-mediated immunity and interferon in malaria and babesia infections, in *NK Cells and Other Natural Effector Cells,* Herberman, R. B., Ed., Academic Press, New York, 1982, 1491.
3. Lotzová, E. and Savary, C. A., Possible involvement of natural killer cells in bone marrow graft rejection. *Biomedicine,* 27, 341, 1977.
4. Kiessling, R., Hochman, P. S., Haller, O., Shearer, G. M., Wigzell, H., and Cudkowicz, G., Evidence for a similar or common mechanism for natural killer cell activity and resistance to hemopoietic grafts, *Eur. J. Immunol.,* 7, 655, 1977.
5. Lotzová, E., Hemopoietic histocompatibility: genetic and immunological aspects, *Compend. Immunol.,* 3, 468, 1983.
6. Lotzová, E., Savary, C. A., and Pollack, S. B., Prevention of rejection of allogeneic bone marrow transplants by NK 1.1 antiserum, *Transplantation,* 35, 490, 1983.
7. Lotzová, E. and Savary, C. A., Natural resistance to foreign hemopoietic transplants: a possible model of leukemia surveillance, in *13th Int. Cancer Congr., Part C, Biol. Cancer Part 2,* Alan R. Liss, New York, 1983, 125.
8. Mangan, K. F., Hartnett, M. E., Matis, S. A., Winkelstein, A., and Abo, T., Natural killer cells suppress human erythroid stem cell proliferation in vitro, *Blood,* 63, 260, 1984.
9. Hansson, M., Beran, M., Andersson, B., and Kiessling, R., Inhibition of in vitro granulopoiesis by autologous and allogeneic human NK cells, *J. Immunol.,* 129, 126, 1982.
10. Arai, S., Yamamoto, H., Itoh, K., and Kumagai, K., Suppressive effect of human natural killer cells on pokeweed mitogen-induced B cell differentiation, *J. Immunol.,* 131, 651, 1983.
11. Abruzzo, L. V. and Rowley, D. A., Homeostasis of the antibody response: immunoregulation by NK cells, *Science,* 222, 581, 1983.

12. Pistoia, V., Nocera, A., Ghio, R., Leprini, A., Perata, A., Pistone, M., and Ferrarini, M., PHA-induced human T cell colony formation: enhancing effect of large granular lymphocytes, *Exp. Hematol.*, 11, 249, 1983.
13. Tyson, C. J. and Jenkin, C. R., The cytotoxic effect of haemocytes from the crayfish *(Parachaeraps bicarinatus)* on tumour cells of vertebrates, *Aust. J. Exp. Biol. Med. Sci.*, 52, 915, 1974.
14. Valembois, P., Roch, P., and Boiledieu, D., Natural and induced cytotoxicities in sipunculids and annelids, in *Phylogeny of Immunological Memory*, Manning, M. J., Ed., Elsevier/North-Holland, 1980, 47.
15. Decker, J. M., Elmholt, A., and Muchmore, A. V., Spontaneous cytotoxicity mediated by invertebrate mononuclear cells toward normal and malignant vertebrate targets: inhibition by defined mono- and disaccharides, *Cell. Immunol.*, 59, 161, 1981.
16. Roder, J. C., Karre, K., and Kiessling, R., Natural killer cells, *Prog. Allerg.*, 28, 66, 1981.
17. Luquet, G. and Leclerc, M., Spontaneous and induced cytotoxicity of axial organ cells from *Asterias rubens* (Asterid-echinoderm), *Immunol. Lett.*, 6, 339, 1983.
18. Hostetter, R. K. and Cooper, E. L., Coelomocytes as effector cells in the earthworm immunity, *Immunolog. Commun.*, 1, 155, 1972.
19. Linthicum, D. S., Stein, E. A., Marks, D. H., and Cooper, E. L., Electron-microscopic observations of normal coelomocytes from the earthworm, *Lumbricus terrestris*, *Cell. Tiss. Res.*, 185, 315, 1977.
20. Hinuma, S., Abo, T., Kumagai, K., and Hata, M., The potent activity of fresh water fish kidney cells in cell-killing. I. Characterization and species-distribution of cytotoxicity, *Dev. Comp. Immunol.*, 4, 653, 1980.
21. Pettey, C. L. and McKinney, E. C., Effect of decreased environmental temperature on spontaneous cytotoxicity in the nurse shark, *Fed. Proc. Fed. Am. Soc. Exp. Biol.*, 39, 934, 1980.
22. Sharma, J. M. and Coulson, B. D., Presence of natural killer cells in specific-pathogen-free chickens, *J. Natl. Cancer Inst.*, 63, 527, 1979.
23. Yamada, A., Hayami, M., Yamanouchi, K., and Fujiwara, K., Detection of natural killer cells in Japanese quail, *Int. J. Cancer*, 26, 381, 1980.
24. Leibold, W., Janotte, G., and Peter, H. H., Spontaneous cell-mediated cytotoxicity (SCMC) in various mammalian species and chickens: selective reaction pattern and different mechanisms, *Scand. J. Immunol.*, 11, 203, 1980.
25. Fleischer, B., Effector cells in avian spontaneous and antibody-dependent cell-mediated cytotoxicity, *J. Immunol.*, 125, 1161, 1980.
26. Herberman, R. B., Brunda, M. J., Domzig, W., Fagnani, R., Goldfarb, R. H., Holden, H. T., Ortaldo, J. R., Reynolds, C. W., Riccardi, C., Santoni, A., Stadler, B. M., Taramelli, D., Timonen, T., and Varesio, L., Immunoregulation involving macrophages and natural killer cells, in *Immune Regulation: Evolutionary and Biological Significance*, Ruben, L. N. and Gershwin, M. E., Eds., Marcel Dekker, New York, 1980, 139.
27. Herberman, R. B. and Holden, H. T., Natural cell-mediated immunity, *Adv. Cancer Res.*, 27, 305, 1978.
28. Kiessling, R. and Haller, O., Natural killer cells in the mouse: an alternative immune surveillance mechanism?, *Contemp. Top. Immunobiol.*, 8, 171, 1978.
29. Shellam, G. R., Gross-virus-induced lymphoma in the rat. V. Natural cytotoxic cells are non-T cells, *Int. J. Cancer*, 19, 225, 1977.
30. Oehler, J. R., Lindsay, L. R., Nunn, M. E., and Herberman, R. B., Natural cell-mediated cytotoxicity in rats. I. Tissue and strain distribution, and demonstration of a membrane receptor for the Fc portion of IgG, *Int. J. Cancer*, 21, 204, 1978.
31. Potter, M. R. and Moore, M., Organ distribution of natural cytotoxicity in the rat, *Clin. Exp. Immunol.*, 34, 78, 1978.
32. DeJong, W. H., Steerenberg, P. A., Ursem, P. S., Osterhaus, A. D. M. E., Vos, J. G., and Ruitenberg, E. J., The athymic nude rat. III. Natural cell-mediated cytotoxicity, *Clin. Immunol. Immunopathol.*, 16, 163, 1980.
33. Reynolds, C. W., Timonen, T., and Herberman, R. B., Natural killer (NK) cell activity in the rat. I. Isolation and characterization of the effector cells, *J. Immunol.*, 127, 282, 1981.
34. Lotzová, E., Savary, C. A., Khan, A., and Stringfellow, D. A., Stimulation of natural killer cell cytotoxicity in two random-bred strains of athymic rats by interferon-inducing pyrimidinones, *J. Immunol.*, 132, 2566, 1984.
35. Lotzová, E., Savary, C. A., Gray, K. N., Raulston, G. L., and Jardine, J. H., Natural killer cell profile of two random-bred strains of athymic rats, *Exp. Hematol.*, in press.
36. Datta, S. K., Gallagher, M. T., and Trentin, J. J., Natural killer cell-mediated cytotoxicity versus lymphoma in hamsters, *Prog. Exp. Tumor Res.*, 23, 180, 1979.
37. Tsang, K. Y., Gnagy, M. J., Yamamura, Y., and Fudenberg, H. H., Detection of natural killer cell-mediated cytotoxicity in hamsters, using Raji target cells, *Clin. Immunol. Immunopathol.*, 21, 332, 1981.

38. Teale, D. M., Rees, R. C., Clark, A., and Potter, C. W., Detection and characterization of natural killer cells in Syrian golden hamsters, *Eur. J. Cancer Clin. Oncol.*, 19, 537, 1983.
39. Altman, A. and Rapp, H. J., Natural cell-mediated cytotoxicity in guinea pigs: properties and specificity of natural killer cells, *J. Immunol.*, 121, 2244, 1978.
40. Arnaud-Battandier, F., Bundy, B. M., and Nelson, D. L., Natural killer cells in guinea pig spleen bear Fc receptors, *Eur. J. Immunol.*, 8, 400, 1978.
41. Nunn, M. E., Herberman, R. B., and Holden, H. T., Natural cell-mediated cytotoxicity in mice against non-lymphoid tumor cells and some normal cells, *Int. J. Cancer*, 20, 381, 1977.
42. Rees, R. G., Reynolds, C. W., and Herberman, R. B., Rat natural killer cell activity against lymphoid and nonlymphoid tumor cells and normal rat cell lines, *Cancer Res.*, 43, 4248, 1983.
43. Lotzová, E. and McCredie, K. B., Natural killer cells in mice and man and their possible biological significance, *Cancer Immunol. Immunother.*, 4, 215, 1978.
44. Tagliabue, A., Befus, A. D., Clark, D. A., and Bienenstock, J., Characteristics of natural killer cells in the murine intestinal epithelium and lamina propria, *J. Exp. Med.*, 155, 1785, 1982.
45. Puccetti, P., Santoni, A., Riccardi, C., and Herberman, R. B., Cytotoxic effector cells with the characteristics of natural killer cells in the lungs of mice, *Int. J. Cancer*, 25, 153, 1980.
46. Zöller, M., Andrighetto, G., and Heyman, B., Natural and antibody-dependent killer cells in the thymus, *Eur. J. Immunol.*, 12, 914, 1982.
47. Kumagai, K., Itoh, K., Suzuki, R., Hinumi, S., and Saitoh, F., Studies of murine large granular lymphocytes. I. Identification as effector cells in NK and K cytotoxicities, *J. Immunol.*, 129, 388, 1982.
48. Itoh, K., Suzuki, R., Umezu, Y., Hanaumi, K., and Kumagai, K., Studies of murine large granular lymphocytes. II. Tissue, strain, and age distributions of LGL and LAL, *J. Immunol.*, 129, 395, 1982.
49. Eremin, O., Wilson, A. B., Coombs, R. R. A., Ashby, J., and Plumb, D., Antibody-dependent cellular cytotoxicity in the guinea pig: the role of the Kurloff cell, *Cell. Immunol.*, 55, 312, 1980.
50. Revell, P. A., The Kurloff cell, *Int. Rev. Cytol.*, 51, 275, 1977.
51. Maximow, A. A. and Bloom, W., *A Textbook of Histology*, 4th ed. W. B. Saunders, Philadelphia, 1942, 46.
52. Hu, J., Starkey, J. R., and Prieur, D. J., A lack of natural killer cell activity in domestic cats, *Fed. Proc., Fed. Am. Soc. Exp. Biol.*, 41, 802, 1982.
53. Tompkins, M. B., Huber, K., and Tompkins, W. A. F., Natural cell-mediated cytotoxicity in the domestic cat: properties and specificity of effector cells, *Am. J. Vet. Res.*, 44, 1525, 1983.
54. Betton, G. R., Natural cell-mediated cytotoxicity in the canine, in *The Canine as a Biomedical Research Model: Immunological, Hematological, and Oncological Aspects*, Shifrine, M. and Wilson, F. D., Eds., Technical Information Center, U.S. Department of Energy, Oak Ridge, Tenn., 1980, 99.
55. Shek, W. R., Schultz, R. D., and Appel, M. J. G., Natural and immune cytolysis of canine distemper virus-infected target cells, *Infect. Immun.*, 28, 724, 1980.
56. Krakowka, S., Natural killer cell activity in adult gnotobiotic dogs, *Am. J. Vet. Res.*, 44, 635, 1983.
56a. Lotzová, E., et al., in preparation.
57. Koren, H. S., Amos, D. B., and Kim, Y. B., Natural killing and antibody-dependent cellular cytotoxicity are independent immune functions in the Minnesota miniature swine, *Proc. Natl. Acad. Sci. U.S.A.*, 75, 5127, 1978.
58. Kim, Y. B., Huh, N. D., Koren, H. S., and Amos, D. B., Natural killing (NK) and antibody-dependent cellular cytotoxicity (ADCC) in specific pathogen-free (SPF) miniature swine and germfree piglets. I. Comparison of NK and ADCC, *J. Immunol.*, 125, 755, 1980.
59. Johnson, D. R. and Jondal, M., Herpesvirus ateles and herpesvirus saimiri transform marmoset T cells into continuously proliferating cell lines that can mediate natural killer cell-like cytotoxicity, *Proc. Natl. Acad. Sci. U.S.A.*, 78, 6391, 1981.
60. Clark, E. A. and Sturge, J. C., Phylogeny of NK cell reactivity against human and nonhuman primate lymphoblastoid cell lines: evolving and conserved target antigens, *J. Immunol.*, 126, 1981.
61. Sharma, J. M. and Okazaki, W., Natural killer cell activity in chickens: target cell analysis and effect of antithymocyte serum on effector cells, *Infect. Immun.*, 31, 1078, 1981.
62. Lam, K. M. and Linna, T. J., Protection of newly-hatched chickens from Marek's disease (JMV) by normal spleen cells from older animals, in *Advances in Comparative Leukemia Research 1977*, Bentvelzen, P., Hilgers, J., and Yohn, D. S., Eds., Elsevier/North Holland, 1978, 111.
63. Huh, N. D., Kim, Y. B., Koren, H. S., and Amos, D. B., Natural killing and antibody-dependent cellular cytotoxicity in specific-pathogen-free miniature swine and germ-free piglets. II. Ontogenic development of NK and ADCC, *Int. J. Cancer*, 28, 175, 1981.
64. Herberman, R. B., Nunn, M. E., and Lavrin, D. H., Natural cytotoxic reactivity of mouse lymphoid cells against syngeneic and allogeneic tumors. I. Distribution of reactivity and specificity, *Int. J. Cancer*, 16, 216, 1975.

65. Nunn, M. E., Djeu, J. Y., Glaser, M., Lavrin, D. H., and Herberman, R. B., Natural cytotoxic reactivity of rat lymphocytes against syngeneic Gross virus-induced lymphoma, *J. Natl. Cancer Inst.*, 56, 393, 1976.
66. Dahl, C. A., Natural cytotoxicity in the mouse embryo. I. Evidence for the presence of natural cytotoxic function in the yolk sac of the 10-day mouse embryo, *J. Immunol.*, 125, 1924, 1980.
67. Dahl, C. A., Natural cytotoxicity in the mouse embryo: characterization of yolk sac-associated natural cytotoxic cells and their activity, *Eur. J. Immunol.*, 13, 747, 1983.
68. Koo, G. C., Peppard, J. R., and Hatzfeld, A., Ontogeny of NK-1⁺ natural killer cells. I. Proportion of NK-1⁺ cells in fetal, baby, and old mice, *J. Immunol.*, 129, 867, 1982.
69. Habu, S., Kasai, M., and Nagai, Y., The glycolipid asialo-GM-1 as a new differentiation antigen of fetal thymocytes, *J. Immunol.*, 125, 2284, 1980.
70. Holden, H. T., Herberman, R. B., Santoni, A., and Nunn, M. E., Natural cell-mediated cytotoxicity in nude mice, in *Use of Athymic (Nude) Mice in Cancer Research*, Houchens, D. P. and Ovejera, A. A., Eds., Gustav Fischer, New York, 1978, 81.
71. Nair, M. P. N., Schwartz, S. A., Fernandes, G., Pahwa, R., Ikehara, S., and Good, R. A., Suppression of natural killer (NK) cell activity of spleen cell by thymocytes, *Cell. Immunol.*, 58, 9, 1981.
72. Savary, C. A. and Lotzová, E., Suppression of natural killer cell cytotoxicity by splenocytes from Corynebacterium parvum-injected bone marrow-tolerant and infant mice, *J. Immunol.*, 120, 239, 1978.
73. Cudkowicz, G. and Hochman, P. S., Do natural killer cells engage in regulated reactions against self to ensure homeostasis?, *Immun. Rev.*, 44, 13, 1979.
74. Lotzová, E., Savary, C. A., and Stringfellow, D. A., Modulation of murine NK cell cytotoxicity *in vitro* and antitumor activity *in vivo* by low molecular weight interferon inducers, in *Cancer: Etiology and Prevention*, Crispen, R. G., Ed., Elsevier, Amsterdam, 1983, 199.
75. Koo, G. C., Peppard, J. R., and Mark, W. H., Natural killer cells generated from bone marrow culture, *J. Immunol.*, 132, 2300, 1984.
76. Luini, W., Boraschi, D., Alberti, S., Aleotti, A., and Tagliabue, A., Morphological characterization of a cell population responsible for natural killer activity, *Immunology*, 43, 663, 1981.
77. Fried, W., Gurney, W., and Swatek, M., The effect of strontium-89 on the stem cell compartment of the spleen, *Radiat. Res.*, 29, 50, 1966.
78. Bennett, M., Baker, E. E., Eastcott, J. W., Kumar, V., and Yonkosky, D., Selective elimination of marrow precursors with the bone-seeking isotope ^{89}Sr: implications for hemopoiesis, lymphopoiesis, viral leukemogenesis, and infection, *J. Reticuloendothel. Soc.*, 20, 71, 1976.
79. Haller, O. and Wigzell, H., Suppression of natural killer cell activity with radioactive strontium: effector cells are marrow dependent, *J. Immunol.*, 118, 1503, 1977.
80. Kumar, V., Mellen, P. F., and Bennett, M., Marrow dependence of natural killer cells, in *NK Cells and Other Natural Effector Cells*, Herberman, R. B., Ed., Academic Press, New York, 1982, 329.
81. Haller, O., Kiessling, R., Orn, A., and Wigzell, H., Generation of natural killer cells: an autonomous function of the bone marrow, *J. Exp. Med.*, 145, 1411, 1977.
82. Lotzová, E., Savary, C. A., Stringfellow, D. A., Drewinko, B., Gray, K. N., Raulston, G. L., and Jardine, J. H., Analysis of natural killer cell activity in random-bred Rowett athymic rats, in *Immune-Deficient Animals, 4th Int. Workshop Immune-Deficient Animals*, S. Karger, Basel, 1984, 53.
83. Uksila, J., Lassilo, O., Hirvonen, T., and Toivanen, P., Development of natural killer cell function in the human fetus, *J. Immunol.*, 130, 153, 1983.
84. Abo, T., Cooper, M. D., and Balch, C. M., Postnatal expansion of the natural killer and killer cell population in humans identified by the monoclonal HNK-1 antibody, *J. Exp. Med.*, 155, 321, 1982.
85. Abo, T., Miller, C. A., Gartland, G. L., and Balch, C. M., Differentiation stages of human natural killer cells in lymphoid tissues from fetal to adult life, *J. Exp. Med.*, 157, 273, 1983.
86. Antonelli, P., Stewart, W., II, and Dupont, B., Distribution of natural killer cell activity in peripheral blood, cord blood, thymus, lymph nodes, and spleen and the effect of in vitro treatment with interferon preparation, *Clin. Immunol. Immunopathol.*, 19, 161, 1981.
87. Kaplan, J., Shope, T. C., Bollinger, R. O., and Smith, J., Human newborns are deficient in natural killer activity, *J. Clin. Immunol.*, 2, 350, 1982.
88. Lubens, R. G., Gard, S. E., Soderberg-Warner, M., and Stiehm, E. R., Lectin-dependent T-lymphocyte and natural killer cytotoxic deficiencies in human newborns, *Cell. Immunol.*, 74, 40, 1982.
89. Lotzová, E., Savary, C. A., Gutterman, J. U., and Hersh, E. M., Modulation of natural killer cell-mediated cytotoxicity by partially purified and cloned interferon α, *Cancer Res.*, 42, 2480, 1982.
90. Pross, H. F. and Bains, M. G., Studies of human natural killer cells. I. In vivo parameters affecting normal cytotoxic function, *Int. J. Cancer*, 29, 383, 1982.
91. Fernandes, G. and Gupta, S., Natural killing and antibody-dependent cytotoxicity by lymphocyte subpopulations in young and aging humans, *J. Clin. Immunol.*, 1, 141, 1981.

Chapter 5

TISSUE AND ORGAN DISTRIBUTION OF NK CELLS

Craig W. Reynolds and Jerrold M. Ward

TABLE OF CONTENTS

I. INTRODUCTION

In the last 10 years, a number of laboratories have investigated the cellular characteristics and functions of natural killer (NK) cells. These studies have suggested that NK cells may be important in mediating resistance to microbial and virus infection,[1-7] immunosurveillance to primary tumors[8,9] and their metastases,[9-13] as well as resistance to bone marrow transplantation.[14,15] Recently, it has also been shown that the major cell responsible for these functions is the large granular lymphocyte (LGL). These studies have demonstrated that most, if not all, NK and antibody-dependent cell-mediated cytotoxicity (ADCC) in the human,[16-18] rat,[18,19] and mouse[20,21] is associated with the LGL. LGL have also been shown to kill a wide range of tumor cells in vitro, including bone marrow and virus-infected targets,[22,23] as well as inhibit the development of in vitro bone marrow colony-forming units (CFU).[24] Furthermore, the adoptive transfer of these cells has been shown to reconstitute NK activity and to inhibit the development of artificial lung metastases.[9,13,25] These results clearly indicate that the major effector cell for both NK and ADCC is the LGL. However, until very recently, little information was available regarding the tissue distribution and histological localization of these cells in lymphoid and nonlymphoid organs. The purpose of the present manuscript is to summarize the available information regarding (1) organ distribution of NK activity and LGL, (2) tissue distribution of LGL, and (3) distribution patterns of LGL following adoptive transfer. This information should provide a foundation for further examination of the in vivo function of NK cells as well as the potential usefulness of NK cell adoptive transfer.

II. ORGAN DISTRIBUTION OF NK ACTIVITY AND LGL

In rodents, as well as in man, the highest levels of NK activity are normally found in the blood and spleen.[26-28] Lower activity is usually found in lymph node and peritoneal cells, although some investigators have found extremely high levels of activity in these organs.[29] Substantial NK activity has also been reported in lungs,[30-32] liver,[32] intestinal epithelium, and lamina propria.[33,34] Low NK cell activity is consistently found in bone marrow with virtually no NK cell activity detectable in unfractionated thymus.[26-29] Recently, some reports have suggested that substantial NK activity may be present in the thymus;[35] however, the presence of inhibitory cells may serve to mask this function in vitro.[36] In addition, human or rat thoracic duct lymphocytes are reported to be devoid of NK activity.[37,38]

In general, the organ distribution of ADCC activity is similar to that for NK.[39,40] Recently, however, it has been suggested that ADCC activity may be present in thoracic duct cells in the absence of NK activity.[38] We have also recently found high levels of both NK and ADCC in the peripheral blood, while there is comparatively less ADCC activity in spleen and peritoneal cells.[40a] We are presently investigating the reason(s) for this discrepancy. In particular, we are interested in studying whether the organ distribution of NK and ADCC activity reflects a differential distribution of effector cells or different regulatory mechanism at various organ sites.

These previous results suggested that the distribution pattern for NK and ADCC activity is distinct from mature T cells, B cells, or monocytes. In contrast, the organ distribution for LGL is very similar to the distribution of NK and ADCC activity.[19] A summary of these results in euthymic rats is found in Table 1. It can be seen that, with the exception of the lungs, there is an excellent correlation between percent cytotoxicity and percent LGL. The low NK activity from lung cells probably reflects a suppression of LGL function by adherent suppressor cells, since other studies have shown that high levels of NK activity are present in nonadherent mononuclear cells from the lungs.[30-32]

Table 1
LGL FREQUENCY AND ORGAN DISTRIBUTION OF NK ACTIVITY IN EUTHYMIC RATS[a]

Organ	Median LU 20%/10^7 cells[b]	Median % LGL
Peripheral blood	18.2	7.0
Spleen	10.7	4.0
Peritoneal cavity	6.4	3.0
Bone marrow	4.5	<0.5
Lymph nodes	1.1	1.0
Thymus	0.0	<0.5
Lungs	0.0	7.0

[a] Rats were 8 to 10 weeks of age.
[b] 4-hr ^{51}Cr-release assay against YAC-1 targets.

Table 2
LGL FREQUENCY AND ORGAN DISTRIBUTION OF NK ACTIVITY IN ATHYMIC (NUDE) RATS[a]

Organ	Median LU 20%/10^7 cells[b]	Median % LGL
Peripheral blood	93.4	22.0
Spleen	71.8	4.0
Lymph nodes	13.4	2.0
Peritoneal cavity	0.9	1.5
Bone marrow	<1.0	<1.0

[a] Rats were 6 to 12 weeks of age.
[b] 4-hr ^{51}Cr-release assay against YAC-1 targets.

Similar organ distribution studies in athymic (nude) rats have demonstrated three- to fivefold increased levels of NK activity and LGL in the blood and spleen (Table 2).[32,41] These results suggest that the organ distribution for NK activity and LGL is very similar in both athymic and euthymic animals. The studies of Luini et al.[20] and Itoh et al.[42] in the mouse would support this hypothesis. These studies also demonstrate a very good correlation between NK activity and LGL percentages in both athymic and euthymic mice (PBL > spleen > lymph node > thymus).

In conclusion, the major organs which have been examined for NK activity are the peripheral blood, spleen, lymph nodes, bone marrow, peritoneal cavity, and thymus. Within these organs there is a very good correlation between NK activity and percent of LGL. Some nonlymphoid organs such as the lungs, liver, and intestine also contain both NK activity and LGL, although the frequency of cytotoxic cells in unfractionated cell suspensions is generally quite low.

III. TISSUE DISTRIBUTION OF LGL

The recent identification of monoclonal antibodies (MoAb) which react selectively with the LGL population has allowed for a rather detailed analysis of the distribution of LGL within both lymphoid and nonlymphoid organs. We have recently studied the distribution of LGL in athymic rats using the MoAb OX-8. Although in euthymic rats this MoAb reacts with >90% of thymocytes and 30 to 40% of peripheral T cells,[43] it is also found on most rat NK cells (>80%)[44] and isolated peripheral blood LGL in both athymic and euthymic animals.[45] Based on these observations, we examined the histological distribution of OX-8-positive cells in lymphoid and nonlymphoid organs of the T cell-deficient nude rat by the avidin-biotin-peroxidase complex (ABC) immunocytochemical technique.[46,47] A summary of these data from hematopoietic organs is presented in Figure 1. The highest percentage of OX-8-positive cells (15%) was found in the lymph node paracortex undergoing interdigitating cell hyperplasia (IDC-H). Appreciable numbers of OX-8-positive cells were also seen in the PALS area of the spleen (6%), bronchial-associated lymphoid tissues (BALT) (5%), lymph node medulla (5%), and splenic red pulp (4%). Very few positive cells (<1%) were found in splenic and lymph node germinal centers or in the bone marrow. A number of pieces of evidence support the presumption that these OX-8-positive cells are LGL: (1) nude rats have few if any mature OX-8-positive T cells, (2) the distribution of OX-8-positive cells is quite different than the distribution of Ia or sIg-positive macrophages or B cells, and

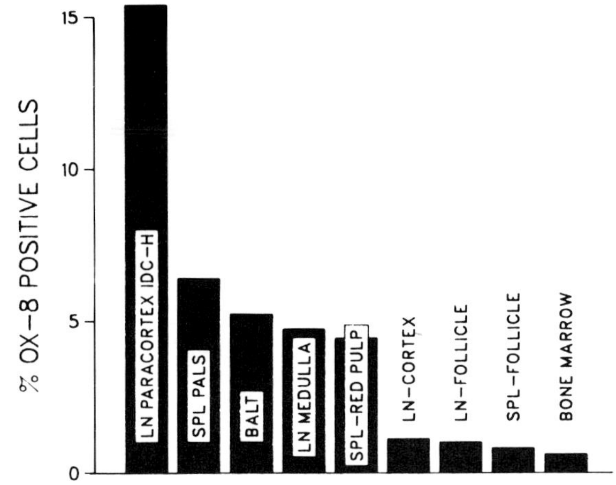

FIGURE 1. Histologic distribution of OX-8-positive lymphocytes in hematopoietic tissues of nude rats.

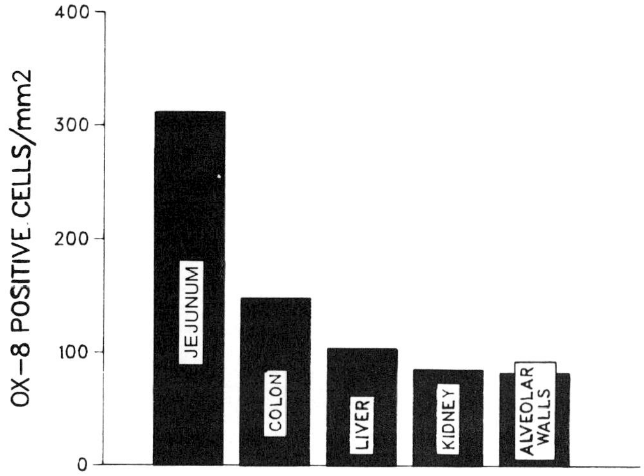

FIGURE 2. Histologic distribution of OX-8-positive lymphocytes in nonhematopoietic tissue of nude rats.

(3) polymorphonuclear leukocytes were OX-8-negative. In addition, the majority of OX-8-positive cells were large lymphoid cells with reniform or irregularly shaped nuclei, a morphology consistent with that of LGL.

In addition to the lymphoid organs, OX-8-positive cells were scattered in the lamina propria and epithelium of the small and large intestine (Figure 2), stomach, and cecum (data not shown). Almost all intraepithelial lymphocytes (IEL) within the intestine of the nude rat were OX-8-positive. Occasional positive lymphocytes with reniform nuclei were also noted in the hepatic sinusoids, interstitium of the kidney, and alveolar walls of the lungs (Figure 2). A few positive cells were also present in the subepithelial and basal layers of the esophagus, skin, uterus, prostate, vagina, preputial or clitoral gland, mammary gland, and urinary bladder (data not shown). OX-8-positive cells in nonlymphoid parenchymal organs, such as liver and kidney, correlated with the presence of capillaries, sinuses, or sinusoids, a finding which should not be unexpected inasmuch as LGL are found in appreciable numbers in the peripheral blood of nude rats.[44]

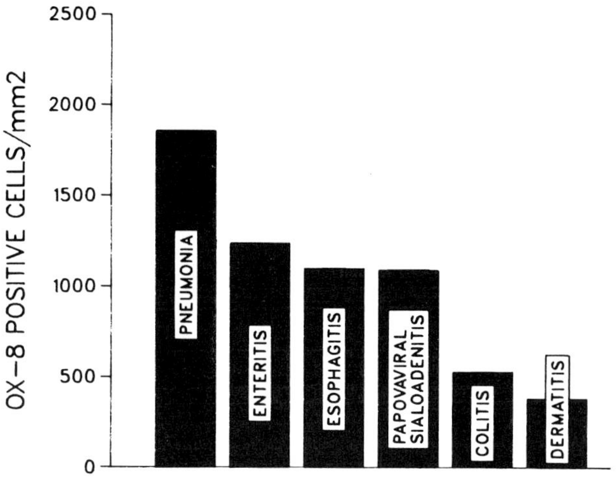

FIGURE 3. Histologic occurrence of OX-8-positive lymphocytes in inflammatory lesions of nude rats.

Large numbers of OX-8-positive cells with reniform nuclei were also found in association with enteritis, suppurative pneumonia, acute esophageal ulcers, papovaviral sialoadenitis, and gastric lesions in some nude rats (Figure 3). Many areas of inflammatory skin lesions also had foci of OX-8-positive cells. In all of the above lesions, OX-8-positive cells were found within the epithelial and submucosal layers in greater than normal numbers. The observations of a large number of LGL in inflammatory lesions and in nonlymphoid organs would support the hypothesis that these cells may play an important role in the first line of defense against infectious agents.[2]

Similar types of immunohistological studies have also been done with human lymphoid tissues using the Leu-7 (HNK-1) MoAb.[48,49] By serial sections, the distribution of Leu-7-positive cells in various tissues was found to be distinctly different than that of T cells, B cells, or Ia-positive cells. In contrast to the nude rat studies, however, Leu-7-positive cells were found in the highest numbers in the germinal centers of secondary follicles in lymph nodes, spleens, and tonsil. The reason for this difference between the rat and human studies is not yet clear, but may reflect the reactivity of the Leu-7 MoAb in some individuals with a substantial number of non-LGL cells.[50,51] The observed variation in Leu-7 staining of lymphoid germinal centers from different individuals would be consistent with this hypothesis.[48] In addition, the OKM1 MoAb, which reacts with monocytes and >60% of LGL, was found by the same authors to react mainly with cells in the interfollicular areas of tonsil and adenoids, in the paracortex and sinuses of lymph nodes, and in the red pulp and periarteriolar sheaths of spleen, but not in the germinal centers. This distribution is more similar to the OX-8 staining in nude rats and further supports the suggestion that most, if not all, of the Leu-7-positive cells in germinal centers are not mature LGL.

In summary, the immunocytochemical localization of LGL reactive with various MoAb suggests that the lymphoid tissues with the greatest density and percentage of reactive cells are those tissues with the highest NK activity. In addition, however, large numbers of LGL are observed in sites not normally associated with high NK activity: the BALT, normal epithelial tissues, inflammatory lesions, and lymph nodes undergoing IDC-H.

Foci of OX-8-positive LGL might also represent either sites of LGL proliferation or prominent areas of LGL immigration. These areas include the paracortex of the lymph node, BALT, interfollicular areas of Peyer's patches, and the periarteriolar lymphoid sheath of the spleen. Any of these areas should be considered as germinative tissues or LGL immigration sites. Further studies are now underway to determine the function of these LGL and to examine the mechanism(s) responsible for their accumulation in large numbers.

IV. DISTRIBUTION PATTERN OF LGL FOLLOWING ADOPTIVE TRANSFER

An alternative means of analyzing the distribution of NK cells is to examine the localization of LGL following adoptive transfer. We have recently completed a series of studies which examine this issue in both normal and tumor-bearing rats.[47,52] For these studies, peripheral blood LGL or T cells were isolated by Percoll gradient centrifugation, labeled with ^{111}In-oxine, and then transferred intravenously (i.v.) or intraperitoneally (i.p.) into syngeneic F344 recipients. At various times following transfer, the animals were sacrificed and a variety of organs removed and counted for remaining radioactivity. The results in Figure 4 demonstrate that following i.v. injection, the majority of ^{111}In-labeled LGL and T cells were found initially in the lungs, blood, and liver. A substantial proportion of these cells, however, left the blood and lungs within the first 24 hr following transfer and accumulated in the liver and spleen.

A number of significant differences were noted in these studies between the distribution patterns for LGL and T cells. LGL were found in higher numbers (two- to fivefold) in the lungs (Figure 4) and remained in this organ for a longer period of time. LGL were also found in higher numbers in the blood and liver at 24 and 48 hr following transfer. In contrast, peripheral blood T cells accumulated more rapidly in the spleen, although at 24 hr approximately equal numbers of LGL and T cells were found at this site. No significant differences were seen in the localization of LGL and T cells in lymph nodes (Figure 4), small intestine, or kidneys (data not shown).

This distribution pattern for adoptively transferred LGL and T cell was not significantly altered in tumor-bearing animals (data not shown). In addition, results from these studies demonstrated that an appreciable number of both LGL (2.5%) and T cells (1.5%) were found in small subcutaneous transplantable syngeneic mammay tumors (Figure 4).

When radiolabeled LGL and T cells were adoptively transferred i.p., only a small percentage of either cell population migrated from the peritoneal cavity within 24 hr (data not shown). In addition, a more rapid decrease in the total counts recovered following i.p. injection suggests that the turnover rate for LGL and T cells was more rapid in the peritoneal cavity than in other organs.

These results demonstrate a distinctive distribution pattern for LGL that is parallel to the proportion of endogenous LGL in the various organs. This distribution is easily distinguishable from that of T cells (Figure 4), thymocytes, or monocytes (data not shown).

V. CONCLUSIONS

The studies discussed in this review clearly demonstrate that both NK activity and LGL are present in both lymphoid and nonlymphoid organs. In most cases, the organ distribution of NK activity and LGL is very similar. In addition, the tissue distribution of LGL in nude rats and human lymphoid tissues is clearly different than that of T cells, B cells, or monocytes. Adoptive transfer studies also demonstrated a localization pattern for LGL which was distinct from that of thymocytes, monocytes, or T cells. Taken together, these studies further support the hypothesis that NK cells are a population of lymphocytes with distinct morphological, functional, and distribution characteristics.

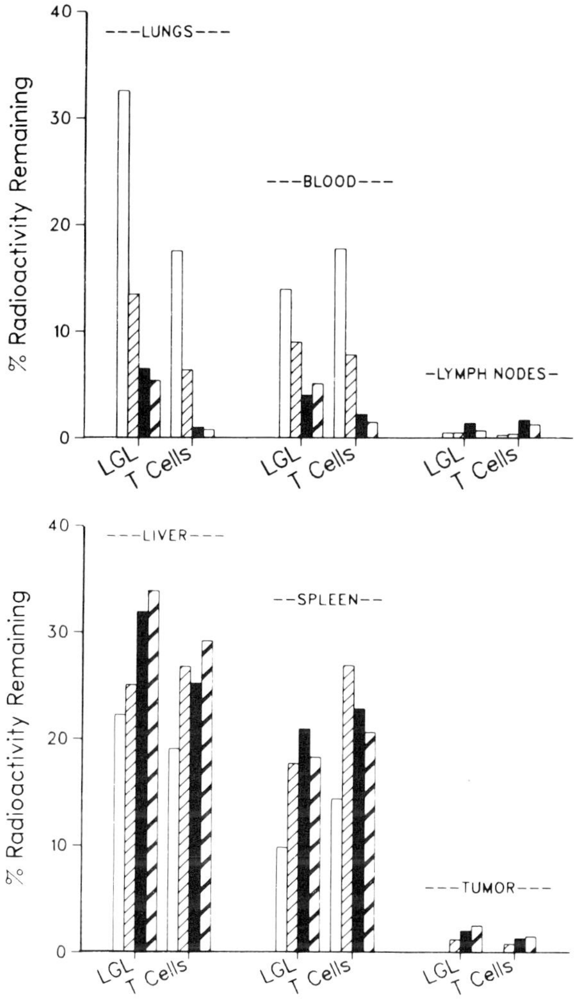

FIGURE 4. Distribution of adoptively transferred ^{111}In-labeled LGL and T cells in syngeneic F344/NCR rats □ 0.5 hr, ▨ 2 hr, ■ 24 hr, and ▨ 48 hr following i.v. transfer.

ACKNOWLEDGMENTS

We wish to thank Mr. John Wine, Ms. Hilda Porter, and Ms. Della Reichardt for their excellent technical assistance; Ms. Rosemary Riggs for her exceptional supervisory animal care; and Drs. Robert Wiltrout and Ronald Herberman for their scientific input.

REFERENCES

1. Santoli, D., Trinchieri, G., and Leifn, F. S., Cell-mediated cytotoxicity against virus-infected target cells in humans. I. Characterization of the effector lymphocytes, *J. Immunol.,* 121, 526, 1978.
2. Lopez, C., Kirkpatrick, D., and Fitzgerald, P., The role of NK (HSV-1) effector cells in resistance to Herpesvirus infections in man, in *NK Cells and Other Natural Effector Cells,* Herberman, R. B., Ed., Academic Press, New York, 1982, 1445.
3. Welsh, R. M., Jr., Zinkernagel, R. M., and Hallenbeck, L. A., Cytotoxic cells induced during lymphocytic choriomeningitis virus infection of mice. II. Specificities of the natural killer cells, *J. Immunol.,* 122, 475, 1979.
4. Brooks, C. G., Rees, R. C., and Leach, R. H., High nonspecific reactivity of normal lymphocytes against mycoplasma-infected target cells in cytotoxicity assays, *Eur. J. Immunol.,* 9, 159, 1979.
5. Trischmann, T., Tanowitz, H., Wittner, M., and Bloom, B. R., *Trypanosoma cruzi:* role of the immune response in the natural resistance of inbred strains of mice, *Exp. Parasitol.,* 45, 160, 1978.
6. Hatcher, F. M. and Kuhn, R. E., Natural killer (nk) cell activity against extracellular form of *Trypanosoma cruzi,* in *NK Cells and Other Natural Effector Cells,* Herberman, R. B., Ed., Academic Press, New York, 1982, 1091.
7. Attallah, A. M., Lewis, F. A., Urritia-Shaw, A., Folks, T., and Yeatman, T. J., Natural killer cells (NK) and antibody-dependent cell-mediated cytotoxicity (ADCC) components of *Schistosoma mansoni* infection, *Int. Arch. Allergy Appl. Immunol.,* 63, 351, 1980.
8. Haller, O., Hansson, M., Kiessling, R., and Wigzell, H., Role of nonconventional natural killer cells in resistance against syngeneic tumor cells in vivo, *Nature (London),* 270, 609, 1977.
9. Warner, J. and Dennert, T., Effects of a cloned cell line with NK activity on bone marrow transplants, tumour development and metastasis in vivo, *Nature,* 300, 31, 1982.
10. Gorelik, E., Wiltrout, R. H., Okumura, K., Habu, S., and Herberman, R. B., Role of NK cells in the control of metastatic spread and growth of tumor cells in mice, *Int. J. Cancer,* 30, 107, 1982.
11. Riccardi, C., Santoni, T., Barlozzari, T., Puccetti, P., and Herberman, R. B., In vivo natural reactivity of mice against tumor cells, *Int. J. Cancer,* 25, 475, 1980.
12. Hanna, N. and Fidler, I., Role of natural killer cells in the destruction of circulating tumor emboli, *J. Natl. Cancer Inst.,* 65, 801, 1980.
13. Barlozzari, T., Reynolds, C. W., and Herberman, R. B., In vivo role of natural killer cells: involvement of large granular lymphocytes in the clearance of tumor cells in anti-asialo GM_1-treated rats, *J. Immunol.,* 131, 1024, 1983.
14. Lotzová, E. and Savary, C. A., Parallelism between the effects of cortisone acetate on hybrid resistance and natural killing, *Exp. Hematol.,* 9, 766, 1981.
15. Miller, S. C., Gallagher, M. T., Datta, S. K., and Trentin, J. J., Development of natural killer cell activity and genetic resistance to bone marrow transplantation with age: effect of neonatal thymectomy, *Scand. J. Immunol.,* 13, 105, 1981.
16. Timonen, T., Ranki, A., Saksela, E., and Hayry, P., Human natural cell-mediated cytotoxicity against fetal fibroblasts. III. Morphological and functional characterization of the effector cells, *Cell. Immunol.,* 48, 121, 1979.
17. Timonen, T., Ortaldo, J. R., and Herberman, R. B., Characteristics of human large granular lymphocytes and relationship to natural killer and K cells, *J. Exp. Med.,* 153, 569, 1981.
18. Timonen, T., Reynolds, C. W., Ortaldo, J. R., and Herberman, R. B., Isolation of human and rat natural killer cells, *J. Immunol. Methods,* 51, 269, 1982.
19. Reynolds, C. W., Timonen, T., and Herberman, R. B., Natural killer (NK) cell activity in the rat. I. Isolation and characterization of the effector cells, *J. Immunol.,* 127, 282, 1981.
20. Luini, W., Boraschi, D., Alberti, S., Aleotti, A., and Tagliabue, A., Morphological characterization of a cell population responsible for natural killer activity, *Immunology,* 43, 663, 1981.
21. Kumagai, K., Itoh, K., Suzuki, R., Hinuma, S., and Saitoh, F., Studies of murine large granular lymphocytes. I. Identification as effector cells in NK and K cytotoxicity, *J. Immunol.,* 129, 388, 1982.
22. Ortis de Landaźuri, M., Lopez-Botet, M., Timonen, T., Ortaldo, J. R., and Herberman, R. B., Human large granular lymphocytes: spontaneous and interferon-boosted NK activity against adherent and nonadherent tumor cell lines, *J. Immunol.,* 127, 1380, 1981.
23. Rees, R. C., Reynolds, C. W., and Herberman, R. B., Rat natural killer cell activity against lymphoid and nonlymphoid tumor cells and normal rat cell lines, *Cancer Res.,* 43, 4248, 1983.
24. Hansson, M., Beran, M., Andersson, B., and Kiessling, R., Inhibition of in vitro granulopoiesis by autologous allogeneic human NK cells, *J. Immunol.,* 129, 126, 1982.
25. Barlozzari, T., Reynolds, C. W., Wiltrout, R., and Herberman, R. B., Direct evidence for the role of NK cells in the inhibition of tumor metastases, *J. Immunol.;* 134, 2783, 1985.
26. Herberman, R. B., Nunn, M. E., and Lavrin, D. H., Natural cytotoxic reactivity of mouse lymphoid cells against syngeneic and allogeneic tumors. I. Distribution of reactivity and specificity, *Int. J. Cancer,* 16, 216, 1975.

27. Oehler, J. R., Lindsey, L. R., Nunn, M. E., and Herberman, R. B., Natural cell mediated cytotoxicity in rats. I. Tissue and strain distribution and demonstration of a membrane receptor for the Fc portion of IgG, *Int. J. Cancer,* 21, 204, 1978.
28. Potter, M. R. and Moore, M., Organ distribution of natural cytotoxicity in the rat, *Clin. Exp. Immunol.,* 34, 78, 1978.
29. Lotzová, E. and McCredie, K. B., Natural killer cells in mice and man and their possible biological significance, *Cancer Immunol. Immunother.,* 4, 215, 1978.
30. Pucetti, P., Santoni, A., Riccardi, C., and Herberman, R. B., Cytotoxic effector cells with the characterisitics of natural killer cells in the lungs of mice, *Int. J. Cancer,* 25, 153, 1980.
31. Nolibe, D., Berel, E., Masse, R., and Lafuma, J., Characterization of a major natural killer activity in rat lungs, *Biomedicine,* 35, 230, 1981.
32. Lotzová, E., Savary, C. A., Khan, A., and Stringfellow, D. A., Stimulation of natural killer cells in two random-bred strains of athymic rats by interferon-inducing pyrimidinone, *J. Immunol.,* 132, 2566, 1984.
33. Mayrhofer, G. and Whately, R. J., Granular intraepithelial lymphocytes of the rat small intestine. I. Isolation, presence in T lymphocyte-deficient rats and bone marrow origin, *Int. Arch. Allergy Appl. Immunol.,* 71, 317, 1983.
34. Targan, S., Britvan, L., Kendal, R., Vimadalal, S., and Soll, A., Isolation of spontaneous and interferon inducible natural killer like cells from human colonic mucosa: lysis of lymphoid and autologous epithelial target cells, *Clin. Exp. Immunol.,* 54, 14, 1983.
35. Hansson, M., Kiessling, R., Anderson, B., Kärre, K., and Roder, J., NK cell-sensitive T-cell subpopulations in thymus: inverse correlation to host NK activity, *Nature (London),* 278, 174, 1979.
36. Zöller, M., Andrighetto, G., and Heyman, B., Natural and antibody-dependent killer cells in the thymus, *Eur. J. Immunol.,* 12, 914, 1982.
37. Oldham, R. K., Forbes, J. T., and Niblach, G. D., Natural killer activity in human thoracic duct lymphocytes, *Proc. Am. Assoc. Cancer Res.,* 19, 161, 1978.
38. Zöller, M., Bellgrau, D., Axberg, I., and Wigzell, H., Natural killer cells do not belong to the recirculating lymphocyte population, *Scand. J. Immunol.,* 15, 159, 1982.
39. Santoni, A., Herberman, R. B., and Holden, H. T., Correlation between natural and antibody-dependent cell-mediated cytotoxicity against tumor targets in the mouse. I. Distribution of the reactivity, *J. Natl. Cancer Inst.,* 62, 109, 1979.
40. Chiba, M., Shorter, R. G., Thayer, W. R., Bartnik, W., and ReMine, S., K-cell activity in lamina proprial lymphocytes from the human colon, *Dig. Dis. Sci.,* 24, 817, 1979.
40a. Fukui, and Reynolds, C. W., unpublished observation.
41. Reynolds, C. W., Timonen, T., Holden, H. T., Hansen, C. T., and Herberman, R. B., Natural killer cells activity in the rat. Analysis of effector cell morphology and effect of interferon on natural killer cell function in the athymic (nude) rat, *Eur. J. Immunol.,* 12, 577, 1982.
42. Itoh, K., Suzuki, R., Umezu, Y., Hanaumi, K., and Kumagai, K., Studies on murine large granular lymphocytes. II. Tissue, strain and age distributions of LGL and LAL, *J. Immunol.,* 129, 395, 1982.
43. Brideau, R. J., Carter, P. B., McMaster, W. R., Mason, D. W., and Williams, A. F., Two subsets of rat T lymphocytes defined with monoclonal antibodies, *Eur. J. Immunol.,* 10, 609, 1980.
44. Cantrell, D. A., Robins, R. A., Brooks, C. G., and Baldwin, R. W., Phenotype of rat natural killer cells defined by monoclonal antibodies marking rat lymphocyte subsets, *Immunology,* 45, 97, 1982.
45. Reynolds, C. W., Sharrow, S. O., Ortaldo, J. R., and Herberman, R. B., Natural killer (NK) activity in the rat. II. Analysis of surface antigens on LGL by flow cytometry, *J. Immunol.,* 127, 2204, 1981.
46. Ward, J. M., Argilan, F., and Reynolds, C. W., Immunoperoxidase localization of large granular lymphocytes in normal tissues and lesions of athymic nude rats, *J. Immunol.,* 131, 132, 1983.
47. Reynolds, C. W., Ward, J. M., Wiltrout, R. H., and Herberman, R. B., Tissue distribution and in vivo localization of rat LGL, in *Proc. Int. Symp. Natural Killer Activity Regul.,* Excerpta Medica, Amsterdam, 1984, 9.
48. Si, L. and Whiteside, T. L., Tissue distribution of human NK cells studied with the anti-Leu-7 monoclonal antibody, *J. Immunol.,* 130, 2149, 1983.
49. Banerjee, D. and Thibert, R. F., Natural killer-like cells found in B cell compartments of human lymphoid tissues, *Nature (London),* 304, 270, 1983.
50. Lipinski, M., Braham, K., Caillaud, J. M., Carlu, C., and Tursz, T., HNK-1 antibody detects an antigen expressed on neuroectodermal cells, *J. Exp. Med.,* 158, 1775, 1983.
51. Lanier, L. L., Le, A. M., Phillips, J. H., Warner, N. L., and Babcock, G. F., Subpopulations of human natural killer cells defined by expression of the Leu-7 (HNK-1) and Leu-11 (NK-15) antigens, *J. Immunol.,* 131, 1789, 1983.
52. Reynolds, C. W., Denn, A. C., III, Barlozzari, T., Wiltrout, R. H., Reichardt, D. A., and Herberman, R. B., Natural killer activity in the rat. IV. Distribution of large granular lymphocytes (LGL) following intravenous and intraperitoneal transfer, *Cell. Immunol.,* 86, 371, 1984.

Chapter 6

GENETIC CONTROL OF NK CELL ACTIVITY IN RODENTS

Edward A. Clark

TABLE OF CONTENTS

I. INTRODUCTION

The phenotype "NK cell activity" is defined operationally: in vitro cytolytic activity of lymphoid effector cells against certain standard tumor target cell lines, where sharing of major histocompatibility complex (MHC) molecules between effector and target cells is not required. Because NK cell activity is not as discrete a phenotype as, for example, protein polymorphisms, it has been difficult to clearly define the genes controlling NK cells; however, some progress has been made. Pertinent studies through 1979 have been reviewed.[1] There are also several good Swedish Ph.D. theses reviewing this area.[2,3] Here, I briefly review earlier studies but focus on more recent results. Most of the work has been done using mice because of the availability of a large number of inbred strains, congenic-resistant and recombinant-inbred lines, and mutant stocks.[4] I will refer to studies using other species when appropriate. This review is meant to be selective and illustrative of key findings.

Genes may influence or control any number of steps in the NK cell pathway (Figure 1). Our knowledge of the genes affecting these various steps is still quite fragmentary. NK cell frequencies clearly differ in inbred strains of mice,[5] suggesting gene control of overall NK cell numbers. NK cells migrate to and reside in distinct regions of lymphoid tissues[6,7] but nothing is known about the genes or gene products influencing this migration. The factors activating NK cells have begun to be identified and some are known to be under distinct gene control.[8] The genes controlling the receptors on NK cells for regulatory signals are not known. Finally, there may be genes affecting NK cell recognition structures, lytic activity, and regulatory activity. Identification of a single gene that clearly controlled any one of these steps would be a significant contribution. As we shall see, even when a gene has a number of pleiomorphic effects which includes an effect on NK cells, it may help us to better understand NK cells.

II. INBRED STRAINS OF MICE

Inbred strains of mice differ considerably in their levels of "endogenous" NK cell activity.[1,9] The strain distribution patterns (SDP) observed of "high", "intermediate", and "low" strains depends on the target cell and assay system used.[1,9,10] The effect of target cell genotype on SDP has not been rigorously tested using, e.g., normal tissue targets from backcross progeny, but a trend toward lower activity against syngeneic or H-2-identical targets has been observed.[1,9,10] Thymocyte target cells taken from "NK high" strains like CBA tend to be less susceptible than targets taken from "NK low" strains;[11] this may be a reflection of the relative amount of interferon (IFN) present in high and low strains which might act to reduce target susceptibility.

Kiessling and Welsh[10] have reported that the genetic control of susceptibility of target cells differs for thymocytes vs. peritoneal cell targets. Killing of peritoneal cells was clearly lower in syngeneic combinations than in allogeneic combinations; considerable "autoreactivity" to thymocytes was observed and thymocyte target sensitivity depended on the NK levels of the donor strain. Unlike with peritoneal cells, the genotype of the thymocyte target did not affect the SDP. As discussed below, when 18-hr assays rather than short-term assays are used to measure natural cytotoxicity, very different SDP are seen.[8,12] The gene control of NK activity in mice recently infected naturally with pathogens is similar to that of "endogenous" NK activity.[13]

NK activity in mouse strains against YAC-1 target cells ranges from a low in, e.g., A/J mice, of <0.01 lytic units (LU)/million spleen cells to >5 to 10 LU/million spleen cells in SM/J mice.[14] Similar SDP are observed whether NK activity or antibody-dependent cell-mediated cytotoxicity (ADCC) are measured.[15] When the NK levels of F_1 mice of "NK low" and "NK high" strains are compared to parental levels, they are

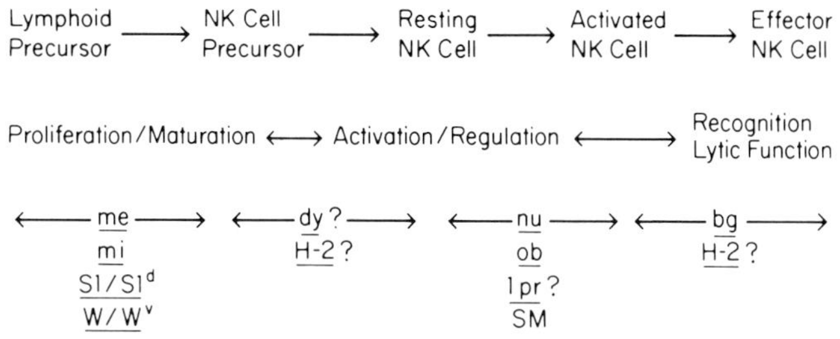

FIGURE 1. Possible sites where genes may influence NK cell differentiation and activity. At early stages of differentiation the genes motheaten *(me)*, microphthalmia (mi), steel anemia *(Sl)*, and dominant spotting anemia *(W)* may influence NK cell development. Genes affecting later stages include dystrophy *(dy)*, nude *(nu)*, obese *(ob)*,, lymphoproliferation *(lpr)*, beige *(bg)*.

the same for most combinations as the "NK high" parent, suggesting *dominant inheritance.* Certain strain combinations, however, yield different results: for example, (B10 × DBA/2)F_1 mice have much higher NK levels than either parent, suggesting *gene complementation.*[13,16,17] The complementation is between a non-*H-2* gene on the B10 background and an *H-2D* end gene from DBA/2 mice.[13] (A/J × SM/J)F_1 mice have intermediate NK levels between parent strains, unlike (NZB × SM/J)F_1 which have the SM/J high phenotype.[17a] This intermediate phenotype, reflecting *gene dosage,* has also been observed in (LEW × BN)F_1 rats.[18] A final pattern is the *recessive* inheritance of "NK high" phenotype in, e.g., (W/Fu × BN)F_1 rats.[19]

When "NK high" F_1 mice are either backcrossed to their "NK low" parent or intercrossed, the NK phenotypes of the progeny range from low to high without any clear segregation into low, intermediate, and high groups.[1,20] These results indicate that, not surprisingly, NK activity is under polygenic control. The number of genes involved is not clear, and given the current difficulty in measuring a discrete NK phenotype, these data should not be overinterpreted.

In order to better identify the genes controlling NK activity in mice, we have crossed two strains with very pronounced differences in NK activity: "NK low" A/J, and "NK high" SM/J mice,[14] and examined the NK activity of F_2 intercross progeny (Figure 2). A range of NK activities was observed in these mice, suggesting polygenic control. Furthermore, a clear correlation between NK and ADCC activity was evident, which formally demonstrates that NK and K cells are under common polygenic gene control. In this and other crosses with SM/J,[14] no effect of *H-2* genotype was demonstrable. The genes influencing NK activity in SM/J mice appear to affect NK activation rather than NK cell numbers (Figure 1).

During the past 3 years, we have attempted to cross the "NK high" gene(s) of SM/J onto the A/J background to create an A.SM "NK high" congenic line. We have used the cross-intercross method of Snell (see Reference 4) because F_1 mice had intermediate NK levels: "NK high" F_2 progeny were backcrossed to A/J parents (Generation 3, 5, 7, etc.) and then intercrossed and tested for NK activity (Generation 4, 6, 8, etc.). "NK high" generation 12 mice have been brother-sister mated and these mice consistently give NK activity intermediate between A/J and SM/J. However, analysis of the segregating G12 intercross progeny suggest more than one locus is involved. Further progeny testing and crossing is in progress. We are very close to establishing an "NK low" and "NK high" strain pair for further genetic and serologic studies.

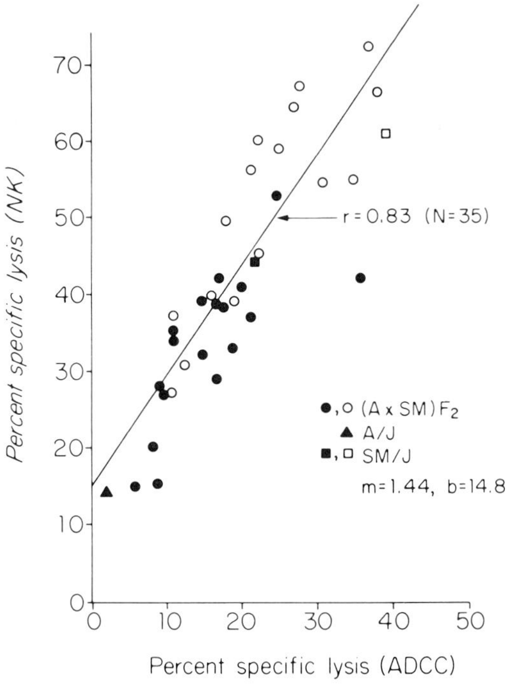

FIGURE 2. Clear correlation of NK cell activity (YAC-1 targets) and K cell activity (Thy-1 antibody coated SL-2 targets) in segregating F_2 progeny formally demonstrates that NK cells and K cells are under common gene control. Open and closed figures are two distinct experiments.

III. *H-2* GENE CONTROL OF NK CELLS

Nearly a decade ago Petranyi and co-workers[20,21] showed that genes linked to the *H-2* complex influence NK activity: F_1 × "NK low" backcross progeny of the heterozygous *H-2*$^{a/b}$ genotype had significantly higher NK activity than did homozygous mice. Using a series of *H-2* congenic and intra *H-2* recombinant mice, Harmon and co-workers[22] identified a gene controlling both NK activity and hybrid tumor resistance mapping within or near the *H-2D* region. This result clearly suggested that NK cells and hybrid resistance were under common gene control: the same *H-2D*^{d}-associated region controlling NK activity had been previously shown by Cudkowicz,[23] Cudkowicz and Bennett,[24] and others[1,25] to control F1 resistance to tumor grafts or resistance to allogeneic or *H-2*^{b} into (*H-2*^{b} × *H-2*^{d})F_1 bone marrow grafts (the *Hh-1* locus). The significance of the *Hh-1-H-2D*^{d} gene in NK cell activity is discussed below. These studies were confirmed and extended by Klein and his co-workers in Stockholm.[16,17]

In order for the *H-2D*^{d}-associated gene to exert its effect, another complementary non-*H-2* gene on the B10 background must be present.[13,16] Complementation of certain *I-A* and *I-E* alleles within the *H-2* complex is necessary for certain immune response (Ir) gene-controlled responses.[26] Complementation of an I-E gene and a non-*H-2* gene of the B10 background on Chromosome 4 appears to be necessary for I-J antigen expression.[27] Current speculations suggest that the genes on Chromosome 4 controlling I-J may be encoding the antigen receptor of T suppressor (T_s) cells.[28] This is of great interest to NK cell biologists since a Chromosome 4-linked gene has been reported to affect NK activity as well.[21] Given that some NK cells and some T_s cells in the human share common antigens such as Tp32 (T8),[29] it is tempting to speculate that a similar mechanism functioning for T_s cells and *I-E* and Chromosome 4 genes is operating for NK cells via *H-2D* and Chromosome 4 genes, e.g., controlling NK receptor molecules or interactions with NK cells and self MHC molecules (see below).

Our initial studies of intra-*H-2* recombinants demonstrated that the NK regulatory locus mapped to the right (telomeric) of *H-2S*.[22] Although the *Hh-1* locus had been shown not to map to the *T1a* region,[23] the left (centromeric) boundary of the *NK* locus was not defined by recombination but was positioned left of *T1a* based only on SDP. More recently, Klein[30] has tested a series of *T1a* congenic and intra-*T1a/Qa* recombinant mice to map more precisely the *H2-D*-end-associated loci affected NK cells. Although the differences between "high" and "low" mice were not that clear, based on statistical arguments, the following conclusions are suggested from this study: first, based on *Hh-1* and hybrid tumor resistance allelic genotypes[1,23,25] and NK assays, $H\text{-}2D^d$ and $H\text{-}2D^k$ mice have higher activity than certain $H\text{-}2D^b$ or $H\text{-}2^{dm2}$ mutant mice, which once again implicates $H\text{-}2D^d$. Second, certain $H\text{-}2D^b$ strains have higher NK activity than other $H\text{-}2D^b$ strains. The gene controlling this effect appears to map in or between Qa-2 and Qa-5.[30] T1a region control was ruled out by testing backcross progeny mice of a cross with the following possible NK gene genotypes ($Qa^{high?}$ $T1a^{high?}$ × $Qa^{low?}$ $T1a^{low?}$) F_1 × $Qa^{low?}$ $T1a^{high?}$. High NK activity segregated with heterozygosity at *Qa* independent of *T1a* genotype. This suggests the gene-conferring high NK activity maps to the Qa region. It will be important to confirm and extend this work once antisera for more Qa-2, 4, and 5 allelic products are available and NK phenotyping is easier.

How these Class I genes ($H\text{-}2D^d$, *Qa*) influence NK activity is not known. Given that Class I and Class II molecules appear to be functioning as guides for regulating T cell and B cell responses,[31] it is compelling to postulate that the products of *H-2* NK regulatory loci are serving a similar function. The elucidation of the function of this *H-2* control of NK cells is absolutely vital for understanding NK activation and recognition. Unraveling this *H-2D* control is also important, particularly for convincing those immunologists who persist with the view that NK cells are, e.g., worn out T_s or T cytotoxic (T_c) cells, nonimmune cells, etc.

One simple model is that *H-2* genes somehow control the triggering and subsequent proliferation of NK cells. This idea is supported by the work of Roder and Kiessling,[5] who measured the number of lymphocytes binding to YAC-1 targets (target binding cells) as an indicator of NK cell frequency in inbred strains and backcross progeny mice. $H\text{-}2^{d/b}$ progeny had significantly more target binders than did $H\text{-}2^{b/b}$ progeny.

As mentioned above, the same $H\text{-}2D^d$ gene region controlling NK cells control F_1 hybrid resistance to $H\text{-}2^b$ bone marrow cells.[1,25] Hybrid resistance violates the genetic rule of transplantation, which states that histocompatibility genes are codominantly expressed and that F_1 progeny therefore are universal recipients.[4] Thus, it is important to explain this exceptional phenomenon that Petranyi et al.,[21] Lotzová,[25] and Cudkowicz and Nakamura[32] so tenaciously and thoroughly studied. Snell[33] has suggested that the *H-2D-Hh-1* region-encoded molecules are cell interaction products and that a cytotoxic response results when F_1 host interaction products are mismatched with donor parental interaction products. We extended this model by suggesting that a total mismatch is necessary for triggering a response.[1]

More recently, Kärre[2] has proposed a unifying model for the role H-2 molecules play in NK activation. According to this theory, T cells and NK cells function as distinct but complementary immune surveillance systems, where T cells are induced by altered or nonself MHC, and NK cells are triggered by the absence of self MHC or the inability to fully match self MHC.[1] Apart from the appeal and logic of such a balanced system to ward off clever pathogens that block or interfere with MHC expression, several descriptive phenomena support this model.[2] For example, target cells with low levels of Class I molecules such as thymocytes,[11] bone marrow,[34] and embryonic cells,[35] are generally more susceptible than targets with high levels of Class I antigens; agents such as IFN, which increase Class I expression, lower target cell susceptibility.[36,37] H-2^- variant lines are also more susceptible to NK killing than H-2^+ wild type cells.[37a] *H-2* allelic differences in NK activity could reflect differences in self-self matching.

This model does not explain why *H-2D*-end genes and not *H-2K*-end genes control NK activity. One possibility is that this control reflects an as yet poorly defined but distinct property or function of *H-2D*, e.g., in self-tolerance regulation. *H-2D*-associated genes control the formation of autologous red cell rosettes, a self-recognition phenomenon.[38,39] H-$2D^d$ allogeneic red cells[40] and tumor cells[41] are clearly more immunogenic than H-2K alloantigens. Flaherty and Zimmerman[42] and Boyse and co-workers[43] have found that H-2D but not H-2K associates with the Tla and Lyt 2 molecules. The murine Lyt 2 molecule is expressed on T_s cells and T_c cells and in humans the Lyt 2 homolog T8 or Tp32 is expressed at low concentrations on some NK cells.[29] Recently, we have demonstrated that Tp32 physically associates with Class I molecules.[43a] Thus Tp32 may be involved in stabilizing or assisting Class I interactions of cytotoxic (NK, T_c) and T_s cells.[44] *H-2D*-associated gene products are clearly distinctive from H-2K products and associate with different membrane structures. These phenomena, together with the possible parallel complementation of Chromosome 4 with *I-E* (for I-J+ T_s cells) or, by analogy, *H-2D* region genes (for NK cells) suggest that *H-2D*-associated genes regulate NK cell recognition and activation.

Brickell and co-workers[45] recently reported that mRNA of a Class I gene is highly expressed in H-2^- embryonic cells and is expressed in high concentrations in transformed fibroblasts. They also suggested that this Class I product of the gene may be expressed on teratocarcinoma cells and serve as recognition or regulatory structures for NK cells in immune surveillance of transformed cells. Based on DNA sequence comparisons but not fine mapping studies, they suggest this gene maps to the *Qa/Tla* region. This work needs confirmation and comparisons to known *Qa* and *Tla* gene sequences are necessary before the relationship of this observation to *H-2D*^{d} and *Qa* NK gene control can be determined. The *H-2*-controlled NK phenotype does not correspond to *H-2*-controlled differences in susceptibility to carcinogen-induced tumorigenesis, suggesting *H-2*-controlled NK activity is not playing an obvious role in surveillance of primary tumors.[46]

IV. MUTATIONS INFLUENCING NK CELL ACTIVITY

If experimetns are designed to compare mutant mice with wildtype sex-matched littermate controls, it is relatively straightforward to determine if a given mutation influences NK cell activity. It is quite another matter to interpret the results or determine the site of gene action and other possible pleiotropic effects a mutation may have on the immune system. The general pattern with immunodeficient mice has been that a pioneering investigator discovers a mutation that is "selective" for T cells *(nu)*, B cells *(xid)*, NK cells *(bg)*, etc., which is very useful for the time; but upon further investigation, other effects on the immune system become evident. Thus, it is prudent to be careful interpreting data using mutants.

One group of mutations acts to reduce NK cell activity by affecting hematopoiesis and/or lymphopoiesis and thereby NK cell development (Figure 1). The generation of NK cells is an autonomous function of the bone marrow.[47] Thus, the mutation *mi* (microphthalmia, Chromosome 6), which leads to congenital osteopetrosis, also reduces NK cell activity,[48] probably because of bone replacement of NK cell precursors.

The reduction of NK levels in anemic *Sl/Sl^d* and *W/W^v* mice reflects yet another set of marrow deficiencies which also affect NK cell development.[49] The motheaten mutation (*me,* also Chromosome 6) has a range of pleiotropic effects that impair immune functions including nonresponsiveness to T cell and B cell mitogens and impaired T_c cell and NK cell activity.[49,50] This defect can be cured by treating irradiated motheaten mice with normal wildtype bone marrow, indicating that the major defect in motheaten mice affects progenitor cells in the bone marrow.[51] More recently, a new spontaneous mutation of the *me* locus occurred in C57BL/6J mice, and the allele has been designated "viable motheaten" (*me^v*) because *me^v* homozygotes have a significantly increased life span compared to conventional *me/me* mice.[52] However, viable motheaten mice are still severely immunodeficient and lack both endogenous and inducible NK cell activity, unlike beige *(bg)* mice.[52] Thus, of all the mutants tested, this mutation clearly lacks NK cell activity. Allogeneic fibrosarcomas rejected by heterozygous littermate controls grow rapidly in motheaten mice and at a similar rate as in syngeneic controls.[52] Furthermore, human T leukemia cells which did not grow in nude mice grew in motheaten mice.

As alluded to above, *H-2* genes may influence the proliferation of NK cells.[5] Recently, a mutation has been identified which affects NK cell numbers: mice homozygous for a mutation leading to muscular dystrophy (dy, Chromosome 10) were found to have significantly higher NK cell activity than age- and sex-matched +/+ mice.[53] This increased NK activity correlated with an increase in target binding cells in *dy/dy,* suggesting that the *dy* gene influences NK cell proliferation. Furthermore, unlike normal mouse strains,[11] the thymus of "NK high" dystrophic mice are very sensitive to NK cell-mediated killing. Homozygous dystrophic mice display early thymic atrophy and altered thymic morphology; thus, it is possible that the abnormal NK cell levels and thymic degeneration are somehow related. The authors also noted that thymic cells and muscle cells share common surface antigens such as Thy-1, but what role, if any, NK cells may play in muscle destruction in muscular dystrophy is unclear.

Another group of mutations influencing NK activity are thought to principally affect NK activation or regulation rather than the development of NK cell numbers. These include *nu* (nude, Chromosome 11), *ob* (obese, yet another Chromosome 6 locus), and *lpr* (lymphoproliferation, unassigned autosomal recessive). NK cells can be activated by all types of species-specific IFN[54] and IL-2,[55] and thus any pleiotropic effects which influence IFN, or IL-2 levels, or induction may also affect NK levels. For example, we have reported that the same alloantigens which activate T cells also activate NK cells;[56] this result can be interpreted as evidence of common gene control for T cells and NK cells and/or as evidence of factors being induced by certain alloantigens that trigger T cells and NK cells (e.g., IL-2). Similarly, the high NK cell levels normally seen in nude mice may be related to the high IFN levels seen in nude mice.[57] This is supported by the finding that specific-pathogen free nude mice have somewhat lower NK levels than conventional nude mice.[13] The nude mutation in the rat *(rnu)* also produces increased NK cell activity.[58] However, the increased activity clearly correlated with increases in the *numbers* of large granular lymphocytes suggesting that the *rnu* gene may influence NK cell numbers. Welsh[54] and others[49,59] have found that IFN can cause NK cells to proliferate, which could account for elevated NK numbers in nude rats. Like the *nu* gene, the *lpr* mutation in MRL mice leads to elevated NK cell activity. It is not clear how the lymphoproliferating cells on MRL-*lpr* mice affect NK cells. These cells produce a B cell growth factor[60] but it is not clear if *lpr* cells produce factors affecting NK cells. The effect of *lpr* on NK cells is more pronounced in the arthritic MRL strain than other strains with the *lpr* gene.

Obese (*ob,* Chromosome 6) mice have lower levels of NK cell activity than phenotypically similar diabetic mice.[49] A clear difference between obese and diabetic mice is that young obese mice, unlike young diabetic mice, have elevated plasma hydrocortisone (HC) levels.[61] Thus, the elevated HC may be decreasing NK activity in young obese mice directly or via an intermediary cell.[62]

A third type of mutation, *bg* (beige, Chromosome 13), may affect the efficiency of NK activation or lytic function. Beige is a recessive coat color mutation that has striking similarities to the Chediak-Higashi syndrome in man. It has a number of pleiotropic effects in mice, including increased susceptibility to pneumonitis and cytomegalovirus infections; defective granulocytes chemotaxis and lysosomal enzyme secretion; and giant lysosomal granules in granule-containing cells (see Reference 63). Initial studies of immunologic functions suggested that beige mice had a selective NK cell defect.[64] However, subsequent studies have shown that beige mice have defective T_c[65] cell and B cell[63] activity. Given these results, the numerous studies using beige mice to "prove" a definitive role of NK cells in, e.g., resistance to tumor metastasis, immune surveillance, etc., are suspect. Given the broad pleiotropic effects of beige on granule formation — recall they are beige in color due to formation and clumping of large melanin granules[66] — it is likely that the *bg* gene influences membrane interactions that affect a range of cell types.

Even with this major caveat, I confess I still work with beige mice. They remain a useful model for examining the effect that a single gene has on various phenotypes. For example, we have found that the bg gene has a profound effect on the development of autoimmune disease in SB/Le mice.[63] As with their BXSB offspring, the SB-derived Y chromosome has a locus which accelerates autoimmune disease *(Yaa)*.[67] The bg gene, in contrast "deaccelerates" the autoimmune disease:[63] beige SB/Le males die approximately 250 days later than SB/Le *bg/+* males of the same disease, suggesting that the beige gene makes certain immune cells involved in autoimmunity less efficient. As early as 6 weeks of age, there are dramatic differences in *bg/bg* and *bg/+* mice in immune complex deposition and autoantibody levels.[63,63a] Given the recent findings of abnormal NK levels in certain human autoimmune diseases,[68,69] it is tempting to speculate that NK cells interact with a *Y*-dictated factor to produce the SB/Le autoimmune disease. However, this idea ignores the possible role of other cells influenced by *bg*.

The *bg* gene does not influence NK cell frequency of IFN levels,[64,70] which suggests that beige NK cells respond poorly to IFN or have reduced lytic activity. To assess the possible site of beige action, we[49] and others[71] have examined the NK activity of a series of pigment mutations related to beige.[66] In a limited study, we found that the mutations pale ears (*ep* Chromosome 19), pearl (*pe* Chromosome 13), and ruby eyes (*ru* Chromosome 19) did not affect NK cell activity.[49] In a larger study, Orn et al.,[71] found that the *bg* gene has the most pronounced effect on NK cell activity, but the *ep*, pallid (*pa* Chromosome 2), and reduced pigment (*rp* Chromosome 7) also lead to a significant reduction in NK activity; the sepia (*sea*, Chromosome 1) mutation did not have an effect. There was no clear correlation between the degree of overall lysosomal enzyme defects in the mutants and NK activity, with the exception that the NK normal sepia mice also had normal lysosomal enzyme activities.

As with their mouse homolog, Chediak-Higashi syndrome patients have impaired NK activity.[72] Patients with X-linked B cell immunodeficiencies have been tested for NK cell activity and found to be normal.[73] In contrast, patients with X-linked lymphoproliferative syndrome (XLP) are profoundly NK cell-deficient.[74] This defect appears to be acquired after the clinical expression of the disease, since males at risk for XLP have normal NK activity in spite of having abnormal EBV serologies.[75] Patients with XLP have normal NK cell levels but low activity. Some patients with severe combined immunodeficiency have normal NK levels, while others have low NK activity.[76]

V. GENE CONTROL OF SOME RELATED PHENOTYPES

Natural cytotoxic activity can also be mediated by cells related to NK cells called natural cytotoxic (NC) cells.[12] NC cells have been distinguished from NK cells based on differences in the assay used, target cell susceptibility, cell surface phenotype, and responsiveness to interleukins.[12] NC cells and NK cells are also under distinct but related gene control. The SDP are quite different for NC and NK reactivity.[77-79] Most notably "NK low" A/J,[12] beige,[79] and motheaten[79a] mice have normal NC activity. NC activity is under polygenic control and the "NC high" phenotype is generally dominant. The results of Stutman and Cuttito[77] once again emphasizes the effect the target cell has on the "gene control" observed. For example, for some target cells, nude mice are "NC high" but with other target cells nude mouse NC levels do not differ significantly from normal controls.

Using one cell line, the Meth 113 fibrosarcoma, Stutman and Cuttito[77,78] have identified genes in the *Qa/Tla* region controlling NC activity. Based on the differential NC reactivity of *H-2* and *Qa/Tla* congenic strains, they suggested genes in *Qa/Tla* region control NC cells.[77] In general, the pattern of gene control is reciprocal to that observed by Klein[30] for NK cells; the differences between NC activity of B6 and B6.*Tla*^{a} are quite clear-cut, while the NK activity differences are less dramatic.[30,78] Interestingly, gene complementation between B10 background genes and *Qa/Tla* genes was suggested by Stutman's results: (B10.A × A.SW)F1, were "NC high" unlike the "NC low" phenotype of both parents; unlike with NK activity, this was not observed with (B10.A × B10)F_1 mice. Thus, the picture emerging is that non-*H-2* background genes may complement with *I-E*[27], *H-2D*,[13,16] and *Qa/Tla*[78] to affect immune functions.

A form of in vivo "natural cytotoxicity" has been studied in rats:[80] rats were injected with radiolabeled allogeneic lymphoid cells and levels of radioactivity-different tissues measured after 24 hr., 95 donor-host combinations were examined. This reactivity was controlled by at least 2 genes, 1 of which is linked to the *Rt-1* MHC. Interallelic effects depending on the *Rt-1* donor-host combinations were evident.

Another important related cell type, autoreactive T_c cells, are controlled by *Hh-1-H-2D* region genes. We refer the reader to recent reviews.[32,81] Another very important related system where gene control of natural resistance has been studied in detail is resistance to allogeneic, semiallogeneic, and xenogeneic bone marrow (see Reference 25). Lotzová[25] and Cudkowicz and Bennett,[24] using a number of strain combinations, identified both *H-2*-linked and non-*H-2* "*Hh*" loci, which like *Hh-1* may influence NK activity. This work would be a fruitful area to extend for an eager NK immunogeneticist.

The SJL/JN mouse displays low NK reactivity to a variety of target cells (e.g., 82). Even after treatment with IFN or IFN-inducers, SJL mice are low responders; in this way they resemble *me*^{v} mice. The genes controlling this low responsiveness appear to map outside the *H-2* complex.[82] This low NK activity may be due to the action of an accessory cell which suppresses NK activity.[83]

For a discussion of genes controlling phenotypes related to NK cells, e.g., natural resistance to pathogens and gene control of ecotropic viruses, see Reference 1.

VI. SOMATIC IMMUNOGENETIC APPROACHES

In addition to segregation analyses and analysis of mutants, somatic cell genetic methods have begun to be used to study NK cell regulation. For example, genes controlling γ IFN and the NK cell-associated differentiation antigen in humans have been mapped to Chromosomes 12 and 11, respectively, using mouse-human hybrids.[84,85]

The major use of somatic cell genetics in NK cell biology has been trying to characterize the structures on target cells recognized by NK cells. Recently, Dubey et al.[86] examined the sensitivity of a series of anchorage-independent and low serum-requiring hamster embryo fibroblast mutant lines to killing by human NK cells. Nontumorigenic but transformed mutants that were anchorage-independent or required only low serum levels remained insensitive to NK-mediated lysis like the nontransformed parent line. Only fully tumorigenic lines derived from the mutants were found to be NK-sensitive. Thus, the susceptibility to NK cell killing of sequentially derived clones correlated with tumorigenicity and not transformation.

Another approach has been to attempt to develop sublines, subclones or "variant" lines of "NK cell-susceptible" lines which are "NK cell-resistant".[87-90] For example, Roder et al.[88] treated YAC-1 target cells with a mutagen and then selected clones more resistant to NK killing than the parent line. The presence of mutagen, however, did not change the already high frequency of resistant variants. the frequency of NK cells binding to the resistant and susceptible targets was the same, suggesting that a property distinct from the target binding structures had altered in the resistant cells.[88,89] In other studies, resistant sublines had less binding by NK cells.[87-91] More recently, Wright and Bonavida[90] claimed to have isolated variants resistant to NK cell killing by culturing susceptible targets in NK cytotoxic factors and selecting resistance cells. The resistant clones bound less cytotoxic factor than susceptible cells yet were bound equally well by NK cells. The authors suggested the resistant line lacks receptors for the cytotoxic factor. While these studies are of interest, they are all missing key data from the perspective of a somatic cell geneticist: evidence for selection of mutants rather than epigenetic changes. The effects of protein or RNA synthetic rates, mycoplasma,[92] etc., are difficult to rule out and indeed may account for much of the phenomenlogy.[92] Selection of true stable mutants with defined mutation rates is needed.

ACKNOWLEDGMENTS

I wish to thank Kevin Draves for expert technical assistance. This work was supported by Grant CA34199 from the National Cancer Institute.

REFERENCES

1. Clark, E. A. and Harmon, R. C., Genetic control of natural cell-mediated cytotoxicity and hybrid resistance, *Adv. Cancer Res.*, 31, 227, 1980.
2. Kärre, K., On the immunobiology of natural killer cells, studies of murine NK-cells and their interactions with T-cells and T-lymphomas, Karolinska Institute, Stockholm, 1981.
3. Örn, A., Natural killer cells: studies on genetic, endogeneous and exogenous factors controlling the expression of natural killer cell activity, Uppsala University, No. 390, Uppsala, Sweden. 1981.
4. Hildemann, W. H., Clark, E. A., and Raison, R. A., *Comprehensive Immunognentics,* Elsevier-North Holland, New York, 1980.
5. Roder, J. C. and Kiessling, R., Target-effector interaction in the natural killer cell system. I. Covariance and genetic control of cytolytic and target-cell-binding subpopulations in the mouse, *Scand. J. Immunol.*, 8, 135, 1978.
6. Lusheng, S. and Whiteside, T. L., Tissue distribution of human NK cells studied with anti-Leu-7 monoclonal antibody, *J. Immunol.*, 130, 2149, 1983.
7. Ward, J. M., Argilan, F., and Reynolds, C. W., Immunoperoxidase localization of large granular lymphocytes in normal tissues and lesions athymic nude rats, *J. Immunol.*, 131, 132, 1983.
8. DeMaeyer, E., DeMaeyer-Guignard, J., and Bailey, D. W., Loci with quantitative effect on circulating interferon, *Mouse News Lett.*, 48, 29, 1973.

9. Herberman, R. B. and Holden, H. T., Natural cell-mediated immunity, *Adv. Cancer Res.*, 27, 305, 1978.
10. Kiessling, R. W. and Welsh, R. M., Jr., Killing of normal cells by activated mouse natural killer cells: evidence for two patterns of genetic regulation of lysis, *Int. J. Cancer*, 25, 611, 1980.
11. Hansson, M., Kiessling, R., Andersson, B., Kärre, K., and Roder, J., Natural killer (NK) cell sensitive T-cell subpopulation in the thymus. Inverse correlation to NK activity of the host, *Nature*, 278, 174, 1979.
12. Stutman, O., Paige, C., and Figarella, F. E., Natural cytotoxic cells against solid tumors in mice. I. Strain and age distribution and target cell susceptibility, *J. Immunol.*, 121, 1819, 1978.
13. Clark, E. A., Russell, P. H., Egghart, M., and Horton, M. A., Characteristics and genetic control of NK-cell-mediated cytotoxicity activated by naturally acquired infection in the mouse, *Int. J. Cancer*, 24, 688, 1979.
14. Clark, E. A., Engel, D., and Windsor, N. T., Immune responsiveness of SM/J mice: hyper NK activity mediated by NK1+ Qa-5$^-$ cells, *J. Immunol.*, 127, 2391, 1981.
15. Santoni, A., Herberman, R. B., and Holden, H. T., Correlation between natural and antibody-dependent cell-mediated cytotoxicity against tumor targets in the mouse. I. Distribution of the reactivity, *J. Natl. Cancer Inst.*, 62, 109, 1979.
16. Klein, G. O., Klein, G., Kiessling, R., and Kärre, K., H-2-associated control of natural cytotoxicity and hybrid resistance against RBL-5, *Immunogenetics*, 6, 561, 1978.
17. Klein, G. O., Kärre, K., Klein, G., and Kiessling, R., The genetic regulation of NK-activity: studies of congenic mice with B10 or AKR background, *J. Immunogenet.*, 7, 401, 1980.
17a. Clark, E. A. and Pollack, S. B., unpublished.
18. Reynolds, C. W. and Holden, H. T., Genetic variation in natural killer (NK) activity in the rat, in *NK Cells and Other Effector Cells*, Herberman, R. B., Ed., Academic Press, New York, 1982, 319.
19. Shellam, G. R. and Hogg, N., Gross-virus-induced lymphoma in the rat. IV. Cytotoxic cells in normal rats, *Int. J. Cancer*, 19, 212, 1977.
20. Petranyi, G., Kiessling, R., and Klein, G., Genetic control of "natural" killer lymphocytes in the mouse, *Immunogenetics*, 2, 53, 1975.
21. Petranyi, G. G., Kiessling, R., Povey, S., Klein, G., Herzenberg, L., and Wigzell, H., The genetic control of natural killer cell activity and its association with in vivo resistance against a Moloney lymphoma isograft, *Immunogenetics*, 3, 15, 1976.
22. Harmon, R. C., Clark, E. A., O'Toole, C., and Wicker, L. S., Resistance of H-2 heterozygous mice to parental tumors. I. Hybrid resistance and natural cytotoxicity to EL-4 are controlled by the H-2D-Hh-1 region, *Immunogenetics*, 4, 601, 1977.
23. Cudkowicz, G., Hybrid resistance to parental grafts of hematopoietic and lymphoma cells, in *The Proliferation and Spread of Neoplastic Cells*, Williams & Wilkins, Baltimore, 1968, 661.
24. Cudkowicz, G. and Bennett, M., Peculiar immunobiology of bone marrow allografts. II. Rejection of parental grafts by resistant F_1 hybrid mice, *J. Exp. Med.*, 134, 1513, 1971.
25. Lotzová, E., Hemopoietic histocompatibility: genetic and immunobiological aspects, *Compen. Immunol.*, 3, 468, 1983.
26. Nagy, Z. A., Baxevanix, C. N., Ishii, N., and Klein, J., Ia antigens as restriction molecules in Ir-gene controlled T-cell proliferation, *Immunol. Rev.*, 60, 59, 1981.
27. Hayes, C. E., Klyczek, K. K., Krum, D. P., Whitcomb, R. M., Hullet, D. A., and Cantor, H., Chromosome 4 *Jt* gene controls murine T cell surface I-J expression, *Science*, 223, 559, 1984.
28. Murphy, D. B., Genetic control of I-J determinants — a commentary, *J. Mol. Cell. Immunol.*, 1, 133, 1984.
29. Perussia, B., Fanning, V., and Trinchieri, G., A human NK and K cell subset shares with cytotoxic T cells expression of the antigen recognized by antibody OKT8, *J. Immunol.*, 131, 223, 1983.
30. Klein, G. O., NK-activity against YAC-1 is regulated by two H-2 associated genes, in *NK Cells and Other Natural Effector Cells*, Herberman, R. B., Ed., Academic Press, New York, 1982, 275.
31. Mitchison, N. A., The MHC: still a few loose ends, in *The Immune System Vol. 1*, Steinberg, C. M., and Lefkovits, I., Eds., S. Karger, Basel, 1981, 187.
32. Cudkowicz, G. and Nakamura, I., Genetics of the murine hemopoietic histocompatibility system: an overview, *Transplant. Proc.*, 15, 2058, 1983.
33. Snell, G. D., Recognition structures determined by the *H-2* complex, *Transplant. Proc.*, 8, 147, 1976.
34. Hansson, M. and Kiessling, R., Human fetal thymus and bone marrow cells contain cells for natural killer cells, *Eur. J. Immunol.*, 11, 8, 1981.
35. Stern, P., Gidlund, M., Örn, A., and Wigzell, H., Natural killer cells mediate lysis of embryonal carcinoma cells lacking MHC, *Nature*, 285, 341, 1980.
36. Trinchieri, G., and Santoli, D., Anti-viral activity induced by culturing lymphocytes with tumor-derived or virus-transformed cells, *J. Exp. Med.*, 147, 1314, 1978.

37. Hansson, M., Kiessling, R., Andersson, B., and Welsh, R. M., Effect of interferon and interferon inducers on the NK sensitivity of normal mouse thymocytes, *J. Immunol.*, 125, 2225, 1980.
37a. Kiessling, R., personal communication.
38. Primi, D., Lewis, G. K., Triglia, R., and Goodman, J. W., Rosette formation between murine lymphocytes and erythrocytes. A new locus in the *H-2* region, *J. Exp. Med.*, 149, 1349, 1979.
39. Sia, D. Y. and Parish, C. R., Anti-self receptors. II. Demonstration of *H-2L*-region-restricted receptors on subpopulations of peripheral T and B lymphocytes, *J. Immunol.*, 124, 2366, 1980.
40. Nakashima, C., Clark, E. A., Lake, P., Kato, N., Nagase, F., Mizoguchi, K., Isobe, K., and Saito, M., Evidence for the erythrocyte as the principal antigenic cell type that triggers primary IgM antibody responses to H-2D alloantigens, *Transplantation*, 35, 180, 1983.
41. Malave, I., Fuji, H., and Milgrom, F., Plaque assay with spleen cells forming alloantibodies to $H\text{-}2^a$ and $H\text{-}2^d$ specificities, *Transplantation*, 15, 499, 1973.
42. Flaherty, L. and Zimmerman, D., Surface mapping of mouse thymocytes, *Proc. Natl. Acad. Sci. U.S.A.*, 76, 1990, 1979.
43. Boyse, E. A., Old, L. J., and Stockert, E., An approach to the mapping of antigens on the cell surface, *Proc. Natl. Acad. Sci. U.S.A.*, 60, 886, 1968.
43a. Ledbetter, J. A., Tsu, T., and Clark, E. A., Covalent association between human thymus leukemia-like antigens and CO8 (Tp32) molecules, *J. Immunol.*, 134, 4250, 1985.
44. Reinherz, E. L., Meuer, S. C., and Schlossman, S. F., The delineation of antigen receptors on human T lymphocytes, *Immunol. Today*, 4, 5, 1983.
45. Brickell, P. M., Latchman, D. S., Murphy, D., Willison, K., and Rigby, P. W. J., Activation of a *Qa/T1a* class I major histocompatibility antigen gene is a general feature of oncogenesis in the mouse, *Nature*, 306, 756, 1983.
46. Gronberg, A., Cochran, A. J., Kärre, K., Klein, G., Klein, G. O., and Kiessling, R., Incidence and type of tumors induced by DMBA carcinogenesis in *H-2* congenic strians on a B10 background, *Int. J. Cancer*, 32, 247, 1983.
47. Kiessling, R. and Haller, O., Natural killer cells in the mouse, an alternative immune surveillance mechanism?, *Contemp. Top. Immunobiol.*, 8, 171, 1978.
48. Seaman, W. E., Gindhart, T. D., Greenspan, J. S., Blackman, M. A., and Talal, N., Natural killer cells, bone, and the bone marrow: studies in estrogen-treated mice and in congenitally osteopetrotic (mi/mi) mice, *J. Immunol.*, 122, 2541, 1979.
49. Clark, E. A., Shultz, L. D., and Pollack, S. B., Mutations in mice that influence natural killer (NK) cell activity, *Immunogenetics*, 12, 601, 1981.
50. Shultz, L. D., Sidman, C. L., and Unanuc, E. R., Immunologic dysfunction in motheaten mice: immunodeficiency, autoimmunity, and hyperimmunoglobulinemia in a short-lived mutant, in *Animal Models of Comparative and Development Aspects of Immunity and Disease*, Gershwin, M. R. and Cooper, E. L., Eds., Pergamon Press, Elmsford, N.Y., 1978, 260.
51. Shultz, L. D., Bailey, C. L., and Coman, D. R., Hematopoietic stem cell function in motheaten mice, *Exp. Hematol.*, 11, 667, 1983.
52. Shultz, L. D., Bailey, C. L., Carlson, G. A., Coman, D. R., Evans, R., and Outzen, H. C., Potential of viable motheaten mice for the growth of tumor xenografts, in *Immune-Deficient Animals*, Sordat, B., Ed., S. Karger, Basel, 1983, 224.
53. Semple, J. W. and Szewczuk, M. R., Enhanced natural killer (NK) cell activity and NK-sensitive thymic cells in murine muscular dystrophy, *Cell. Immunol.*, 82, 316, 1983.
54. Welsh, R. M., Natural killer cells and interferon, *CRC Crit. Rev. Immunol.*, 5(1), 55, 1984.
55. Kuribayashi, K., Gillis, S., Kern, D. E., and Henney, C. S., Murine NK cell cultures: effects of interleukin-2 and interferon on cell growth and cytotoxic reactivity, *J. Immunol.*, 126, 2321, 1981.
56. Clark, E. A. and Holly, R. D., Activation of natural killer (NK) cells in vivo with H-2 and non-H-2 alloantigens, *Immunogenetics*, 12, 221, 1981.
57. Minato, N., Reid, L., Cantor, H., Lengyel, P., and Bloom, B. R., Mode of regulation of natural killer cell activity by interferon, *J. Exp. Med.*, 152, 124, 1980.
58. Reynolds, C. W., Timonen, T. T., Holden, H. T., Hansen, C. T., and Herberman, R. B., Natural killer cell activity in the rat. Analysis of effector cell morphology and effects of interferon on natural killer cell function in the athymic (nude) rat, *Eur. J. Immunol.*, 12, 577, 1982.
59. Tai, A. and Warner, N. L., Analysis of recognition patterns of NK cells through use of varying combinations of mouse strains and tumor targets, in *Natural Cell-Mediated Immunity Against Tumors*, Herberman, R. B., Ed., Academic Press, New York, 1980, 257.
60. Prud'homme, G. J., Park, C. L., Fieser, T. M., Kofler, R., Dixon, F. J., and Theofilopoulos, A. N., Identification of a B cell differentiation factor(s) spontaneously produced by proliferating T cells in murine lupus strains of the *1pr/1pr* genotype, *J. Exp. Med.*, 157, 730, 1983.
61. Bray, G. A. and York, D. A., Hypothalamic and genetic obesity in experimental animals: an autonomic and endocrine hypothesis, *Physiol. Rev.*, 59, 719, 1979.

62. Cudkowicz, G. and Hochman, P. S., Do natural killer cells engage in regulated reactions against self to ensure homeostasis?, *Immunol. Rev.*, 44, 13, 1979.
63. Clark, E. A., Roths, J. B., Murphy, E. D., Ledbetter, J. A., and Clagett, J. A., The beige *(bg)* gene influences the development of autoimmune disease in SB/Le male mice, in *NK cells and Other Natural Effector Cells,* Herberman, R. B., Ed., Academic Press, New York, 1982, 301.
63a. Clark, E. A., Draves, K., and Torres, R., Influence of beige gene on autoantibody development and lymphocyte subsets in SB/Le mice, submitted.
64. Roder, J. C., Lohmann-Matthes, M. -L., Domzig, W., and Wigzell, H., The beige mutation in the mouse. II. Selectively of the natural killer (NK) cell defect, *J. Immunol.*, 123, 2174, 1979.
65. Saxena, R. K., Saxena, Q. B., and Adler, W. H., Defective T-cell response in beige mutant mice, *Nature,* 295, 240, 1982.
66. Silvers, W. K., *The Coat Colors of Mice,* Springer-Verlag, New York, 1979.
67. Murphy, E. D. and Roths, J. B., A Y-chromosome associated factor producing accelerated autoimmunity and lymphoproliferation in strain BXSB, *Arthritis Rheum.*, 22, 1188, 1979.
68. Beeighbour, P. A., Reinitz, E., Grayzel, A. I., Miller, A. E., and Bloom, B. R., Studies of human NK cell function in chronic diseases, in *NK Cells and Other Natural Effector Cells,* Herberman, R. B., Ed., Academic Press, New York, 1982, 1241.
69. Merrill, J., Jondal, M., Seeley, J., Ullber, M., and Siden, A., Decreased NK killing in patients with multiple sclerosis: an analysis on the level of the single effector cell in peripheral blood and cerebrospinal fluid in relation to the activity of the disease, *Clin. Exp. Immunol.*, 47, 419, 1982.
70. Welsh, R. M., Jr. and Kiessling, R. W., Natural killer cell response to lymphocytic chorio meningitis virus in beige mice, *Scand. J. Immunol.*, 11, 363, 1980.
71. Örn, A., Hakansson, E. M., Gidlund, M., Ramstedt, U., Axberg, I., Wigzell, H., and Lundin, L.-G., Pigment mutations which also affect lysosomal functions lead to suppressed NK activity, *Scand. J. Immunol.*, 15, 305, 1982.
72. Haliotis, T., Roder, J., Klein, M., Ortaldo, J., Fauci, A. S. and Herberman, R. B., Chediak-Higashi gene in humans. I. Impairment of Natural-Killer function, *J. Exp. Med.*, 151, 1039, 1980.
73. Koren, H. S., Amos, D. B., and Buckley, R. H., Natural killing in immunodeficient patients, *J. Immunol.*, 20, 796, 1978.
74. Sullivan, J. L., Byron, K. S., Brewster, F. E., and Purtilo, D. T., Deficient natural killer activity in X-linked lymphoproliferative syndrome, *Science,* 210, 543, 1980.
75. Seeley, J. K., Bechtold, T., Purtillo, D. T., and Lindsten, T., NK deficiency in X-linked lymphoproliferative syndrome, in *NK Cells and Other Natural Effector Cells,* Herberman, R. B., Ed., Academic Press, New York, 1982, 1211.
76. Peter, H. H., Friedrich, W., Dopfer, R., Muller, W., Kortmann, C., Pichler, W. J., Heinz, F., and Rieger, C. H. L., NK cell function in severe combined immunodeficiency (SCID): evidence of a common T and NK cell defect in some but not all SCID patients, *J. Immunol.*, 131, 2332, 1983.
77. Stutman, O. and Cuttito, M. J., in, *Natural Cell-Mediated Immunity Against Tumors,* Herberman, R. B., Ed., Academic Press, New York, 1980, 187.
78. Stutman, O. and Cuttito, M. J., Genetic control of NC activity in the mouse: three genes located on Chromosome 17, in *NK Cells and Other Natural Effector Cells,* Herberman, R. B., Ed., Academic Press, New York, 1982, 281.
79. Stutman, O. and Cuttito, M. J., Normal levels of natural cytotoxic cells against solid tumors in NK-deficient beige mice, *Nature,* 290, 254, 1981.
79a. Stutman, O., personal communication.
80. McNeilage, L. J., Heslop, B. F., Heyworth, M. R., and Gutman, G. A., Natural cytotoxicity in rats: strain distribution and genetics, *Cell. Immunol.*, 72, 340, 1982.
81. Nakamura, I. and Cudkowicz, G., Fine specificity of auto- and alloreactive cytotoxic T-lymphocytes: heteroclitic cross-reactions between mutant and original H-2 antigens, *Curr. Top. Micro. Immunol.*, 99, 51, 1982.
82. Kaminsky, S. G., Nakamura, I., and Cudkowicz, G., Selective defect of natural killer and killer cell activity against lymphomas in SJL mice: low responsiveness to interferon inducers, *J. Immunol.*, 130, 1980, 1983.
83. Ricardi, C., Santoni, A., Barlozzari, T., Cesarini, C., and Herberman, R. B., Suppression of natural killer (NK) activity by splenic adherent cells of low NK-reactive mice, *Int. J. Cancer,* 28, 811, 1981.
84. Schröder, J., Nikinmaa, B., Kavathas, P., and Herzenberg, L. A., Fluorescence-activated cell sorting of mouse-human hybrid cells aids in locating the gene for the Leu 7 (HNK-1) antigen to human chromosome 11, *Proc. Natl. Acad. Sci. U.S.A.*, 80, 3421, 1983.
85. Trent, J. M., Olson, S., and Lawn, R. M., Chromosomal localization of human leukocyte, fibroblast, and immune interferon genes by means of *in situ* hybridization, *Proc. Natl. Acad. Sci. U.S.A.*, 79, 7809, 1982.

86. Dubey, D. P., Staunton, D. E., Smith, B. L., Yunis, E. J., and Sager, R., Lysis of Chinese hamster embryo fibroblast mutants by human natural cytotoxic (NK) cells, *Proc. Natl. Acad. Sci. U.S.A.*, 80, 7303, 1983.
87. Durdik, J. M., Beck, B. N., Clark, E. A., and Henney, C. S., Characterization of a lymphoma cell variant selectively resistant to natural killer cells, *J. Immunol.*, 125, 683, 1980.
88. Roder, J. C., Beaumont, T. J., Kerbel, R. S., Haliotis, T., and Kozbor, D., Selective natural killer resistance in a clone of YAC lymphoma cells, *Proc. Natl. Acad. Sci. U.S.A.*, 78, 6396, 1981.
89. Kimber, I., Moore, M., and Roberts, K., Variance in resistance to natural and antibody-dependent cellular cytotoxicity and to complement-mediated lysis among K562 lines, *Int. J. Cancer*, 32, 219, 1983.
90. Wright, S. C. and Bonavida, B., YAC-1 variant clones selected for resistance to natural killer cytotoxic factors are also resistant to natural killer cell-mediated cytotoxicity, *Proc. Natl. Acad. Sci. U.S.A.*, 80, 1688, 1983.
91. Gronberg, A., Kiessling, R., Eriksson, E., and Hansson, M., Variants from an MLV-induced lymphoma selected for decreased sensitivity to NK lysis, *J. Immunol.*, 127, 1734, 1981.
92. Wayner, E. A. and Brooks, C. G., Induction of NKCF-like activity in mixed lymphocyte-tumor cell culture: direct involvement of mycoplasma infection of tumor cells, *J. Immunol.*, 132, 2135, 1984.

Chapter 7

PHENOTYPE, FUNCTIONAL HETEROGENEITY, AND LINEAGE OF NATURAL KILLER CELLS

Sylvia B. Pollack*

TABLE OF CONTENTS

* Supported by USPHS Grant CA-32553 from the National Institutes of Health and DOE Contract 225 (AT 06-79EV10270).

I. INTRODUCTION

Natural killer (NK) cells are functionally defined as white blood cells with the ability to recognize and lyse certain normal and malignant cell types in the absence of any overt immunization. Although other leukocytes such as neutrophils and monocytes can express "natural" (i.e., nonimmune) cytotoxicity, NK cells appear to be a distinct population of cells with lymphoid morphology that contain, at least in humans, characteristic large, azurophilic granules. In this chapter three interrelated aspects of NK cells will be considered — phenotypic characterisitcs, functional heterogeneity, and possible lineage(s). Since the mid-1970s when NK cells were first recognized to be different from classical cytotoxic cells, intensive efforts have been made to characterize the effector cell type or types. Despite these efforts, no single definition of NK cells has emerged, i.e., NK cells are phenotypically and functionally heterogeneous.

Studies with antibody directed to cell surface components have indicated a strong association of T cell markers with NK cells. However, markers associated with other cell types (macrophages or granulocytes) are also present on some NK cells. One marker that seems to be present on most, if not all, human NK cells is the Fc receptor (FcR) for immunoglobulins, although the FcR is not involved in the functional activity of NK cells.

In addition to the heterogeneity of surface markers associated with NK cells, it has also become apparent that NK are heterogeneous with respect to target cell preference. Populations of NK cells that have specificity for certain prototype targets such as the YAC-1 murine lymphoma line or the K562 myeloid human line are not necessarily the same effector cells that lyse other targets such as bone marrow cells, thymocytes, or herpes virus-infected fibroblasts. However, when we consider that the main role of NK cells may be to control differentiation of hemopoietic and other rapidly proliferating cells, diversity and redundancy may be desirable features of this homeostatic system. The multiplicity of roles for naturally cytotoxic cells (reviewed elsewhere in this book) may require that different cell types have NK activity. Indeed, as will be discussed below, it may be that cells of several lineages are able to function as NK cells.

A variety of techniques have been used in the studies reviewed here. Phenotypic characterization of NK cells has been done by depletion of effector cells with antibody and complement or by monolayer absorption (panning), or by enrichment for NK cells by panning, or with the fluorescence activated cell sorter (FACS). Functional heterogeneity has been demonstrated in studies using panels of target cells and in cold target inhibition studies. Genetic models, which are considered elsewhere in this volume, as well as studies on natural cytotoxicity to bone marrow transplants, virus-infected targets, and the activity of cloned lines of NK cells are outside the scope of this chapter, but are also relevant to the questions of heterogeneity of NK cells.

II. PHENOTYPE OF NK CELLS

Data on murine NK cells will be considered first and then that on human NK cells. It will become apparent that there are differences between endogenous, or unstimulated, NK cells and those which have been stimulated or activated in some manner. We will focus first on endogenous NK cells.

A. Murine

Murine NK cells were originally described by Herberman et al.[1] and Kiessling et al.[2] in 1975. Both groups reported that cells with natural cytotoxic activity were negative for the expression of FcR and for the T cell-associated marker Thy-1. Both of these conclusions were modified with subsequent analysis. It was found that FcR are present on some but not all murine NK cells.[3] These FcR appear to be of relatively low avidity. Mattes et al.[4] found that Thy-1 is expressed on some NK cells, although in lower amounts than on T cells. This was demonstrated by two approaches: (1) by depletion of Thy-1-bearing cells with two rounds of lysis with Thy-1.2 antibody and complement and (2) by selection of Thy-1$^+$ cells with the FACS. NK activity measured as the ability to lyse YAC-1 targets was found in both Thy-1$^+$ and Thy-1$^-$ subpopulations.

Other T cell-associated antigens have also been detected on murine NK cells. We evaluated the expression of T cell-associated antigens on NK cells of C57BL/6 mice by cytotoxic depletion experiments with alloantisera prepared against the Thy-1, Lyt-1, Lyt-2, and Ly 5 antigens.[5] In these experiments we found that NK activity to the YAC-1 target was not affected by antisera to the Thy-1, Lyt-1, or Lyt-2 antigens, but was depleted with anti-Ly-5 and C, confirming the reports of Cantor et al.[6] and Kasai et al.[7] that NK cells are Ly-5$^+$. This antigen, however, is expressed on most lymphohemopoietic cells.[8] Koo et al.,[9] using a protein A binding assay, also detected the presence of Lyt-1 on a subpopulation of NK cells.

A more quantitative estimate of the expression of various cell surface markers on murine NK cells was achieved by using the technique of target cell binding.[10] B cell-depleted spleen cells were labeled with various antisera and fluorescent antimouse immunoglobulin, allowed to react with YAC-1 target cells, and the resulting cell conjugates and free cells examined under the fluorescence microscope. These studies showed that lymphocytes which bound to YAC-1 were negative for Lyt-1 and Lyt-2. Approximately 60% of the cells were positive for Thy-1, 77% for Qa-4, 79% for Qa-5, and 94% for Ly-5. These authors concluded that the best phenotypic distinction between murine NK cells and cytotoxic T lymphocytes (CTL) was based on the presence of Qa-4 and FcR for IgG2b. Both of these markers are present on NK cells, but absent from CTL. In cytotoxic depletion experiments with monoclonal antibodies (MoAb), Seaman et al.[11] confirmed that NK cells express the T200 antigen (Ly-5) but lacked detectable Lyt-1 or ThB, an antigen found on thymocytes and peripheral B cells but not mature T cells.[12]

In addition to T cell-associated antigens, a number of NK-specific or NK-associated antigens have been reported. The first of these was the NK 1.1 antigen described by Glimcher et al.[13] This alloantigen was originally detected as a contaminant in conventionally produced Lyt-1 alloantiserum. By immunizing (BALB/c × C3H)F_1 hybrid mice with CE/J spleen cells, an antiserum was obtained that lacked activity to Lyt-1 but had specific activity for NK cells. NK 1.1 antiserum and complement does not deplete CTL activity. We used NK 1.1 antiserum to positively select for NK cells with the fluorescence activated cell sorter and were able to recover all of the NK activity in the NK 1.1$^+$ population, whereas the NK 1.1$^-$ population was devoid of activity.[14] This antiserum will also deplete NK activity in vivo.[15] NK 1.1 currently appears to be the most specific of the available alloantisera for murine NK cells, although other antisera have been developed. Despite numerous attempts to produce monoclonal anti-NK 1.1 antibodies, stable lines have not been produced to date.

Burton and Winn[16] prepared an antisera that depleted NK activity by immunizing CE mice with C3H spleen cells. This antiserum was originally designated as NK 1.2. However, subsequent analyses revealed that the activity was to an antigen that segregates independently from NK 1.[17] We had detected a similar activity in our studies using antisera from NZB mice immunized with BALB/c spleen cells and designated the alloantigen NK 2.1.[18] The strain distribution of NK-2.1 is very similar to that found with the anti-"NK 1.2" sera.[18] Thus, we suggest that the designation NK-1 be reserved for the antigens detected with (C3H × BALB/c) anti-CE sera and that the antisera called NK-1.2 or NK-2.1 be simply called NK-2 until further analyzed. That convention will be used in this chapter.

Seaman et al.[11] produced two MoAb to cell surface antigens expressed on murine NK cells by immunization of rats with mouse spleen and thymus membranes. The antigens recognized by the MoAb H11 and 7.2 are also expressed on T cells. Meruelo et al.[19] have described another NK-associated antigen, Ly-11.2, detected with the allo-antisera (A.AL × BALB.B)F_1 anti-B10.A(4R). Ly-11.2 appears to be present on cells that are susceptible to oncogenic viruses.

Another NK-associated antigen is the neutral glycolipid asialo GM1. Young et al.[20] and Kasai et al.[21] demonstrated the presence of this antigen on murine NK cells using rabbit antiasialo GM1 serum and complement in cytotoxic depletion experiments. However, the expression of asialo GM1 is not limited to NK cells: it is also expressed on some T cells including the precursors of cytotoxic cells and IL-2-producing (helper T ?) cells.

Cloned lines or cultured murine NK cell lines generally express both T cell-associated antigens and NK-associated antigens. NK clones are discussed in detail in Chapter 9, Volume II and will be mentioned only briefly here. It should be noted that such stimulated lines often express a greater number and/or higher density of antigens than do endogenous NK cells. Dennert et al.[23] reported that their cloned NK lines were positive for Thy-1.2, T200, asialo GM1, and asialo GM2. The lines were negative for Lyt-1 and Lyt-2. Kuribayashi et al.[24] cultured Thy-1-depleted spleen cells from poly-I:C-stimulated mice in IL-2. The cells expressed NK activity and were positive for Thy-1 and asialo GM1, but were negative for Lyt-2. However, there is a great deal of heterogeneity among cloned NK lines. Brooks et al.[25] described five cloned NK lines that were positive for asialo GM1, Qa-5, and NK 2 and were negative for Mac-1, a macrophage differentiation antigen; two of the lines were also positive for Lyt-2. The activity of all lines was blocked by anti-Ly-5. Although greater than 90% of IL-2 cultured NK cells were positive for the expression of Thy-1.2 as detected by immunofluorescence, these cells were resistant to lysis with Thy-1 and complement.[26] In addition, these cultured NK cells were negative for the expression of surface Ig and FcR. A cloned NK line described by Galli et al.[27] had receptors for IgE. These cells were morphologically more similar to basophils than to lymphocytes.

Another type of naturally cytotoxic cell, termed the NC cell, has been described by Paige et al.[28] and Stutman and colleagues.[29] NC cells differ from NK cells most notably in their preference for different targets (discussed below), in their ontogeny, and in their expression of cell surface antigens. NC cells do not express Thy-1, Lyt-1, Lyt-2, NK 1, asialo GM1, Qa-1, Qa-4, Qa-5, surface Ig, or FcR. The results with Qa-2 and Qa-3 have been somewhat equivocal. A summary of the phenotypic characteristics of NK cells, activated or cultured NK cells, and NC cells is given in Table 1.

B. Human

Analysis of the phenotype of human NK cells has paralleled that of murine cells with a few notable differences. From the earliest report by Jondal and Pross[30] in 1975, it has been consistently demonstrated that human NK cells have FcR. This observation was confirmed by Bakas et al.,[31] Cooper et al.,[32] Kay et al.,[33] West et al.,[34] and Bolhuis.[35] With further study, however, it became apparent that not all FcR-positive cells mediate NK. Indeed, NK activity seemed to be mediated mostly by T gamma cells, i.e., T cells with receptors for IgG.[36] However, even this was not an absolute categorization. Jondal and Merrill,[37] using the single cell binding assay, found that (1) 55% of target-binding cells had FcR for IgG ($Fc_\gamma R$). These cells were responsible for 60% of the total killing observed; (2) 24% of target-binding cells had FcR for IgM ($Fc_\mu R$). These cells were responsible for 17% of the total killing. It is of interest that cells with the Fc_γ receptor also include cytotoxic and suppressor T cells and K cells that mediate ADCC. Although there was originally some thought that human NK cells expressed receptors for C3,[38] this has now been shown to not be the case.[39]

Table 1
COMPARISON OF PHENOTYPIC MARKERS ON ENDOGENOUS NK, ACTIVATED, OR CULTURED NK AND NC CELLS

Antigen/marker	Endogenous NK	Activated/cultured NK	NC
Thy-1	+/−	+	−
Lyt-1	−	−	−
Lyt-2	−	−/+	−
Ly-5 (T200c/)	+	+	N.D.
Qa4	+	N.D.	−
Qa5	+	+	−
NK-1	+	+	−
NK-2	+	+/−	−
LY-11	+	N.D.	−
FcR	+/−	?	−
Asialo GM1	+	+	+/−
Mac-1	+	+	?

Note: N.D. = not determined.

It is abundantly clear that human NK cells bear a number of T cell-associated antigens, including the E receptor (the receptor for sheep erythrocytes,[40,41]) and some T cell-associated antigens detected with MoAb of the OKT and Leu series. Zarling and Kung[42] studied the expression of OKT3 (a pan-T cell marker), OKT4 (helper T), OKT8 (suppressor/cytotoxic T), and OKM1 (macrophage) on NK cells by cytotoxic depletion and found that only anti-OKM1 caused a significant decrease in cytotoxic activity. These results were extended in experiments using the large granular lymphocyte (LGL) fraction of human peripheral blood lymphocytes (PBL).[43] Although expression of the different markers varied among subpopulations of NK (LGL) cells, at least some of the cells were positive for OKT8, OKT10, and Lyt-3, whereas no reactivity was detected with OKT3, OKT4, OKT6 (a thymocyte marker), or OKT11 (an E receptor marker). Three other MoAb to human T lymphocytes were tested in cytotoxic depletion experiments by Fast et al.[44] Antigen 9.3 was present on CTL but absent from NK cells. Antigen 10.2 was also present on CTL and on about one half the NK cells. In contrast, antigen 9.6 (the E receptor) was found on all NK cells. However, when human PBL were first separated into E rosette-positive (E^+) and E rosette-negative (E^-) subpopulations, NK activity was found in both the E^-, $OKM1^+$, $OKT3^-$, and the E^+, $OKM1^-$, $OKT3^-$ fractions.[45] Thus both "non-T" and "T" type NK cells can be defined. Similarly, Perussia et al.[46] found that 30 to 50% of human NK cells were $OKT8^+$. The expression of this T cell antigen was at a lower density than on cytotoxic T cells, however.

Recently several MoAb have been described which react more or less specifically with human NK cells. Abo and Balch[47] raised a monoclonal IgM antibody to a membrane antigen from the cultured T cell line HSB-2. The antigen-detected, designated HNK-1 (Leu-7), was present on 15% of normal blood lymphocytes. $HNK\text{-}1^+$ cells separated with the FACS were nonadherent, surface Ig^-, and included both E rosetting and E nonrosetting cells. Most $HNK\text{-}1^+$ cells expressed the Fc_γ receptor. Some, but not all, $Leu\text{-}7^+$ cells in germinal centers of lymph nodes also express DR antigens.[48] Another MoAb to human NK cells, designated B73.1, was prepared by Perussia et al.[49,50] B73.1, which recognizes the FcR, reacts with about 15% of the lymphocytes in human peripheral blood. The $B73.1^+$ subset does not bear the markers typical of mature T or B cells. $B73.1^+$ subset does not bear the markers typical of mature T or B cells. B73.1

also reacts with neutrophils. Another antibody which detects FcR and reacts with essentially all NK cells that lyse K562 is Leu-11a (NKP-15).[51] Extensive analyses of the coexpression of Leu-11a, Leu-7 (HNK-1), and a series of T cell-associated antigens by Lanier et al.[52] revealed that expression of Leu-11a and of the T cell antigens Leu-1 (pan T and a B cell subset), Leu-4 (pan T), and Leu-3a (helper T) was mutually exclusive. However, a subset of Leu-11a$^+$ cells that also expressed a low concentration of Leu-2a (associated with cytotoxic/suppressor T cells) was detected. In contrast, Leu-7 was often coexpressed with Leu-1 and Leu-4 and 40% of Leu-7$^+$ cells were also Leu-2a$^+$. In studies on the functional activity of the Leu-7$^{+/-}$ Leu-11$^{+/-}$ subsets, the Leu-11a$^+$, 7$^-$ cells were found to have the most activity, whereas the Leu-11a$^-$, 7$^+$ cells were only weakly lytic. Thus antibodies that detect NK-associated FcR, e.g., Leu-11a and B73.1 appear to be the most specific reagents currently available for human NK cells. These antibodies do not block NK function, however, indicating that the FcR are not involved in binding or lysis of targets.

Several anti-NK antibodies have been prepared by immunizing mice with human lymphocytes enriched for NK cells by density centrifugation on Percoll to obtain the LGL fraction. One of these is the 13.1 antibody described by Newman.[53] This antibody is very similar, both in its preparation and reactivity, to the NK 8 antibody described by Nieminen et al.[54] Both are of the IgG1 subclass. Whereas the 13.1 antigen is found on all peripheral blood mononuclear cells, the NK8 antigen is detected on 33% of peripheral blood LGL cells but not on monocytes, granulocytes, or other lymphocytes. Rumpold et al.[55] have described a monoclonal IgM antibody (VEP13) which was also raised by immunizing mice with cells enriched for LGL. With fluorescence, VEP13 reacts with 21% of PBL and more than 90% of the granulocytes, but not with B cells, monocytes, erythrocytes, platelets, thymocytes, or immature bone marrow cells. Treatment of human peripheral blood with VEP13 and complement reduced the NK activity against a variety of susceptible target cells. In coexpression studies it was found that 85% of VEP13$^+$ cells also expressed M1, 82% expressed T10, 48% expressed Leu-2a, 2% expressed human Lyt-3, and 6% were positive for HLA-DR antigens. Leu-1, Leu-3A, and T6 were not detected on VEP13$^+$ cells. Several other antibodies that react with human NK cells have been prepared by immunizing with either cytotoxic T lymphocytes[56] or with Con A activated blast cells.[57,58]

Ault and Springer[59] reported that the Mac-1 antigen, which is detected with a rat MoAb directed against murine macrophages and granulocytes, was expressed on human NK cells as well as on neutrophils and monocytes. Numerous reports have confirmed the presence of OKM1 on a subset of NK cells (e.g., see Reference 60 and discussion below). Other antigens that have been detected on human NK cells include β-2-microglobulin[61] and a B cell antigen.[62] As mentioned above, HLA-DR or DS (Ia) antigens have also been detected on some NK cells, e.g., see Reference 43.

By 1979, the difference between fresh human NK cells and cultured cells was already appreciated.[63] Both fresh and cultured cells showed NK activity in the E receptor-negative populations, but fresh NK cells were also highly active in the E receptor-positive population, whereas cultured E$^+$ cells were only weakly active. Both fresh and cultured cells expressed FcR and were sensitive to treatment with anti-T cell serum and complement. Fresh NK cells were unaffected by treatment with anti-Ia-like serum and complement while cultured effector cells were somewhat diminished in treatment, indicating that at least some cultured cells were Ia$^+$. Krensky et al.,[64] however, found that human cell lines maintained in vitro that had NK activity against K562 and lymphoblastoid targets possessed the sheep red blood cell (SRBC) receptor but lacked other T cell markers such as Lyt-3 and OKT3. Natural killer activity correlated with the presence of Mac-1 on cells in these long-term lines. Hercend et al.[65] studied a panel of cloned NK cell lines and found that each line had a unique phenotype. HNK-1 was present on only 1 of 8 lines tested. The expression of OKT1, T4, T3, T8, T11, T12, and Mo1 were also evaluated. The heterogeneity and expression of T cell- and macrophage-associated antigens was reflected in heterogeneity of target cell preference as will be discussed below. Some cloned T cell lines have also been shown to exhibit NK-like activity.[66] These cloned T cell lines expressed Leu-1, a pan T antigen, and Leu-2, a marker of suppressive/cytotoxic T cells.

Cells with NK-like activity have also been generated in human mixed lymphocyte cultures (MLC). This cytotoxicity to NK-sensitive targets has been termed anomolous killing or AK[67] or simply NK-like killing. Zarling and Kung[42] reported that endogenous NK, poly-I:C-activated NK or MLC-activated NK-like cells were not affected by treatment with OKT3 or OKT8 MoAb and complement, whereas both of these antibodies depleted cytotoxic T lymphocyte activity. OKM1 MoAb and C reduced endogenous NK and poly-I:C activated NK activity. The NK-like activity is found in both the blast population and the small-medium lymphocyte fraction.[68] After expansion of the blast cell populations in IL-2, it was found that cells with NK-like activity were insensitive to treatment with either OKT4 or OKT8 and complement. A cloned human NK line derived from a 6-day MLC by Kornbluth et al.[69] reacted with MoAb 9.6, which recognizes the E receptor, and with monoclonal 3A1, which also reacts with thymocytes and E rosette-forming cells. The line was also positive for OKT10, 7.2, HLA-DR determinants, and T200, the leukocyte common antigen analogous to Ly5 in the mouse. The line was negative for Leu-1, Leu-4, OKT3, Leu-2a, OKT8, Leu-3a, OKT4, and HNK-1 (Leu-7). Observations on the phenotypes of cultured or cloned human NK cells and their comparison with endogenous NK are summarized in Table 2.

C. Other

Although the vast majority of studies on the phenotype of NK cells have been done with either murine or human cells, several other species have been examined. Rat NK cells have FcR for IgG[70] and are resistant to treatment with C and anti-T cell serum or anti-Ig.[71] Reynolds et al.[72] have characterized the LGL fraction of rat spleen and found that essentially all of the cells with NK activity expressed the T cell-associated antigens W3/W13, OX8, and asialo GM1, as well as the leukocyte antigen C-C. A few of these rat LGL expressed Ia, surface immunoglobulin, Thy-1, or W3/25. Guinea pig NK cells have been characterized only to the extent to say that they are FcR-positive nonadherent cells.[73,74] Chicken NK cells have been reported to be resistant to both anti-T and anti-B cell serum.[75]

III. FUNCTIONAL HETEROGENEITY

It is readily apparent from the data presented above that there is a great deal of phenotypic heterogeneity among NK cells. The functions ascribed to NK cells have been as diverse as the phenotypic markers. Many of these aspects of heterogeneity of function are dealt with in other chapters in this book, i.e., the role of NK cells in the response to tumors, bone marrow grafts, hybrid resistance, antiviral responses, and graft-vs.-host reactions. Here we will concentrate on heterogeneity detected by using different targets and/or different phenotypic markers, mainly in in vitro assays. These observations have important implications for the function of NK cells, their lineage, and regulation.

A. Murine

One of the first indications of heterogeneity among murine naturally cytotoxic cells came from the work of Stutman et al.,[76] who reported that NC cells which lyse methylcholanthrene-induced fibrosarcoma targets differed from the NK cells which lyse YAC-1 and other lymphomas. NC cells are present at birth and activity does not de-

Table 2
EXPRESSION OF CELL SURFACE MARKERS ON HUMAN NK CELLS: COMPARISON OF ENDOGENOUS, ACTIVATED, AND CELL LINE (CLONED) NK[a]

Marker	Endogenous[b]		Activated[b]		Cloned[b]	
FcR	+		+			
Leu-11a	+	(51,52)				
B73.1	+	(49,50)				
3G8	+					
E Receptor	+	(40)				
Lyt-3	−/+	(42,55,86)			−	(64)
OKT11a	+/−	(41,43)				
9.6	+	(44)				
Pan-T						
Leu-1	−	(52,55)			−/+	(66,69)
Leu-4	−	(52)			−	(69)
OKT3	−	(42,43,45)	−	(42)	−	(64,69)
3A1	+	(113)			+	(66)
10.2	±	(44)				
Helper T						
OKT4	−	(42,43)			−	(68,69)
Leu-3a	−	(52,55)			−	(69)
9.3	−	(44)				
Suppressor/cytotoxic T						
OKT8	+/−	(42,43,46)	−	(42)	−	(68,69)
Leu-2a	+	(52,55)			+/−	(66,69)
Thymocyte						
OKT6	−	(43,55)				
OKT10	+	(43,55)			+	(66)
Macrophage/monocyte						
OKM1	+	(42,45,55,60)	+	(42)		
Mac-1	+	(59)	+	(64)		
NK						
Leu-7 (HNK-1)	+	(47)				
13.1 (T200)	+	(53)				
NK-8	+	(54)				
Other						
Leu-10 (HLA-Dc/DS)	+	(43)				
OK11 (Ia)			+	(63)		
VEP10 (Ia)	+					
VEP13	+	(55)				
7.2 (Ia)					+	(69)

[a] Cell surface markers are listed as +/− or −/+ when there have been both positive and negative reprots, whereas ± indicates low level of expression.
[b] Numbers in parentheses indicate References.

crease with age, in contrast to conventional NK cell activity, which does not appear until 4 weeks of age and which decreases after 10 to 11 weeks of age. NC cells also appear to be under different genetic regulation than NK cells. NC activity is present in beige mice, whereas NK activity is low or absent. Similarly, NC activity is present in SJL mice while NK activity is low. As mentioned above, there are also phenotypic differences between NC and NK cells, the most notable being the presence of Qa4, Qa5, NK 1, and NK 2 on NK cells, and their absence from NC cells. NC cells are also resistant to treatment with Ly-11.2 and asialo GM1 and complement, whereas NK cells are susceptible to both.[77] The original distinction that NC cells lyse solid tumor targets while NK cells lyse lymphoid targets has not turned out to be absolute. Indeed, it is now clear that cells of solid tumors can be lysed by both NK and NC cells. On the basis of the differential sensitivity of NK and NC cells to lysis with Qa5 and complement, Lattime et al.[78] separated target cells into 3 groups: (1) an NK-sensitive group of target cells which were sensitive to $Qa5^+$ NK effector cells, (2) NC-sensitive cells which are lysed by $Qa5^-$ effector cells that are not augmented in activity by poly I:C, and (3) a group of NC- and NK-susceptible targets which are lysed by both $Qa5^+$ and $Qa5^-$ effectors.

We[79] have detected heterogeneity among NK cells using the two alloantisera NK 1.1 and NK 2.1. Nylon wool-nonadherent C57BL/6 spleen cells were treated with complement and either NK 1.1 or NK 2.1 antisera and tested for NK activity against a panel of tumor targets in 6 and 19 hr ^{51}chromium (^{51}Cr)-release assays. Both antisera were effective in depleting NK activity to the murine lymphoma targets YAC-1, RBL-5, and L5178C127v, against the melanoma B16 and against the Chang human polyploid liver line. However, NK activity to the lymphona FBL-3 and the human erythroleukemia K562 were significantly reduced by treatment with NK 2.1 and complement but not by treatment with NK 1.1. In each case, similar patterns of NK activity were observed at both the 6 and 19 hr time points, suggesting that the effector cells were NK, since NC activity is not detectable in short-term, 4 to 6 hr assays.

Several different classification schemes for murine NK cells have been set forth on the basis of differences in target cell preference, the effects of ^{89}Sr, and the presence of phenotypic markers. Kumar et al.[80] found that in vivo treatment of mice with the bone marrow-seeking isotope ^{89}strontium (^{89}Sr) ablated NK activity against YAC-1. However, NK activity to another lymphoma target, EL-4, was not affected, suggesting that NK cells can be divided into bone marrow-dependent and bone marrow-independent subpopulations. These results were extended by Lust et al.,[81] who demonstrated that the population of NK cells that were insensitive to ^{89}Sr (which they term NK_B) were unaffected by the beige mutation and were not lysed by NK 2 antiserum and complement. Although these NK_B cells seemed to preferentially lyse nonlymphoma targets, they did lyse several lymphoma targets, notably EL-4 and FLD-3. Our results comparing susceptibility to NK 1 vs. NK 2 antisera suggest that murine NK cells which lyse K562 and FBL-3 are in the NK_B category. The other group of NK cells defined by Lust et al. (NK_A) were sensitive to ^{89}Sr, were reduced in mice bearing the beige mutation, and were susceptible to treatment with NK 2 plus C.

Minato and colleagues[82] categorized murine NK cells into four subgroups based on the expression of the T cell-associated antigens, Thy-1, Lyt-2, Qa-5, and Ly-5, and the responses of these subgroups to interferon (IFN) and interleukin 2 (IL-2). A subpopulation of cells that had the Thy-1^-, Lyt-2^-, Qa-5^+, Ly-5^+ phenotype and that were regulated by IFN but not by IL-2 corresponded most closely to the classic NK cells that lyse YAC-1. A second subgroup, with a Thy-1^+, Lyt-2^-, Qa-5^+, Ly-5^+ phenotype, also lysed YAC-1 but could be regulated by both IFN and IL-2. NK_A cells have properties of both these two subgroups described by Minato et al.[82] A third subgroup had the typical phenotype of CTL (Thy-1^+, Lyt-2^+, Qa-5^-, Ly-5^+) and did not spontaneously lyse YAC-1. This population was regulated by IL-2 but not IFN. A fourth subgroup was positive for only the Ly-5 antigen of the four tested and was present predominantly in the bone marrow. This group of cells lysed YAC-1 but was not regulated by either IFN or IL-2. Both the third and fourth subgroups were present in beige mutant mice, whereas the first two were absent. The distinction between NK_A cells and NK_B cells was further explored in experiments by Burton et al.[83] NK_A cells were susceptible to treatment with anti-NK-2 antibody and complement, whereas lytic activity for nonlymphoma targets was not affected.

These studies on heterogeneity of murine NC cells are summarized in Table 3. It is apparent that there are two broad subpopulations: the "conventional" NK cells and

Table 3
HETEROGENEITY OF MURINE NATURALLY CYTOTOXIC CELLS

	Thy-1	Lyt-2	Qa5	Ly-5	NK-1/2	bg	Regulated by IFN	Regulated by IL-2	Sensitivity to ^{89}Sr	Prototype target	Refs.
NK	+/−	−	+	+	+	$\downarrow$	+	+	+	YAC-1	1—10,80
NK_A	+/−				+				+	YAC-1 EL-4	81
NK_I	−	−	+	+		$\downarrow$	+	−		YAC-1	82
NK_T	+	−	+	+		$\downarrow$	+	+		YAC-1	82
NC	−	−	−	+	−	=	−			METH A WEHI 164	76,77
NK_B	−				−/+	=			−	FLD-3	81
NK_M	−	−	−	+		=	−	−			82

NC cells. However, there is heterogeneity within these populations, and other populations have been described which do not fit precisely into either the NK or NC category. Studies with cloned lines of NK cells reviewed in Chapter 9, Volume II lend further support to the heterogeneity of phenotype and function among NK cells.

B. Human

Similar heterogeneity has been detected among human effector cells for natural cytotoxicity, both with regard to target cell preference and to phenotypic markers. Immunoabsorption of human PBL on monolayers of the NK-sensitive targets K562 or HSB revealed target cell preference among the NK cells.[84] PBL recovered from a K562 monolayer were significantly more depleted in activity against K562 than in anti-HSB activity and conversely. D'Amore and Golub[85] studied the specificity of NK cells at the single cell level using a double target binding assay. They found that fewer than 5% of Percoll density gradient purified NK cells were capable of simultaneously binding two different NK-sensitive targets, K562 and MOLT-4.

Further recent evidence for the heterogeneity of human NK cells comes from the studies of Fitzgerald et al.,[86] comparing the lysis of K562 and Herpes virus-infected fibroblasts. Although NK activity to uninfected fibroblasts, to HSV-1-infected fibroblasts, and to K562 were all found in the LGL fraction of PBL, competition studies revealed that while both the infected and uninfected fibroblast targets competed for lysis with each other, K562 cells competed only poorly. The converse was also true in that unlabeled K562 cells competed well against Cr-labeled K562 but poorly against HSV-1-infected or -uninfected fibroblasts. Analysis of the NK cells that killed the different targets using panning or complement depletion experiments revealed that the majority of NK cells with specificity for HSV-infected targets bore an Ia framework antigen, while NK cells with specificity for K562 were Ia-negative. The majority of K562 effectors were recognized by antibodies to the E rosette receptor (Lyt 3 and OKT11a), whereas NK activity to HSV-infected targets was much less sensitive to these antibodies. OKM1, OKT10, and Leu-7 (HNK-1) were found on some but not all of the cells that lysed both the fibroblast and K562 targets. Thus, there is phenotypic heterogeneity within functional subgroups of NK cells. Fitzgerald et al. concluded that there are at least three subpopulations of effector cells: one that kills the infected or uninfected fibroblasts, one that kills K562 cells, and one that may be able to kill all targets. These studies on the heterogeneity of NK cells in normal donors were further substantiated by studies with cells from patients having a variety of immune deficiencies. Patients with aplastic anemia generally had low NK activity to HSV-infected targets but normal activity to K562. In contrast, normal NK to HSV targets was detected in patients with acute lymphocytic leukemia, severe combined immunodeficiency, acute myelocytic leukemia, and AIDS, while these patients had low activity to K562. These data suggest the presence of separate, independently regulated NK subpopulations. It should be noted, however, that not all virus-infected cells are lysed by effectors different from those that lyse K562. Ault and Wiener[87] found that measles virus-infected HeLa cells competed well against killing of K562. Moreover, there was a strong correlation between NK to the virus-infected targets and K562.

The experiments discussed above illustrate that a major factor in detecting NK heterogeneity is the susceptibility of the target to lysis. Gidlund et al.[88] have shown that susceptibility to natural killing is a function of the stage of differentiation of the human cell lines K562 and U937 and/or a mouse line, GM86. When each of these lines was treated with inducers to become more differentiated, they decreased in susceptibility to NK lysis. Blazar et al.[89] showed that induction of EBV expression increased the sensitivity to NK lysis in human lymphoid lines.

Further evidence for heterogeneity of NK cells has come with studies using MoAb. Zarling et al.[41] demonstrated the presence of OKT11a and OKM1 on separate subpopulations of NK cells, both of which lysed K562 targets. Abo et al.[90] differentiated two distinct subsets of human $HNK1^+$ cells: an $HNK1^+T3^-M1^+$ population and an $HNK1^+T3^+M1^-$ subpopulation. The $T3^-$ cells were highly cytotoxic for K562, whereas the $T3^+$ cells were only weakly cytotoxic. The majority of $HNK1^+$ cells in the blood were $T3^-$, while the HNK1 cells of bone marrow are mainly $T3^+M1^-$. Abo et al.[90] suggested that these subsets of cells represent different stages of NK cell differentiation. The recent studies by Lanier et al.,[52] discussed above, comparing the expression of two NK antigens, Leu 7 (HNK-1) and Leu 11a also illustrate the phenotypic heterogeneity of NK cells even when only one target is being considered. Fast et al.[91] have shown that functional heterogeneity of NK cells can be revealed by treatment of human PBL with very low doses of trypsin (5 μg/mℓ). Trypsinized effector cells bound normally to a series of NK-sensitive targets yet were unable to lyse certain of the targets (e.g., K562 and MOLT-4), whereas lysis of other targets such as Jurkat and Daudi was not significantly affected. Analysis of the trypsin-sensitive cell surface structures implicated the involvement of T200 glycoproteins that were indistinguishable from the T cell form of T200 but different from the monocyte form.

Another potential source of apparent heterogeneity among NK cells arises from arming the cells with specific antibody via effector cell FcR. Comparison of NK cells with the K cells that mediate antibody-dependent cellular cytotoxicity (ADCC) are considered in another chapter in this volume. For our purposes it is important to remember that NK cells bear Fcγ receptors. Thus the possibility of ADCC is often present and must be ruled out if one is to speak only of NK activity. Koren and Williams[92] were able to make this distinction experimentally using competitive inhibition. Their studies indicate that NK cells bear receptors for NK target determinants as well as having FcR, whereas K cells bear only FcR. The presence of simultaneously occurring immunoglobulin-dependent and -independent natural cytotoxicity was also observed by Pape et al.[93] ADCC could be completely inhibited by the addition of aggregated IgG to the assay but NK was unaffected.

A further aspect of the heterogeneity of NK cells lies at the level of different regulatory mechanisms for NK cells. The metabolic and cellular regulators of NK are outside the scope of this chapter. At this point it is clear that heterogeneity of NK cells exists. However, the molecular and functional basis for this heterogeneity is only beginning to be understood. It will be necessary to isolate target antigens and effector cell receptors to have an understanding of the basis of heterogeneity. Many unanswered questions remain, including: (1) how much does the apparent heterogeneity reflect the stage of differentiation of the NK cells themselves vs. a clonal distribution of target antigen receptors on NK cells? (2) How does the stage of differentiation of the target cells and their susceptibility to the lytic event affect lysis?

IV. LINEAGE

Given the phenotypic and functional heterogeneity of naturally cytotoxic cells, it is not surprising that there is no single unifying sceme regarding their lineage. It has been suggested that NK cells are in the T cell lineage, that they are closely related to the myeloid series, or that they comprise a separate, unique lineage. There is the additional possibility that natural cytotoxicity is an activity expressed by cell types of different lineages at certain stages of their differentiation.

To date, the strongest case has been made for a close association of NK cells with the T cell lineage. The presence of T cell-associated antigens on both human and murine NK cells has been repeatedly reported (cf. Tables 1 and 2). In addition, it has become clear that the thymus has some regulatory role in NK function, but the nature of that role is not yet known.[94] A proportion of murine NK cells do express Thy-1, although at a lower density than CTL.[4] Qa-4 and Qa-5 are present on NK[9] but not on NC[29] cells. In most cases Lyt-1 and Lyt-2 have not been detected on endogenous murine NK cells,[5,10] although Koo et al.[9] reported the presence of Lyt-1 on a subpopulation of NK cells. Studies on cloned NK lines have also supported the notion that NK cells are related to T cells. For example, Brooks et al.[95] have detected the presence of T cell-associated antigens on cloned NK lines, and conversely[96] the presence of NK-1 and NK-2 alloantigens on cloned antigen-dependent CTL lines.

In studies on fetal thymocytes Habu et al.[97] found that the expression of asialo GM1, which was detected on day 13 of gestation, decreased as the expression of the T cell markers Thy-1, Lyt-1, and Lyt-2 increased. The cells positive for asialo GM1 on day 13 werc negative for the expression of Thy-1 and conversely Thy-1+ cells were negative for asialo GM1. This lack of coexpression of NK and T cell markers in the fetal thymus suggested to Habu and Okumura[98] that NK and T cells may share a common precursor but follow different developmental pathways. Koo et al.[99] compared the expression of NK 1 and the receptor for peanut agglutinin (PNA) on prothymocytes and splenic NK cells. The PNA receptor is characteristic of cells of the T lineage and was present on prothymocytes but not detectable on splenic NK cells. This experiment argues against the identity of T and NK cells. However, since splenic NK cells are mature postmitotic cells,[100] cycling NK1$^+$ cells of the bone marrow should be tested for PNA receptors to confirm this conclusion.

In studies on human NK cells, several T cell-associated antigens were regularly detected, including the receptors for sheep erythrocytes and antigens associated with cytotoxic suppressor cells, i.e., OKT8 and Leu-2a. However, as discussed above, there is heterogeneity of expression of these antigens among the NK population. It should be noted that in studies on the tissue distribution of Leu-7 (HNK-1)-positive cells the presence of Leu7 cells in the thymus was "extremely rare".[48]

If it could be shown that all cells with NK activity express some T markers at some stage of their differentiation, a compelling argument might be made for a T lineage for NK cells. However, several things mitigate against this conclusion. One is the finding that some antigens previously thought to be exclusively expressed on T cells, for instance Lyt-1, may also be expressed on other cell types, such as B cells.[101] Phenotypes are notoriously plastic and antigenic expression can be modulated by many factors. Thus, the sensitivity of the detection method is of paramount importance. Moreover, antigens associated with the myeloid series are also detected on NK cells (cf. Tables 1 and 2). For example, Kay and Horowitz[102] fractionated human PBL into E receptor-positive and E-negative subpopulations by E rosetting. The populations were further fractionated into FcR^+ and FcR^- by adherence to immobilized complexes. The NK activity was found in two fractions, the E^+FcR^+ and the E^-FcR^+ subpopulations. Characterization of these populations with a series of MoAb, including OKT3, OKT4, OKT5, OKT8, OKT10, M1, and OK11 revealed that the E^+FcR^+ NK population was strongly positive for the M1 antigen expressed on cells of the myeloid lineage. M1 was also expressed on the E^-FcR^+ NK subpopulation. On the basis of these results, these authors argued for a myeloid origin of NK cells. Zarling and Kung[42] reached the same conclusion based on their studies with MoAb to T and myeloid antigens. Another MoAb that reacts with human NK cells, VEP13, was found by Rumpold et al.[103] to cross-react with granulocytes and cells with T markers. The MoAb 3G8, that detects FcR on human neutrophils[104] also reacts with human NK cells. Another indication that NK cells may be related to the myeloid lineage comes from the studies of Galli et al.[27] with a cloned line of NK cells that express an IgE receptor and have a morphology reminiscent of basophils. It is also interesting that pigment mutations that affect lysosomes generally lead to a decreased expression of NK activity.[105]

However, other studies suggest that NK cells may be neither of the T nor myeloid lineage, but constitute a separate lineage. For instance, in the studies by Haller and Wigzell[106] with ^{89}Sr-treated mice, all other cell types except NK recovered. Whether this is due to preferential depletion of a stem cell for the NK lineage, or to an effect on an accessory cell necessary for the maturation of NK cells, or on NK cells themselves is not known. It has been reported that strontium causes degranulation of NK cells.[107] Several groups have reported the generation of NK or NK-like cells from cultured bone marrow.[108,109] Although such studies have not yet answered the question of lineage of NK cells, this approach will be very useful. In studies with bone marrow transplant patients, Lopez et al.[110] found that four patients with severe combined immunodeficiency had normal NK cells, suggesting that NK is not of lymphoid lineage. Although there was some correlation with presence of cells of the monocyte-granulocyte lineage, this was variable and led these authors to conclude that NK cells are in a distinct lineage separate from either the lymphoid or myeloid. Abo et al.[111] interpreted their results on the coexpression of HNK1, T3, and M1 antigens on NK cells from fetal tissue, adult bone marrow or spleen, and peripheral blood to be most compatible with a separate differentiation pathway for NK cells, i.e., neither T nor monocyte. The same conclusion was reached by Ferrarini and Grossi.[112] After reviewing the data which suggest that NK cells are a subset of mature T cells, are immature T cells, or are in the myeloid lineage, they argue that the results are best explained by NK cells constituting a separate lineage. Similarly, Ortaldo[113] concluded that the data are not strong enough to assign NK cells to one lineage but are most compatible with the expression of various antigens during differentiation of a separate lineage.

It is, of course, possible that several populations from different lineages are involved in the phenomenon we detect as natural cytotoxicity. Rather than restricting our thinking to one cell type, we should consider the possibility that cells of several hemopoietic lineages are able to express NK activity at particular stages of their differentiation by virtue of their expression of surface moieties ("receptors") that allow them to interact with "target" structures on other cells and that this interaction activates the inherent cytotoxic machinery of the effector cells. Although there is no hard evidence for this hypothesis, it is one that is worth testing. If natural cytotoxicity has evolved as a means for surveillance against abnormal hemopoiesis and the development of tumors, it may be that nature has built redundancy into this system and that several lineages are capable of expressing natural cytotoxicity. Thus, even if one is eliminated, e.g., because of bone marrow dysfunction in one cell lineage, the other effectors of natural cytotoxicity would be able to take over the surveillance and regulatory functions. This scheme

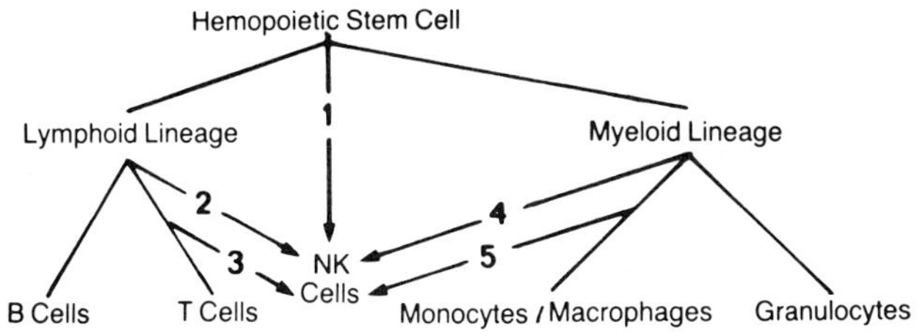

FIGURE 1. Possible lineages of NK cells: (1) a unique lineage, neither lymphoid nor myeloid; (2) an offshoot of the lymphoid lineage, distinct from T or B cells; (3) a branch of the T-cell pathway; (4) an offshoot of the myeloid lineage; (5) a branch of the monocyte/macrophage pathway.

allows both for the apparent preference of some NK cells for certain targets and for the existence of phenotypically different subsets with cytotoxicity for one target.

These possibilities regarding the lineage of NK cells are outlined in Figure 1. There can be no doubt that NK cells share many phenotypic markers with T cells. Similarly, the phenotype data suggest a relationship of NK and myeloid cells. The idea that NK cells constitute a separate lineage is attractive in that it would allow the apparently conflicting data on the expression of T vs. myeloid markers to be reconciled. Finally, we should remain open to the possibility that cells of several lineages can function as naturally cytotoxic cells.

V. CONCLUSIONS

Naturally cytotoxic cells are a diverse population both in terms of their phenotype and their function. Although a number of monoclonal and alloantibodies have been described that react preferentially with NK cells, it has not yet been possible to ascribe one unique feature to NK cells in either the human or mouse. However, this may be an unattainable goal, since there are few unique markers within the hemopoietic system. Although immunoglobulin production is unique to the B cell lineage, other cells can pick up Ig via their FcR and appear to be Ig^+ and T cells may express V region products. As mentioned above, antigens that were thought to be unique to one cell population, such as Lyt-1, have now been shown to be expressed on other lymphoid cells, and antigens such as Thy-1 are expressed on nonlymphoid cells as well as on T cells. However, it is worth persisting in attempts to pinpoint the phenotype and lineage of NK cells more closely, since it is now abundantly clear that naturally cytotoxic cells play important roles in vivo (e.g., see Reference 114). It is likely that studies on the bone marrow, both in vitro and in vivo, will ultimately reveal the lineage(s) of NK cells and their relationship to both lymphoid and myeloid cells.

REFERENCES

1. Herberman, R. B., Nunn, M. E., and Lavrin, D. H., Natural cytotoxic reactivity of mouse lymphoid cells against syngeneic and allogeneic tumors. I. Distribution of reactivity and specificity, *Int. J. Cancer,* 16, 216, 1975.
2. Kiessling, R., Klein, E., and Wigzell, H., "Natural" killer cells in the mouse. I. Cytotoxic cells with specificity for mouse Moloney leukemia cells. Specificity and distribution according to genotype, *Eur. J. Immunol.,* 5, 112, 1975.

3. Kiessling, R. and Wigzell, H., An analysis of the murine NK cell as to structure, function and biological relevance, *Immunol. Rev.*, 44, 165, 1979.
4. Mattes, M. J., Sharrow, S. O., Herberman, R. B., and Holden, H. T., Identification and separation of Thy-1 positive mouse spleen cells active in natural cytotoxicity and antibody-dependent cell-mediated cytotoxicity, *J. Immunol.*, 123, 2851, 1979.
5. Pollack, S. B., Tam, M. R., Nowinski, R. C., and Emmons, S. L., Presence of T cell-associated surface antigens on mruine NK cells, *J. Immunol.*, 123, 1818, 1979.
6. Cantor, H., Kasai, M., Shen, F. W., LeClerc, J. C., and Glimcher, L., Immunogenetic analysis of "natural killer" activity in the mouse, *Immunol. Rev.*, 44, 1, 1979.
7. Kasai, M., LeClerc, J. C., Shen, F. -W., and Cantor, H., Identification of Ly 5 on the surface of "natural killer" cells in normal and athymic inbred mouse strains, *Immunogenetics*, 8, 153, 1979.
8. Scheid, M. P. and Triglia, D., Further description of the Ly5 system, *Immunogenetics*, 9, 423, 1979.
9. Koo, G. C., Jacobson, J. B., Hammerling, G. J., and Hammerling, J., Antigenic profile of murine natural killer cells, *J. Immunol.*, 125, 1003, 1980.
10. Beaumont, T., Roder, J., Elliott, B., Kerbel, R., Dennis, J., Kasai, M., and Okumura, K., A comparative analysis of cell surface markers on murine NK cells and CTL target-effector conjugates, *Scand. J. Immunol.*, 16, 123, 1982.
11. Seaman, W. E., Talal, N., Herzenberg, L. A., Herzenberg, L. A., and Ledbetter, J. A., Surface antigens on mouse natural killer cells: use of monoclonal antibodies to inhibit or to enrich cytotoxic activity, *J. Immunol.*, 127, 982, 1981.
12. Stout, R. D., Yutoku, M., Grossberg, A., Pressman, D., and Herzenberg, L. A., A surface membrane determinant shared by subpopulations of thymocytes and B lymphocytes, *J. Immunol.*, 115, 508, 1975.
13. Glimcher, L., Shen, F. W., and Cantor, H., Identification of a cell-surface antigen selectively expressed on the natural killer cell, *J. Exp. Med.*, 145, 1, 1977.
14. Tam, M. R., Emmons, S. L., and Pollack, S. B., Analysis and enrichment of murine natural killer cells with the fluorescence activated cell sorter, *J. Immunol.*, 124, 650, 1980.
15. Pollack, S. B. and Hallenbeck, L. A., In vivo reduction of NK activity with anti-NK 1 serum: direct evaluation of NK cells in tumor clearance, *Int. J. Cancer*, 29, 203, 1982.
16. Burton, R. C. and Winn, H. J., Studies on natural killer (NK) cells. I. NK cell specific antibodies in CE anti-CBA serum, *J. Immunol.*, 126, 1985, 1981.
17. Burton, R. C., Bartlett, S. P., and Winn, H. J., Alloantigens specific for natural killer cells, in *NK Cells and Other Natural Effector Cells*, Herberman, R. B., Ed., Academic Press, New York, 1982, 105.
18. Pollack, S. B. and Emmons, S. L., NK 2.1: an NK-associated antigen detected with NZB anti-BALB/c serum, *J. Immunol.*, 129, 2277, 1982.
19. Meruelo, D., Paolino, A., Flieger, N., Offer, M., and Dworkin, J., Ly 11.2: a cell surface antiger that may identify murine lymphocytes susceptible to transformation by oncogenic agents, *Fed. Proc. Fed. Am. Soc. Exp. Biol.*, 40, 2717, 1981.
20. Young, W., Hakomori, S., Durdik, J., and Henney, C., Identification of ganglio-n-tetraosylceramide as a new cell surface marker for murine natural killer cells, *J. Immunol.*, 124, 199, 1980.
21. Kasai, M., Iwamori, M., Nagai, Y., Okumura, K., and Tada, T., A glycolipid on the surface of mouse natural killer cells, *Eur. J. Immunol.*, 10, 175, 1980.
22. Beck, B., Gillis, S., and Henney, C. S., Display of the neutral glycolipid ganglio-N-tetraosylceramide (asialo GM1) on cells of the natural killer and T lineages, *Transplantation*, 33, 118, 1982.
23. Dennert, G., Yogeeswaran, G., and Yamagata, S., Cloned cell lines with natural killer activity: specificity, function and cell surface markers, *J. Exp. Med.*, 153, 545, 1981.
24. Kuribayashi, K., Gillis, S., Kern, D. E., and Henney, C. S., Murine NK cell cultures: effects of interleukin-2 and interferon on cell growth and cytotoxic reactivity, *J. Immunol.*, 126, 2321, 1981.
25. Brooks, C., Kuribayashi, K., Sale, G., and Henney, C., Characterization of five cloned murine cell lines showing high cytolytic activity against YAC-1 cells, *J. Immunol.*, 128, 2326, 1982.
26. Ting, C., Yang, S., and Hargrove, M., Effect of interleukin 2 on cytotoxic effectors. II. Long term culture of NK cells, *Cell. Immunol.*, 73, 275, 1982.
27. Galli, S., Dvorak, A., Ishizaka, T., Nabel, G., Simonian, H., Cantor, H., and Dvorak, H., A cloned cell with NK function resembles basophils by ultrastructure and expresses IgE receptors, *Nature*, 298, 288, 1982.
28. Paige, C. J., Figarella, E. F., Cuttito, M. J., Cahan, A., and Stutman, O., Natural cytotoxic cells against solid tumors in mice. II. Some characteristics of the effector cells, *J. Immunol.*, 121, 1827, 1978.
29. Stutman, O., Lattime, E., and Figarella, E., Natural cytotoxic cells against solid tumors in mice: a comparison with natural killer cells, *Fed. Proc.,Fed. Am. Soc. Exp. Biol.*, 40, 2699, 1981.

30. Jondal, M. and Pross, H., Surface markers on human B and T lymphocytes. VI. Cytotoxicity against cell lines as a functional marker for lymphocyte subpopulations, *Int. J. Cancer,* 15, 596, 1975.
31. Bakacs, T., Gergely, P., and Klein, E., Characterization of cytotoxic human lymphocyte subpopulations: the role of Fc-receptor-carrying cells, *Cell. Immunol.,* 32, 317, 1977.
32. Cooper, S. M., Hirsen, D. J., and Friou, G. J., Spontaneous cell-mediated cytotoxicity against Chang cells by nonadherent, non-thymus-derived, Fc receptor-bearing lymphocytes, *Cell. Immunol.,* 32, 135, 1977.
33. Kay, H. D., Bonnard, G. D., West, W. H., and Herberman, R. B., A functional comparison of human Fc-receptor-bearing lymphocytes active in natural cytotoxicity and antibody-dependent cellular cytotoxicity, *J. Immunol.,* 118, 2058, 1977.
34. West, W. H., Cannon, G. B., Kay, D., Bonnard, G. D., and Herberman, R. B., Natural cytotoxic reactivity of human lymphocytes against a myeloid cell line: characterizations of effector cells, *J. Immunol.,* 118, 355, 1977.
35. Bolhuis, R. L. H., Schuit, H. R. E., Nooyen, A. M., and Ronteltap, C. P. M., Characterization of natural killer (NK) cells and killer (K) cells in human blood: discrimination between NK and K activities, *Eur. J. Immunol.,* 8, 731, 1978.
36. Pichler, W. J., Gendelman, F. W., and Nelson, D. L., Fc receptors on human T lymphocytes. II. Cytotoxic capabilities of human Tγ, Tμ, B, and L cells, *Cell. Immunol.,* 42, 410, 1979.
37. Jondal, M. and Merrill, J., Distribution of IgG and IgM receptors on human peripheral natural killer cells measured on the level of the single effector cells, *Eur. J. Immunol.,* 11, 531, 1981.
38. Pross, H. F., Baines, M. G., and Jondal, M., Spontaneous human lymphocyte-mediated cytotoxicity against tumor target cells. II. Is the complement receptor necessarily present on the killer cells?, *Int. J. Cancer,* 20, 353, 1977.
39. Tedder, T. F., Fearon, D. T., Gartland, G. L., and Cooper, M. D., Expression of C3b receptors on human B cells and myelomonocytic cells but not natural killer cells, *J. Immunol.,* 130, 1668, 1983.
40. West, W. H., Boozer, R. B., and Herberman, R. B., Low affinity E-rosette formation by the human K cell, *J. Immunol.,* 120, 90, 1978.
41. Zarling, J. M., Clouse, K. A., biddison, W. E., and Kung, P. C., Phenotypes of human natural killer cell populations detected with monoclonal antibodies, *J. Immunol.,* 127, 2575, 1981.
42. Zarling, J. M. and Kung, P. C., Monoclonal antibodies which distinguish between human NK cells and cytotoxic T lymphocytes, *Nature,* 288, 394, 1980.
43. Ortaldo, J. R., Sharrow, S. O., Timonen, T., and Herberman, R. B., Determination of surface antigens on highly purified human NK cells by flow cytometry with monoclonal antibodies, *J. Immunol.,* 127, 2401, 1981.
44. Fast, L. D., Hansen, J. A., and Newman, W., Evidence for T cell nature and heterogeneity within natural killer (NK) and antibody-dependent cellular cytoxicity (ADCC) effectors: a comparison with cytolytic T lymphocytes (CTL), *J. Immunol.,* 127, 448, 1981.
45. Caraux, J., Serrou, B., and Weigle, W., Natural killer activity: effector cells in purified human T or null cells have different phenotypes defined by monoclonal antibodies, *Cell. Immunol.,* 74, 404, 1982.
46. Perussia, B., Fanning, V., and Trinchieri, G., A human NK and K cell subset shares with cytotoxic T cells expression of the antigen recognized by antibody OKT8, *J. Immunol.,* 131, 223, 1983.
47. Abo, T. and Balch, C. M., A differentiation antigen of human NK and K cells identified by a monoclonal antibody (HNK-1), *J. Immunol.,* 127, 1024, 1981.
48. Si, L. and Whiteside, T. L., Tissue distribution of human NK cells studied with anti-Leu-7 monoclonal antibody, *J. Immunol.,* 130, 2149, 1983.
49. Perussia, B., Starr, S., Abraham, S., Fanning, V., and Trinchieri, G., Human natural killer cells analyzed by B 73.1, a monoclonal antibody blocking Fc receptor functions. I. Characterization of the lymphocyte subset reactive with B 73.1, *J. Immunol.,* 130, 2133, 1983.
50. Perussia, B., Acuto, O., Terhorst, C., Faust, J., Lazarus, R., Fanning, V., and Trinchieri, G., Human natural killer cells analyzed by B73.1, a monoclonal antibody blocking Fc receptor functions. II. Studies of B73.1 antibody-antigen interaction on the lymphocyte membrane, *J. Immunol.,* 130, 2142, 1983.
51. Phillips, J. H. and Babcock, G. F., NKP-15: a monoclonal antibody reactive against purified human natural killer cells and granulocytes, *Immunol. Lett.,* 6, 143, 1983.
52. Lanier, L. L., Le, A. M., Phillips, J. H., Warner, N. L., and Babcock, G. F., Subpopulations of human natural killer cells defined by expression of the Leu-7 (HNK-1) and Leu-11 (NK-15) antigens, *J. Immunol.,* 131, 1789, 1983.
53. Newman, W., selective blockade of human natural killer cells by a monoclonal antibody, *Proc. Natl. Acad. Sci. U.S.A.,* 79, 3858, 1982.
54. Nieminen, P., Paasivuo, R., and Saksela, E., Effect of a monoclonal anti-large granular lymphocyte antibody on the human NK activity, *J. Immunol.,* 128, 1097, 1982.

55. Rumpold, H., Kraft, D., Obexer, G., Bock, G., and Gebhart, W., A monoclonal antibody against a surface antigen shared by human large granular lymphocytes and granulocytes, *J. Immunol.*, 129, 1458, 1982.
56. Hiserodt, J. C., Britran, L. J., and Targan, S. R., Inhibition of human killing by heterologous and monoclonal antibodies, *J. Immunol.*, 129, 2248, 1982.
57. Neville, M. and Hiserodt, J., Inhibition of human antibody-dependent cellular cytotoxicity, cell mediated cytotoxicity, and natural killing by a xenogenic antiserum prepared against "activated" alloimmune human lymphocytes, *J. Immunol.*, 128, 1246, 1982.
58. Devlin, J., Phaneuf, J., and Granger, G., Inhibition of human lectin-dependent cell-mediated cytotoxicity, natural killer-like cytotoxicity, and cytotoxic T-lymphocyte-mediated cytolysis by xenoantisera raised against concanavalin A-stimulated human lymphocytes, *Cell. Immunol.*, 68, 64, 1982.
59. Ault, K. and Springer, T., Cross-reaction of a rat-anti-mouse phagocyte-specific monoclonal antibody (anti-Mac-1) with human monocytes and natural killer cells, *J. Immunol.*, 126, 359, 1981.
60. Breard, J., Reiherz, E., O'Brien, C., and Schlossman, S., Delineation of an effector population responsible for natural killing and antibody-dependent cellular cytotoxicity in man, *Clin. Immunol. Immunopathol.*, 18, 145, 1981.
61. Hokland, M., Heron, I., Berg, K., and Hokland, P., Natural killer cell activity correlates with the amount of β_2-microglobulin on human peripheral blood lymphocytes, *Cell. Immunol.*, 72, 40, 1982.
62. Koide, Y., Takasugi, M., and Billing, R., B cell antigens on effectors for natural cell-mediated cytotoxicity, *Eur. J. Immunol.*, 7, 731, 1977.
63. Ortaldo, J. R., Bonnard, G. D., Kind, P. D., and Herberman, R. B., Cytotoxicity by cultured human lymphocytes: characteristics of effector cells and specificity of cytotoxicity, *J. Immunol.*, 12, 1489, 1979.
64. Krensky, A., Ault, K., Reiss, C., Strominger, J., and Burakoff, S., Generation of long-term human cytolytic cell lines with persistent natural killer activity, *J. Immunol.*, 129, 1748, 1982.
65. Hercend, T., Reinharz, E., Meuer, S., Schlossman, S., and Ritz, J., Phenotypic and functional heterogeneity of human cloned natural killer cell lines, *Nature*, 301, 158, 1983.
66. Sugamura, K., Tanaka, Y., and Hinuma, Y., Two distinct human cloned T cell lines that exhibit natural killer-like and anti-human effector activities, *J. Immunol.*, 128, 1749, 1982.
67. Seeley, J. K., Masucci, G., Poros, A., Klein, E., and Golub, S. H., Studies on cytotoxicity generated in human mixed lymphocyte cultures. II. Anti-K562 effectors are distinct from allospecific CTL and can be generated from NK-depleted T cells, *J. Immunol.*, 123, 1303, 1979.
68. Lopez-Botet, M., Silva, A., Rodriguez, J., and DeLandazuri, M., Generation of T cell blasts with NK-like activity in human MLC: cellular precursors, IL 2 responsiveness and phenotype expression, *J. Immunol.*, 129, 1109, 1982.
69. Kornbluth, J., Flomberg, N., and Dupont, B., Cell surface phenotype of a cloned line of human natural killer cells, *J. Immunol.*, 129, 2831, 1982.
70. Oehler, J. R., Lindsay, L. R., Nunn, M. E., and Herberman, R. B., Natural cell-mediated cytotoxicity in rats. I. Tissue and strain distribution, and demonstration of a membrane receptor for the Fc portion of IgG, *Int. J. Cancer*, 21, 204, 1978.
71. Shellam, G. R., Gross-virus-induced lymphoma in the rat. V. Natural cytotoxic cells are non-T cells, *Int. J. Cancer*, 19, 225, 1977.
72. Reynolds, C. W., Sharrow, S. A., Ortaldo, J. R., and Herberman, R. B., Natural killer activity in the rat. II. Analysis of surface antigens on LGL by flow cytometry, *J. Immunol.*, 127, 2204, 1981.
73. Altman, A. and Rapp, H. J., Natural cell-mediated cytotoxicity in guinea pigs: properties and specificity of natural killer cells, *J. Immunol.*, 121, 2244, 1978.
74. Arnaud-Battandier, F., Bundy, B. M., and Nelson, D. L., Natural killer cells in guinea pig spleen bear Fc receptor, *Eur. J. Immunol.*, 8, 400, 1978.
75. Sharma, J. and Okazaki, W., Natural killer cell activity in chickens: target cell and effect of antithymocyte serum on effector cells, *Infect. Immun.*, 31, 1078, 1981.
76. Stutman, O., Paige, C. J., and Figarella, E. F., Natural cytotoxic cells against solid tumors in mice. I. Strain and age distribution and target cell susceptibility, *J. Immunol.*, 121, 1819, 1978.
77. Lattime, E. C., Pecoraro, G. A., and Stutman, O., Natural cytotoxic cells against solid tumors in mice. III. A comparison of effector cell antigenic phenotype and target cell recognition structures with those of NK cells, *J. Immunol.*, 126, 2011, 1981.
78. Lattime, E. C., Pecoraro, G. A., Cuttito, M., and Stutman, O., Solid tumors are killed by NK and NC populations: interferon inducing agents do not augment NC activity under NK activating conditions, in *NK Cells and Other Natural Effector Cells*, Herberman, R. B., Ed., Academic Press, New York, 1982, 179.
79. Emmons, S. L. and Pollack, S. B., Murine NK cell heterogeneity: subpopulations of C57BL/6 splenic NK cells detected by NK 1.1 and NK 2.1 antisera, in press.

80. Kumar, V., Ben-Ezra, J., Bennett, M., and Sonnenfeld, G., Natural killer cells in mice treated with ^{89}strontium: normal target-binding cell numbers but inability to kill even after interferon administration, *J. Immunol.*, 123, 1832, 1979.
81. Lust, J. A., Kumar, V., Burton, R. C., Bartlett, S. P., and Bennett, M., Heterogeneity of natural killer cells in the mouse, *J. Exp. Med.*, 154, 306, 1981.
82. Minato, N., Reid, L., and Bloom, B. R., On the heterogeneity of murine natural killer cells, *J. Exp. Med.*, 154, 750, 1981.
83. Burton, R. C., Bartlett, S. P., Kumar, V., and Winn, H. J., Studies on natural killer (NK) cells II. Serologic evidence for heterogeneity of murine NK cells, *J. Immunol.*, 127, 1864, 1981.
84. Jensen, P. J. and Koren, H. S., Heterogeneity within the population of NK and K cells, *J. Immunol.*, 124, 395, 1980.
85. D'Amore, P. and Golub, S., Detection of double target binders at the single cell level: an evaluation of the specificity of NK and MLC-induced NK-like cells, *Cell. Immunol.*, 71, 66, 1982.
86. Fitzgerald, P. A., Evans, R., Kirkpatrick, D., and Lopez, C., Heterogeneity of human NK cells: comparison of effectors that lyse HSV-1-infected fibroblasts and K562 erythroleukemic targets, *J. Immunol.*, 130, 1663, 1983.
87. Ault, K. A. and Weiner, H. L., Natural killing of measles-infected cells by human lymphocytes, *J. Immunol.*, 122, 2611, 1979.
88. Gidlund, M., Örn, A., Pattengale, P. K., Jansson, M., Wigzell, H., and Nilsson, K., Natural killer cells kill tumour cells at a given stage of differentiation, *Nature*, 292, 848, 1981.
89. Blazar, B., Patarroyo, M., Klein, E., and Klein, G., Increased sensitivity of human lymphoid lines to natural killer cells after induction of the Epstein-Barr viral cycle by superinfection or sodium butyrate, *J. Exp. Med.*, 151, 614, 1980.
90. Abo, T., Cooper, M., and Balch, C., Characterization of HNK-1$^+$ (Leu-7) human lymphocytes I. Two distinct phenotypes of human NK cells with different cytotoxic capability, *J. Immunol.*, 129, 1752, 1982.
91. Fast, L. D., Beatty, P., Hanson, J. A., and Newman, W., T cell nature and heterogeneity of recognition structures of human natural killer (NK) cells, *J. Immunol.*, 131, 2404, 1983.
92. Koren, H. S. and Williams, M. S., Natural killing and antibody-dependent cellular cytotoxicity are mediated by different mechanisms and by different cells, *J. Immunol.*, 121, 1956, 1978.
93. Pape, G. R., Troye, M., Axelsson, B., and Perlmann, P., Simultaneous occurrence of immunoglobulin-dependent and immunoglobulin-independent mechanisms in natural cytotoxicity of human lymphocytes, *J. Immunol.*, 122, 2251, 1979.
94. Kaiserlian, D., Bardos, P., and Bach, J. -F., Immunoregulation of mouse NK activity by the serum thymic factor (FTS), in *NK Cells and Other Natural Effector Cells*, Herberman, R. B., Ed., Academic Press, New York, 1982, 215.
95. Brooks, C. G., Kuribayashi, K., Sale, G. E., and Henney, C. S., Characterization of five cloned murine cell lines showing high cytolytic activity against YAC-1 cells, *J. Immunol.*, 128, 2326, 1982.
96. Brooks, C. G., Burton, R. C., Pollack, S. B., and Henney, C. S., The presence of NK alloantigens on cloned cytotoxic T lymphocytes, *J. Immunol.*, 131, 1391, 1983.
97. Habu, S., Kasai, M., Nagai, Y., Tamaoki, N., Tada, T., Herzenberg, L. A., and Okumura, K., The glycolipid asialo GM_1 as a new differentiation antigen of fetal thymocytes, *J. Immunol.*, 125, 2284, 1980.
98. Habu, S. and Okumura, K., Cell lineages of NK cell: evidence for T cell lineage, in *NK Cells and Other Natural Effector Cells*, Herberman, R. B., Ed., Academic Press, New York, 1982, 209.
99. Koo, G. C., Cayre, Y., and Mittl, L. R., Comparative study of splenic natural killer cells and prothymocytes, *Cell. Immunol.*, 62, 164, 1981.
100. Miller, S., Production and renewal of murine natural killer cells in the spleen and bone marrow, *J. Immunol.*, 129, 2282, 1982.
101. Manohan, V., Brown, E., Leiserson, W. M., and Chused, T. M., Expression of Lyt-1 by a subset of B lymphocytes, *J. Immunol.*, 129, 532, 1982.
102. Kay, H. D. and Horowitz, D. A., Evidence by reactivity with hybridoma antibodies for a probable myeloid origin of peripheral blood cells active in natural cytotoxicity and antibody-dependent cell-mediated cytotoxicity, *J. Clin. Invest.*, 66, 847, 1980.
103. Rumpold, H., Kraft, D., Obexer, G., Bock, G., and Gebhart, W., Amonoclonal antibody against a surface antigen shared by human large granular lymphocytes and granulocytes, *J. Immunol.*, 129, 1458, 1982.
104. Fleit, H. B., Wright, S. D., and Unkeless, J. C., Human neutrophil Fc_γ receptor distribution and structure, *Proc. Natl. Acad. Sci. U.S.A.*, 79, 3275, 1982.
105. Örn, A., Hakansson, E., Gidlund, M., Ramstedt, U., Axberg, I., Wigzell, H., and Lundin, L. -G., Pigment mutations in the mouse which also affect lysosomal functions lead to suppressed natural killer cell activity, *Scand. J. Immunol.*, 15, 305, 1982.

106. Haller, O. and Wigzell, H., Suppression of natural killer cell activity with radioactive strontium: effector cells are marrow dependent, *J. Immunol.,* 118, 1503, 1977.
107. Neighbour, P. A., Huberman, H., and Kress, Y., Human large granular lymphocytes and natural killing: ultrastructural studies of strontium-induced degranulation, *Eur. J. Immunol.,* 12, 588, 1982.
108. Claesson, M. H. and Olsson, L., Autoreactive natural killer-like cells from agar-cloned murine bone marrow cells, *Nature,* 283, 578, 1980.
109. Klimpel, G. and Klimpel, K., Specificity and characterization of cytotoxic cells generated from alloantigen-stimulated murine bone marrow cells, *J. Immunol.,* 130, 1084, 1983.
110. Lopez, C., Kirkpatrick, D., Fitzgerald, P. A., Ching, C. Y., Pahwa, R. N., Good, R. A., and Smithwick, E. M., Studies of the cell lineage of the effector cells that spontaneously lyse HSV-1 infected fibroblasts (NKCHSV-1), *J. Immunol.,* 129, 824, 1982.
111. Abo, T., Cooper, M. D., and Balch, C. M., Characterization of human NK cells identified by the monoclonal HNK-1 (Leu-7) antibody, in *NK Cells and Other Natural Effector Cells,* Herberman, R. B., Ed., Academic Press, New York, 1982, 31.
112. Ferrarini, M. and Grossi, C. E., Could human large granular lymphocytes represent a new cell lineage?, in *NK Cells and Other Natural Effectors,* Herberman, R. B., Ed., Academic Press, New York, 1982, 257.
113. Ortaldo, J. R., Natural killer cells: a separate lineage?, in *NK Cells and Other Natural Effector Cells,* Herberman, R. B., Ed., Academic Press, New York, 1982, 265.
114. Pollack, S. B., *In vivo* functions of natural killer cells, *Surv. Synth. Pathol. Res.,* 2, 93, 1983.

Chapter 8

TARGET CELL STRUCTURES, RECOGNITION SITES, AND THE MECHANISM OF NK CYTOTOXICITY

Tatsuo Kiyohara, Robert Lauzon, Tina Haliotis, and John C. Roder

TABLE OF CONTENTS

I. INTRODUCTION

Natural killer (NK) cells have been operationally defined as lymphocytes capable of binding to and destroying neoplastic cells of various histogenic origins, virally infected cells, and certain undifferentiated normal cell types with no apparent prior sensitization.[1-3] There is an increasing body of evidence implicating the NK phenomenon as a primary means of host defense against the growth and dissemination of tumor cells, resistance to viral infections, regulation of hemopoiesis, and immune responses.[4,5] Genetic abnormalities associated with impaired NK cell activity in both murine and human systems may predispose to the development of lymphoid malignancies.[6-9] Although most of the evidence to date has been indirect, a recent report by Warner and Dennert[10] showed that adoptive transfer of a NK clone to beige or normal mice provided resistance to (1) radiation-induced thymic leukemia, (2) allogeneic bone marrow transplantation, and (3) development of metastasis following challenge with melanoma tumor cells. Recent data from our laboratory shows that NK-deficient bg/bg mice develop spontaneous tumors at a faster rate ($p < 0.001$) than littermate +/bg mice.[11] In this experiment, groups of 96 bg/bg and 71 +/bg retired breeders were followed carefully for a 3 1/2 year period. All dying mice were autopsied and almost all tumors were confirmed histologically as lymphomas. These data taken together provide compelling evidence supporting the role of NK cells in host surveillance.

The molecular mechanisms governing NK cell recognition and cytolysis of tumor target cells are poorly understood. Some of this obscurity may well result from an inadequate comprehension of the mechanisms underlying cell-cell adhesion. However, it is well established that NK-tumor cell interaction proceeds through several discrete stages including: (1) effector-target cell recognition and binding, (2) triggering and activation of the NK effector cells, (3) release and binding of the lytic factor (NKCF) to "acceptor sites" on the tumor cell surface, and (4) target cell death.[2,12] The triggering of NK cells appears to be followed by Ca^{2+}-dependent programming for lysis.[13,14] In this chapter, we will attempt to review the various aspects of the NK cytolytic reaction and elucidate the multigenic nature of target cell susceptibility.

II. EFFECTOR-TARGET CELL RECOGNITION

Although it is well established that NK-target cell binding is a required event in the NK cytolytic pathway, such a condition is not sufficient to render a target cell susceptible to NK mediated cytotoxicity. The expression of target cell-borne surface determinants represent only one aspect of a multifactorial system conferring NK sensitivity.

A. NK Cell Recognition Receptor

NK cells bind to their targets via a magnesium (Mg^{++}) dependent reaction. The recognition involves a receptor-ligand interaction between a target structure (TS) on the plasma membrane of the target cell and a recognition receptor (RR) on the surface of the NK cell. The characteristics of this RR which are necessary for effector-target cell binding are unknown. However, pretreatment of murine[15] or human[16] NK cells with proteolytic enzymes (trypsin, papain, pronase) eliminated both effector-target binding and cytolysis. These two functions were shown to regenerate concomitantly over a 4-hr period and could be blocked by the protein synthesis inhibitor, cycloheximide. Furthermore, treatment of nontrypsinized cells for 18 hr with concentrations of puromycin or cycloheximide inhibitory to cellular protein synthesis also impeded these two events. It thus appears that the NK-RR is a *de novo* synthesized cell surface protein with a turnover rate similar to that of other plasma membrane proteins.

Earlier reports had implicated a lectin-like mechanism in NK-target cell recognition, owing to the ability of simple sugars to inhibit both murine[17] and human NK cytotoxicity.[18] However, the delineation of the NK cytolytic mechanism into discrete stages, determined by calcium pulsing,[13] has provided compelling evidence that various simple sugars and their phosphorylated derivatives may specifically impede a postbinding lytic step.[19,20] Nonetheless, the role of saccharides in tumor cell recognition cannot be excluded, since one report has clearly demonstrated that (1) mutations conferring resistance to the lectin Concanavalin A (Con A) in Chinese Hamster Ovary (CHO) cells led to a parallel increase in NK cell binding and susceptibility to NK-mediated cytolysis, while (2) inhibitors of lipid-linked oligosaccharide assembly, tunicamycin and 2-deoxyglucose, impaired NK binding and cytolysis of CHO cells.[21] Thus, alterations in the expression of asparagine-linked oligosaccharides are critical in the CHO system of NK-target interaction. In the human system, N-acetylglucosamine and B-gentibiose also inhibited NK binding to some extent.[20] Regardless of their nature, the distribution of NK-RR in the population has also been examined at the clonal level.

Cloned human cell lines displaying NK activity are phenotypically and functionally heterogeneous, as determined by the unique expression of cell surface markers and pattern of reactivity of different clones against a panel of human tumor lines and virally transformed cells.[22] These results provide suggestive evidence for the clonal distribution of a family of NK-RR. A previous report had failed to establish such clonal segregation.[23] However, it appears likely that NK-RR are widely distributed among non-NK leukocytes, since nonlytic murine thymocytes and peritoneal macrophages can preferentially bind to NK-sensitive targets.[24] Furthermore, the NK-RR system appears to be coded for by genes linked to the H-2 complex[25] and such genes are distinct from those coding for T cell receptors.[26] The existence of two separate receptors or receptor families on the same cell, each specific for either T or NK cell functions can also be inferred from recent data provided by Brooks.[27] In this report, antigen-specific cytotoxic T cell clones could be reversibly induced to express NK reactivity analogous to that of splenic NK cells, following culture in high concentrations of interleukin-2 (IL-2) and interferon (IFN)-containing, Con A-activated spleen cell supernatants. This work has also led to the proposal that a proportion of NK cell activity found in the spleen or peripheral blood may be a function of the differentiation state of T cell subsets.

B. Target Cell Structures

TS has been more extensively studied.[28-30] Preincubation of nylon wool-enriched, murine NK cells with detergent-solubilized cell surface proteins of the YAC, T cell lymphoma, prevented subsequent binding to intact YAC target cells.[29] The material was shown to bind to Con A-Sepharose columns, and could be eluted with the specific sugar, suggesting that the TS may be glycosylated. SDS-PAGE analysis revealed the presence of three molecular species tentatively assigned molecular weights of 130, 160, and 240 $\pm$ 10^3 kdaltons. These molecules were distinct from Moloney cell surface antigens (MCSA, gp71, p30) and H-2 antigens and were absent from the surface of NK-insensitive target cells (P815, EL-4, A9HT, YWA). Furthermore, the NK-TS molecules selectively inhibited the binding of NK cells but not that of alloimmune cytotoxic T lymphocytes (CTL) to their respective targets. Additional cell lines lacking surface major histocompatibility complex products (F9, K-562) and Fc, C3, or sheep red blood cell receptors are equally susceptible to NK-mediated cytotoxicity, suggesting that none of these surface determinants serve as the target structure. Human NK-sensitive targets displayed a different array of surface proteins from that of mouse NK-sensitive lines.[28] Obexer et al.[30] have isolated three K-562-derived membrane protein fractions of 200, 120, and 80 kdaltons capable of inhibiting binding of large granular lymphocytes (LGL) to K-562 targets. Two of these molecular species (120 and 80 kdaltons) were also present on other NK-sensitive tumor lines (HL-60, Molt-4), but absent from the NK-resistant target, Reh-6. This study also showed preferential binding of the 80 kdalton surface protein from all three NK-sensitive lines to LGL-enriched lymphocyte populations. Indirect techniques for assessing the NK-TS have also been employed.

Various absorption techniques, whereby NK-enriched populations were depleted on target cell monolayers and subsequently analyzed for their pattern of reactivity against a panel of target cells, have provided suggestive evidence for the existance of multiple target specificities.[31,32] Some of the target structures were shared among all cell lines, whereas others were unique to a given group of targets. The existance of multiple NK-TS has been inferred from other laboratories using interaction analysis,[33] cold target competition assays,[34,35] monolayer adsorptions,[32] and SDS-PAGE fractionated membrane glycoproteins.[29,30]

The widespread occurrence of some common TS among different lines had led to the suggestion that NK-TS represent either (1) highly conserved derepressed fetal or embryonic antigens or (2) differentiation antigens. In some targets, the NK-TS appears to represent immature antigens that are lost upon differentiation. For instance, normal immature thymocytes from neonates[36,37] and bone marrow cells[38] are sensitive to lysis by NK cells. Rapidly proliferating hemopoietic elements from lethally irradiated, bone marrow-reconstituted CBA mice serve as strong cold target competitors in the NK assay.[39] Furthermore, the competitive ability of early regenerating marrow correlates very well with the occurrence of high frequencies of immature cell types of various lineages. There exists an inverse correlation between the NK sensitivity of fetal fibroblasts and the donor age of the fetus.[40] Adult fibroblasts are generally NK-resistant. These findings clearly indicate that TS expression may not always be a consequence of malignant transformation, although such expression may be augmented in tumor targets which are often more sensitive to cytolysis.

C. Differentiation of Target Cells

In murine tumor cell models, undifferentiated embryonal carcinoma cells were highly susceptible to NK cytolysis, whereas their more differentiated endodermal progeny were NK-resistant.[41] In several human tumor cell lines (K-562, U-937, GM-86), an excellent correlation could be established between induction of differentiation and development of NK resistance.[42] These results have been confirmed and extended with differentiation-induced K-562 and HL-60.[43-45] Werkmeister et al.[43] observed (1) selectivity in the relative acquisition of NK resistance, since antibody-dependent cellular cytotoxicity (ADCC), anomalous killing, and monocyte-mediated lysis were not different from that detected in untreated cultures, and (2) a concomitant decrease in TS expression, as assessed by decreased binding ability and cold-target inhibitory capacity. On the other hand, theophylline-induced human melanoma cells (MeWo) were enhanced in NK sensitivity rather than decreased following differentiation.[46] The changes leading to TS modulation during differentiation are poorly understood events. Analysis of several TS-deficient tumor cell variants in the mouse has revealed an inverse correlation between the amount of cell surface sialic acid and NK sensitivity, whereas a positive correlation could be detected between surface asialo-GM2 content and NK sensitivity in two independent reports.[47-50] More recent work by Werkmeister et al.[51] has indicated that decreased TS expression may be secondary to other events in butyrate-induced K-562 clones. An increase in neuraminidase-accessible cell surface sialic acid concomitant with augmented sialotransferase activity in such clones may also contribute to the development of NK resistance. These results raise the possibility that surface sialic acid may mask TS expression. Further work is needed to substantiate the roles of asialo-GM2 and other gangliosides in NK sensitivity.

D. Transferrin Receptors

The transferrin (tf) receptor has recently been proposed as a possible candidate for the TS involved in human NK-target cell recognition.[52] Since NK-sensitive targets encompass rapidly proliferating cell types such as hemopoietic precursors, immature thymocytes, and various tumor cell lines, and since tf receptor expression is directly correlated with the proliferation rate of a cell population,[53,54] one could predict a direct correlation between tf receptor density and NK sensitivity. This study has demonstrated the following: (1) tumor cell lines expressing little or no OKT9-positive cells (monoclonal antibody [MoAb] to the tf receptor) were largely NK-resistant, whereas those which bore the receptor were either sensitive or resistant, indicating the multigenic nature of NK sensitivity; (2) tf receptor-positive tumor lines were very efficient cold-target competitors, and (3) NK cell recognition could be partially inhibited with a trypsin-generated 70,000 mol wt fragment of the tf receptor. Thus, tf receptor recognition may well function as a primary regulatory mechanism of normal hemopoiesis, whereas immunosurveillance against tumor growth and dissemination is perhaps only a consequence of this primary role.

E. Viral Glycoproteins

In the case of certain virally infected target-target cells (HSV-1, HSV-2, EBV), NK recognition may be intimately linked to the expression of viral glycoproteins on the plasma membrane of such infected targets.[55-57] Cells normally resistant to NK cytolysis can be rendered NK-sensitive following infection with HSV-1,[55,58] or a substrain of Epstein-Barr virus.[56] Inhibition of viral protein synthesis during infection prevented normal development of NK susceptibility, and HSV-1 infected lines rendered deficient in the ability to produce glycoprotein C, B, or both, were impaired in their ability to act as cold target inhibitors and in their susceptibility to cytolysis.

F. Genetic Factors

Genetic factors regulating the expression of NK-TS have also been investigated. A somatic cell hybrid between NK-sensitive and -resistant murine tumor lines (YAC-IR/A9HT) did not express NK-TS and consequently failed to bind or be lysed by nylon wool-enriched mouse NK cells.[28] Other murine intraspecies hybrids of high NK/low NK combinations demonstrated a similar pattern of NK resistance.[59] Since alloantigens are normally codominantly expressed in somatic hybrids, while differentiation markers are suppressed, such findings have led to the proposal that NK sensitivity is under regulatory mechanisms governing differentiation. The NK-insensitive phenotype was not a general phenomenon, since hybrids resulting from the fusion of human NK-sensitive (K-562) with NK-resistant (P3H-R1) lines yielded hybrids with intermediate sensitivity.[59] More recent work has attempted to focus on the mechanism of NK resistance in murine somatic hybrids.[60] Somatic fusion of (1) NK-sensitive TS^+ with NK-resistant TS^+ tumor targets, (2) NK-sensitive TS^+ with NK-resistant TS^- targets, or (3) NK-resistant TS^+ with NK-resistant TS^- targets generated hybrids that were NK-resistant. The mechanism of resistance to NK cytolysis was not due to a failure to express surface NK-TS determinants, as assessed by cold target inhibition of YAC-1 tumor cells. In fact, NK recognition determinants were found to be dominantly expressed on all hybrids. Rather, failure of the hybrids to be lysed by NK cells was shown to be a consequence of the dominant expression of a protein synthesis-independent, postrecognition mechanism.[60] These findings clearly illustrate that although TS expression is a necessary step in the NK cytolytic reaction, surface expression of NK-TS does not solely provide the ability of a given cell line to express the NK-sensitive phenotype. Other postbinding counterlytic mechanisms may render target cells NK-resistant.

III. TRIGGERING AND ACTIVATION OF THE NK EFFECTOR CELLS

A. Do Oxygen Intermediates Play a Role?

The release of oxygen intermediates from human LGL is one of the earliest events which are known to occur after binding of NK cells and target cells.[61] Using chemiluminescence and cytochrome C reduction, oxygen intermediates were detected as early as 30 sec after incubation of effector with NK-sensitive (K-562) but not NK-insensitive targets (P815). Low NK responders produced less chemiluminescence than high NK responders and the HNK-1$^+$ cells were thought to be responsible for this chemiluminescence reaction. Following our initial report, we[62] and others,[63] found that not only HNK-1$^+$ NK cells but also Mo2$^+$ monocytes are essential for this reaction since (1) treatment of Percoll-enriched LGL populations with anti-Mo2 and complement abrogates chemiluminescence and (2) passage of peripheral blood lymphocytes over nylon wool prior to Percoll fractionation also decreases chemiluminescence by 80 to 90%. Monocytes alone at low concentrations do not respond to NK-sensitive targets but synergize with NK cells in the chemiluminescence response. We do not know yet which cell type actually produces the oxygen intermediates. In any event, the radicals generating chemiluminescence may not be essential for cytolysis since chronic granulomatous disease patients have normal NK cytolysis but fail to generate any detectable chemiluminescence.[62,64] In normal donors, on the other hand, hydroxyl scavengers block NK cytolysis in direct proportion to their chemical reaction constants.[65,66] Therefore, further studies are in order to resolve these issues.

B. Transmembranous Glycoprotein

The suggestion that the state of the lipid bilayer and the organization of cytoskeleton are crucially important for NK-cytolysis was originally based on pharmacological inhibitor experiments.[15,67] It was found that (1) pretreatment of murine effector cells with respiratory inhibitors such as DNP and NaN3 markedly inhibited NK cytolysis; (2) pretreatment of murine effector cells with iodoacetate, an inhibitor of the glycolytic pathway, also inhibited NK cytolysis and therefore, the energy necessary for cytolysis may be derived from both glycolysis and oxidative phosphorylation; (3) dimethyl-sulfoxide (DMSO), a dipolar solvent and a free radical scavenger, inhibited both binding and lysis of YAC targets by murine effector cells; (4) Cytochalasin B, a microtubule disruptor, also inhibited NK-cytolysis. These events are superficially quite similar to the activation of T cells by plant lectins. Some of the actual triggering molecules on the NK cell have also been uncovered.

LY5 and T-200 are T cell-associated antigens which are found on murine NK cells[68-72] and various hematopoietic cells.[69] T-200 antigen is a transmembranous glycoprotein which is composed of two domains. The first domain is protease-resistant and exposed to the cell surface. The other domain faces inward on the cytoplasmic side of the plasma membrane and has a phosphoserine residue.[73] MoAb (13.1) directed against this T-200/Ly5.1 antigen blocked NK cytolysis.[74,75] By using the Ca^{++} pulse technique, it was found that antibody 13.1 blocked the phase after binding and before the calcium-dependent step.[14] Therefore, T-200 may be involved in the calcium-independent triggering stage, prior to calcium-dependent programming for lysis. A chymotrypsin-like protease inhibitor, tosylphenylalanyl chloromethylketone (TPCK), is known to block this triggering stage of NK cytolysis.[76]

The relationship between effector-target binding and the triggering stage of NK cytolysis is obscure, but two interesting results have recently been obtained using the F2.5 MoAb which recognizes the human antigen equivalent to murine T-200. This antibody blocked NK cytolysis against K-562 tumor cells with no influence on influenza virus-specific CTL-cytolysis.[77] Binding of NK and K-562 cells was also reduced (35%). This suggests that the NK RR and the triggering structure are closely related. The other report showed that nonlytic conjugates of human LGL and Raji cells changed into lytic conjugates by addition of antitarget antibody or Con A without any change in frequency of originally cytolytic conjugates.[78] This result shows us that bound and nonlytic NK-target conjugates need appropriate triggering signals before proceeding on to NK cytolysis. T-200 is the best candidate to date which connects the binding and triggering phase in NK cytolysis.

C. Phospholipid Methylation

There are two kinds of methyl transferases which catalyze methylation of phosphatidylethanolamine (PE) in the cytoplasmic membrane, and these enzymatic activities are important in activating cellular function. When the substrate of these enzymes, PE, is catalyzed into its intermediate product, monomethylphosphatidylethanolamine (MPE), it becomes depressed into the membrane and increases membrane fluidity.[79] In the human NK cytolytic reaction, uptake of 1-methyl-^{3}H-methionine into phospholipid was increased compared to controls with no targets added. On the other hand, pretreatment of Percoll-enriched human LGL with the methyl transferase inhibitor 3-deazaadenosine remarkably inhibited NK cytolysis of K-562.[80] This suggests that methylation of phospholipid is required in NK cytolysis. Using the Ca^{++} pulse technique and 5′-deoxyisobutylthio-3′-deazaadenosine (deaza-SIBA), an inhibitor of transmethylation, it was shown that transmethylation may be involved in the triggering stage before Ca^{++}-dependent programming for lysis.[76]

D. Calcium and Calmodulin

Calcium is required in cytolysis mediated by NK cells,[81] ADCC, alloreactive CTL,[82] and anomalous killer cells generated in mixed lymphocyte culture (MLC). However, the site of action of Ca^{++} in NK cytolysis is poorly understood. It could be involved with calmodulin in the regulating of Ca^{++}-ATPase activity associated with phospholipid methylation in cell membranes.[83] Calmodulin is a major intracellular, calcium-binding-protein of 148 amino acids in length. It can modulate various enzymatic activities including Ca^{++}/Mg^{++} ATPase, myosin light chain kinase, cyclic nucleotide phosphodiesterase, and many others. Calmodulin inhibitors such as trifluoperazine, naphthalene sulfonamides or fluphenazine (FP) all inhibited NK cytolysis.[76,84,85] Binding of FP pretreated CBA effector cells to YAC-1 cells was also inhibited from 20 to 60% ($p < 0.02$). Therefore, calmodulin may be involved in the very early stages of the NK cytolytic pathway. Calmodulin-dependent lysis was not NK-specific. T lymphocytes, derived from both MLC and by Con A stimulation, also revealed depressed cytolytic activity against P815 tumor targets after FP treatment. Tumoricidal activity by activated macrophages and ADCC activities were also inhibited.[85]

E. Cyclic Nucleotides

Cyclic nucleotides are the second messengers which were first expected to be involved in the triggering of NK cytolysis.[86] Pretreatment of nylon wool column-passed spleen cells from CBA mice with prostaglandin E_1 (PGE_1), an activator of adenylate cyclase; theophylline, an inhibitor of phosphodiesterase activity and dibutyryl cAMP itself, significantly inhibited NK cytolysis, whereas binding of NK cells to the target was not affected. In contrast to the inhibitory effects of cAMP elevating agents, dB-cGMP and carbamylcholine caused a significant acceleration in the rate of lysis and could compete with inhibitor doses of dB-cAMP to reduce the level of suppression. Similar results have been reported in the human system.[87] Therefore, the cAMP/cGMP ratio was thought to be important in regulating NK cytolysis.

F. Lysosomal Enzymes

The lysosomal enzyme inhibitor, chloroquine, inhibited the lytic phase of NK cytolysis when either murine[67] or human effectors[76] were pretreated. In addition, lysosome-defective, beige,[8] and other mutants[88] were deficient in NK lytic function, although some lysosomal mutants were shown to have normal NK function.[89] These results suggest that some lysosomal constitutents may be important in NK cytolysis.

IV. THE LETHAL HIT

A. Secretion and Degranulation

Monensin is a carboxylic acid ionophore which interrupts the vesicular traffic of Golgi-derived vacuoles to the cell surface. This reagent caused an accumulation of cytoplasmic vesicles in LGLs and inhibited NK cytolysis.[90] Therefore, Golgi-derived products may be carried to the NK cell surface for delivery to target cells. The relationship between these vesicles and the characteristic NK granules is not known. However, after a 1 hr incubation of effector and target cells, NK cell granules gathered at the contact site and NK cell microvilli appeared to be pushed into cytoplasmic pouches of the target cell.[91] It is interesting to note that all of the human T cell-derived clones including NK, ADCC, and allospecific killers, have granules, whereas noncytotoxic ones do not.[92] This relationship does not hold up in the mouse, where noncytolytic clones are often granulated as well.[93] Further evidence that secretion may be important can be summarized as follows: (1) pretreatment of LGL with Sr^{2+} led to degranulation and a concomitant loss of cytolytic activity;[94] (2) a calcium flux across the membrane is necessary for both cytolysis and secretion as shown by inhibition with verapamil,[13,42,95] a Ca^{2+} channel blocker; (3) reagents which inhibit cytolysis (cAMP, PGE1, theophylline, histamine)[86] also block lysosome secretion in other cells[96] at the same concentrations, and, conversely, agents which increase lysosomal discharge ([cGMP], carbamylcholine) augment NK cytolysis;[86,87] (4) secretion is energy dependent, and DNP and CCCP, uncouplers of oxidative phosphorylation, block both NK cytolysis[15] and secretion; and (5) Chediak-Higashi (CH) patients and beige mice carry a recessive mutation which selectively impairs both the lethal hit stage of NK-mediated cytolysis[8,9] and the secretion of lysosomal enzymes in the kidney and into the phagolysosome of leukocytes.[97] In addition, the secretion of plasminogen activator, a neutral serine protease, from CH LGL was impaired.[98] Since HNK-1^+ LGL from CH patients have a single giant granule rather than many small granules,[99] it is likely that lack of secretion may also explain this genetic NK insufficiency. Neither monocytes nor T cells from these patients exhibited giant granules, and both effector-cell types had normal cytolytic function.[9] It seems likely, therefore, that the giant granules in NK may be linked to the functional defect in CH patients.

B. The Lytic Moiety

At least three possible candidates for the lytic moiety in NK cytolysis have been proposed. Lysosomal protease was the first suggestion since serine esterase inhibitors (phenylmethylsulfonylfluoride, diisofluorophosphate) blocked NK cytolysis.[15] Later studies using more specific inhibitors revealed that this was an early rather than late event in NK cytolysis.[76] Lysophosphatidylcholine, a detergent-like product of phospholipid metabolism was also proposed as the lytic moiety since inhibitors of phospholipase A_2, (tetracaine, mepacrine, Rosenthal's inhibitor, corticosteroid) blocked NK cytolysis.[80] A more specific and naturally occurring phospholipase A_2, C, D, inhibitor, lipimodulin, also blocked postbinding NK cytolysis.[100] The third suggestion was that a specific lytic molecule was released from NK cells and bound to specific acceptor sites on the target cell membrane.[2,101] The first evidence in support of this hypothesis was demonstrated by Wright and Bonavida.[102] Using a miniaturized Marbrook system, they observed that murine or human lymphocytes stimulated with phytohaemagglutinin (PHA) or Con A released a factor which lysed NK-sensitive targets. The factor was termed natural killer cytotoxic factor (NKCF) and could also be induced by coculturing effector and target cells for approximately 24 to 48 hr.[103] Some NKCF is produced by unstimulated cultures of human peripheral mononuclear cells but lectin or NK-sensitive target cells enhanced this NKCF production.[104] In the murine system, NKCF-producing cells were Thy-1,2-negative, asialo-GM_1-positive. Spleen cells from nu/nu produced high levels of NKCE, whereas bg/bg produced very low levels.[103] Similarly, in the human system fractions highly enriched for NK cells by Percoll fractionation synthesized high levels of NKCF.[105] The target specificity of NKCF closely paralleled that of NK cells as determined in screening panels of NK-sensitive and -resistant targets. The YAC-R clone, selected for resistance to NKCF, was also resistant to cytolysis mediated by NK cells.[106]

The mechanism of NKCF production is not well understood. Serine-dependent protease is though to play some role in release or the activation of production of this factor since 1×10^{-6} M 1-1-tosylamide-2-phenylethylchloromethyl ketone (TPCK) and 5×10^{-4} *M* acetyl-L-tyrosineethylester (ATEE) blocked NKCF production from murine spleen cells.[107] One of the problems to be solved in the future is the biochemical sturcture of NKCF. In this respect, it is interesting to note that a transplantable NK leukemia in F344 rats produced high levels of NKCF.[108] Preliminary studies have shown that 25 to 50 m*M* α-methyl-D-mannoside, D-galactose, or *N*-acetyl-D-galactosamine inhibit the lytic activity of NKCF, thereby suggesting that NKCF may be glycosylated and bind to lectin-like receptors on the tumor cell.[102]

C. The Acceptor Site for NKCF

Recent results with variants of the YAC cell line have led to the inference of an acceptor site on the target cell which binds to NKCF.[101] In general, there are two classes of YAC variants: those that possess target structures (TS^+) but lack acceptor sites (Acc^-) and those which lack both determinants. The third class (TS^-, Acc^+) has not yet been described. As shown in Table 1, both class 1 and 2 variants resist NK-mediated cytolysis, but are susceptible to lysis by other effector cells such as alloimmune CTL. The first YAC variant described, YAC-6-28, was obtained by mutagenesis and cloning.[101] This NK^R line bound to NK cells as measured in a conjugate assay or by its ability to compete with parental YAC cells in a ^{51}Cr-release assay. Since the line was recognized by NK cells, it was not surprising that NKCF was recovered in cocultivation experiments.[109] The fact that YAC-6-28 failed to deplete NKCF in absorption experiments confirmed that it lacked acceptor sites (Acc^-) for NKCF and this is the most plausible explanation of the basis of its resistance to NK-mediated cytotoxicity. An additional class I YAC variant, YAC-R15.1, was selected by Wright and Bonavida[106] by prolonged culture in the presence of NKCF.

Class 2 variants were selected by many cycles of exposure to NK cells in vitro followed by in vivo passage in NK-bearing mice.[47] NK^R variants of this type, such as YAC-Acc10, were not recognized by NK cells (TS^-) and therefore did not induce the production of NKCF when cocultured with NK cells.[109] In addition, YAC-Acc10 failed to absorb NKCF, and we assume therefore that it lacks acceptor sites (Acc^-). The nature of the acceptor for NKCF is not known, but preliminary results show that (1) pretreatment of targets with phosphorylated sugars had no effect on NKCF binding to target cells; (2) interference of target cell glycosylation with tunicamycin inhibited NKCF binding.[104] Therefore, carbohydrate in the acceptor site is thought to play some role in NKCF binding.

Table 1
TWO CLASSES OF YAC VARIANTS

	YAC parent	Class 1		Class 2
		YAC-6-28[a]	YAC-R15.1[b]	YAC-Acc10[c]
NK cytolysis	+	−	−	−
CTL cytolysis	+	+	+	+
NK conjugates	+	+	+	−
NK competition	+	+	ND	−
Induce NKCF	+	+	+	−
Absorb NKCF	+	−	−	−
NKCF lysis	+	−	−	−
Phenotype	TS^+ Acc^+	TS^+ Acc^-	TS^+ Acc^-	TS^- Acc^-

[a] Data from Reference 101.
[b] Data from Reference 106.
[c] Data from Reference 47.

V. TARGET CELL DEATH

A. Membrane Lesions

Recent electron microscopic observations have revealed membrane lesions on target cell membranes after NK-target cell interaction.[110,111] When an NK clone and YAC-1 cells were coincubated, two types of membrane lesions were detected, type 1 (T1) membrane lesions with inner diameters of 16 ± 2 nm, outer diameters of 26 ± 2 nm and type 2 (T2) membrane lesions with inner diameters of 6 to 7 nm. The number of these two types of lesions were increased in proportion to the increase of NK cytolytic activity assessed from ^{51}Cr-release assays. Detergent extraction of membranes revealed that these two types of target membrane lesions were formed by insertion of tubular complexes. Similar complexes could be seen when NK cells were incubated with erythrocytes in the presence of Con A. Therefore, T_1 and T_2 were thought to be NK-cell products. At high magnification, axially sectioned T1 appeared to form a 15 nm wide transmembrane channel at its binding site. It is hypothesized that vesicles from NK cells are associated with proteins (perforins), and capable of polymerizing into tubular complexes (polyperforins) of T1 and T2 on tumor cell surfaces and these subsequently lead to the death of the tumor cell. It is not known, however, if target cell death results from colloid osmosis or if it resembles internal disintegration (apoptosis).[112,113]

VI. RECYCLING

When an effector cell lyses, a sensitive target cell is detached from it and initiates killing of another target. This recycling phenomenon was demonstrated for NK cells by Ullberg and Jondal[114] using a combination of a single cell cytotoxicity assay in agarose[115] with estimations of the maximal NK potential (V_{max} from enzymatic kinetic analysis) derived from ^{51}Cr-release assays.[116] Approximately 10% of nylon wool-passed human peripheral lymphocytes had the ability to bind to NK-sensitive targets.[114] Of these, some 50% would normally go on to kill T cell targets (Molt-4 and 1301) and some 20% would kill K-562. Estimated number of killed target cells by a single effector cell, i.e., the maximal recycling capacity in the 3 hr test period was calculated as follows: 2.8 (Molt-4), 1.4 (1301), and 3.8 (K-562). Human leukocyte IFN augmentation of NK cytolysis against K-562 target cells was due to recruitment of new effector cells and recycling.[117] On the other hand, Sr^{++}, a cation known to cause degranulation of granulocytes, inhibited NK activity. The recovery of NK-CMC (cell-mediated cytotoxicity) after treatment of this cation was also shown to result from the reactivation of NK cells rather than recruitment of new effectors.[94] The mechanisms of detachment from lysed targets and reactivation are as yet unknown.

VII. PARTICIPATION OF SACCHARIDES IN NK CYTOLYSIS

As was discussed earlier in this chapter, some monosaccharides (D-mannose, D-galactose, *N*-acetylglucosamine, D-glucose) inhibited murine NK activity.[17] Phosphorylated sugars (mannose-6-phosphate, fructose-1 and 6-phosphate) were more potent inhibitors in the human NK system.[18,20] These results suggest that a lectin-like substance may play a role in the NK cytolytic pathway. There are two examples of animal lectins which could serve as models. One known as galactose binding protein was isolated from mammalian liver acetone powder.[118] This lectin is an endogenous receptor of liver cells and binds to circulating asialoglycoprotein via galactose or *N*-acetylgalactosamine. The ligand (asialoglycoprotein) is endocytosed via liver cell surface structures, termed "Coated Pits".[119]

Another well-known animal lectin is the fibroblast lysosomal enzyme assimilation apparatus. Lysosomal enzyme-derived mannose-6-phosphate or fucose-6-phosphate is recognized by this lectin and bound ligand is endocytosed into the fibroblast from the extracellular environment.[120] The inhibition of NK cytolysis by various simple sugars suggested that lectin-like structures were present on either the effector cell or target cell surface. Using penta-mannose attached to the seed lectin, Gelonin, Forbes et al.[18] demonstrated binding sites for mannose-6-phosphate on F-265 cells and K-562 cells. However, the relationship of this binding site to the acceptor site for NKCF is unknown and a clear demonstration of lectin-like receptors which mediate NK cytolysis has not yet been made.

The genetic regulation of NK cytolysis via simple sugars has recently been approached by Gorczynski and co-workers[121] using a spleen fragment culture system adapted to statistical analysis. In this study, a variety of monosaccharides were found to inhibit NK activity of B10 mice, with no apparent effect on B10 anti-B10-D2 allospecific cytotoxic T cell activity. Sugar inhibition patterns were subsequently compared among different congenic strains and showed a poor correlation between B10 and B10-D10 ($r = 0.49$, $p > 0.05$), but a very high correlation between the F_1 hybrid with either parental strains (B10: $r = 0.84$; B10.D2: $r = 0.88$). From this data, it was concluded that genes regulating carbohydrate recognition involved in NK cytolysis are inherited and expressed codominantly.

VIII. SUMMARY

NK cells are clearly important in host defense and homeostatic regulation. Our current view of the NK cytolytic pathway is summarized in the stimulus secretion model shown in Figure 1. The TS glycoprotein has been isolated and described[28,29] and the NK receptor is known to be a *de novo* synthesized protein.[15] Step 1 involves a Mg^{2+}-dependent, calmodulin-controlled contact between the target and effector.[13,85] Step 2: following the interaction, four necessary events are triggered including the generation of O_2,[61] an influx of Ca^{2+},[13] the transmethylation of membrane phospholipids, and the activation of phospholipase A_2 (PL-A_2).[80] Step 3: secretion of NK-lymphotoxin begins by an energy dependent process.[15] Step 4: the lytic molecules have been isolated[103] and may bind to acceptor sites on the target membrane and thereby deliver the lethal hit.[108,109] Target cell death is thought to result from colloid osmotic lysis which occurs due to the insertion of channel-forming proteins in the target cell membrane.[110] Neutral

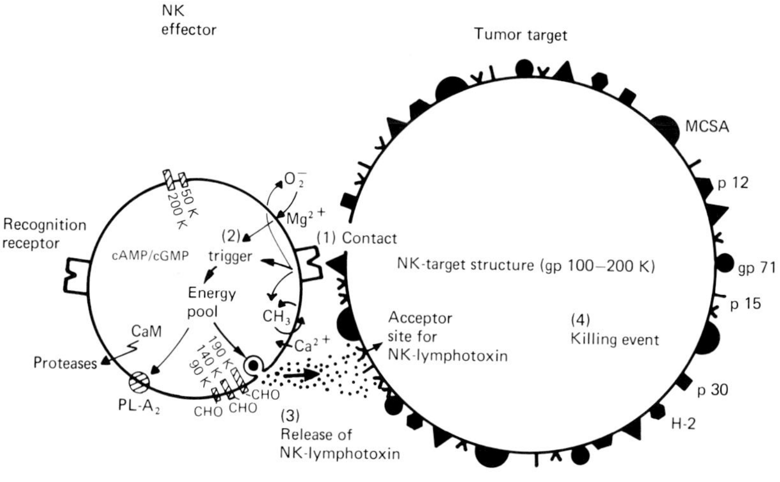

FIGURE 1. Stimulus-secretion model of NK cytolysis. The YAC tumor cell expresses a number of antigens at the cell surface including the retrovirus proteins p12, p15, p30, gp71, and Moloney cell surface antigen (MCSA); class I major histocompatibility complex encoded glycoproteins (H-2) and a glycoprotein recognized by natural killer (NK) cells, referred to as NK-TS. The existence of an acceptor site for NK cytotoxic factor, referred to as NK lymphotoxin, is inferred from data with NK-TS$^+$ mutants which resist NK cytolysis. The four steps which occur at the NK effector level include (1) recognition of a tumor cell, (2) triggering, (3) stimulation of lymphotoxin release, and (4) target cell destruction. The generation of oxygen radicals such as O_2^-, or more importantly, OH^-; the transmethylation of membrane phospholipids (CH_3); the influx of calcium, and the role of calmodulin (CaM), phospholipase-A_2 (PL-A_2), cyclic AMP/cyclic GMP ratios, energy metabolism, and the role of other surface proteins (50 K, 200 K; 90 K, 140 K, 190K) including the NK recognition receptor, are discussed in the summary.

serine proteases are also released[98] and seem to be necessary to NK cytolysis[67,98] but there is no evidence yet to show that this event is stimulus-coupled. Antibodies against 190, 140, and 90K effector cell glycoproteins block the lethal hit stage[122] and it is therefore presumed that these molecules lie in close proximity to the secretory vesicles. MoAb against 200K and 50K effector cell proteins also block cytolysis.[14,75] While great strides have been made, more work is clearly necessary before we fully understand the biochemical and genetic aspects underlying NK cytolysis.

Note Added in Proof

Three recent findings have shown that:

1. Murine NK cells rearrange and express the B chain gene of the T cell receptor (Yanagi et al., *Nature,* 314, 631, 1985).
2. A mannosidase-sensitive triggering structure on NK cells is coupled to transmethylation of membrane phospholipids (Kiyohara et al., *J. Immunol.,* 135, 659, 1985).
3. Tumor cell susceptibility to NK cytolysis is coded by two separate genetic elements (Lauzon and Roder, *Cell. Immunol.,* 94, 85, 1985).

REFERENCES

1. Roder, J. C. and Haliotis, T., Do NK cells play a role in anti-tumor surveillance?, *Immunol. Today,* 8, 96, 1980.
2. Roder, J. C., Kärre, K., and Kiessling, R., Natural killer cells, *Prog. Allerg.* 28, 66, 1981.
3. Roder, J. C. and Pross, H. F., The biology of the human natural killer cell, *J. Clin. Immunol.,* 2, 249, 1982.
4. Hanna, N., Natural killer cell-mediated inhibition of tumor metastasis in vivo, *Surv. Synth. Pathol. Res.,* 2, 68, 1983.
5. Abruzzo, L. V. and Rowley, D. A., Homeostasis of the antibody response: immuneregulation by NK cells, *Science,* 222, 581, 1983.
6. Talmadge, J. E., Meyers, K. M., Prieur, D. J., and Starkey, S. R., Role of natural killer cells in tumor growth and metastasis in beige mice, *Nature,* 284, 622, 1980.
7. Kärre, K., Klein, G. O., Kiessling, R., Klein, G., and Roder, J. C., Low natural *in vivo* resistance to syngeneic leukemias in natural killer-deficient mice, *Nature,* 284, 624, 1980.
8. Roder, J. C. and Duwe, A., The beige mutation in the mouse selectively impairs natural killer cell function, *Nature,* 278, 451, 1979.
9. Roder, J. C., Haliotis, T., Klein, M., Korec, S., Jett, J., Ortaldo, J., Herberman, R. B., Katz, P., and Fauci, A. S., A new immunodeficiency disorder in humans involving NK cells, *Nature,* 284, 553, 1980.
10. Warner, J. F. and Dennert, G., Effects of a cloned cell line with NK activity on bone marrow transplants, tumor development and metastasis in vivo, *Nature,* 300, 31, 1982.
11. Haliotis, T., Ball, J. K., Dexter, D., and Roder, J. C., Spontaneous tumors and induced primary oncogenesis in NK deficient beige mice, *Int. J. Cancer,* 35, 505, 1985.
12. Roder, J. C. and Lauzon, R., THe mechanism of NK cell cytotoxicity, *Surv. Synth. Pathol. Res.,* 2 (5), 82, 1983.
13. Hiserodt, J., Britvan, L. J., and Targan, S. R., Characterization of the cytolytic reaction mechanism of the human natural killer (NK) lymphocytes. Resolution into binding, programming and killer cell-independent steps, *J. Immunol.,* 129, 1782, 1982.
14. Targan, S. R. and Newman, W., A definition of a "trigger" stage in the NK cytolytic reaction sequence by a monoclonal antibody to the glycoprotein T-200, *J. Immunol.,* 131, 1149, 1983.
15. Roder, J. C., Kiessling, R., Biberfield, P., and Anderson, B., Target-effector interaction in the natural killer (NK) cell system. II. The isolation of NK cells and studies on the mechanism of killing, *J. Immunol.,* 121, 2509, 1978.
16. Kay, D. H., Bonnard, G. D., West, H. W., and Herberman, R. B., A functional comparison of human Fc-receptor-bearing lymphocytes active in natural cytotoxicity and antibody-dependent cellular cytotoxicity, *J. Immunol.,* 118, 2058, 1977.
17. Stutman, O., Dien, P., Wisun, R., and Lattime, E., Natural cytotoxic cells against solid tumors in mice: blocking of cytotoxicity by D-mannose, *Proc. Natl. Acad. Sci. U.S.A.,* 77, 2895, 1980.
18. Forbes, J. T., Bretthauer, R. R., and Oeltmann, T. N., Mannose-6-fructose and fructose-6-phosphates inhibit human natural cell-mediated cytotoxicity, *Proc. Natl. Acad. Sci. U.S.A.,* 78, 5797, 1981.
19. Vose, B. M., Harding, M., White, W., Moore, M., and Gallagher, J., Effect of simple sugars on natural killing: evidence against the involvement of a lectin-like mechanism in target recognition, *Clin. Exp. Immunol.,* 51, 517, 1983.
20. Werkmeister, J., Roder, J. C., Curry, C., and Pross, H. F., The effect of unphosphorylated and phosphorylated sugar moieties on human and mouse natural killer cell activity: is there selective inhibition at the level of target recognition and lytic acceptor site?, *Cell Immunol.,* 80, 172, 1983.
21. Pohajdak, B., Wright, J. A., and Greenberg, A. J., An oligosaccharide biosynthetic defect in concanavalin A resistant Chinese hamster ovary (CHO) cells that enhances NK reactivity in vitro and in vivo, *J. Immunol.,* 133, 2423, 1984.
22. Hercend, T. et al., Phenotypic and functional heterogeneity of human cloned natural killer cell lines, *Nature,* 301, 158, 1983.
23. Dennert, G., Yogeeswaran, G., and Yamageta, S., Cloned cell lines with natural killer activity. Specificity, function and cell surface markers, *J. Exp. Med.,* 153, 545, 1981.
24. Piontek, G. E., Gronberg, A., Ahrlund-Richter, L., and Kiessling, R., NK-patterned binding expressed by non-NK mouse leukocytes, *Int. J. Cancer,* 30, 225, 1982.
25. Roder, J. C. and Kiessling, R., Target-effector interaction in the natural killer cell system. I. Covariance and genetic control of cytolytic and target-cell-binding subpopulations in the mouse, *Scand. J. Immunol.,* 8, 135, 1978.
26. Binz, A., Fenner, M., Frei, D., and Wigzell, H., Two independent receptors allow selective target lysis by T cell clones, *J. Exp. Med.,* 157, 1252, 1983.

27. Brooks, C. G., Reversible induction of natural killer cell activity in cloned murine cytotoxic T lymphocytes, *Nature,* 305, 155, 1983.
28. Roder, J. C., Ahrlund-Richter, L., and Jondal, M., Target-effector interaction in the human and murine nature killer system. Specificity and xenogeneic reactivity of solubilized natural killer target structure complex and its loss in a somatic cell hybrid, *J. Exp. Med.,* 150, 471, 1979.
29. Roder, J. C., Rosen, A., Fenyo, E. M., and Troy, E. A., Target-effector interaction in the natural killer cell system. The isolation of target structures, *Proc. Natl. Acad. Sci., U.S.A.,* 76, 1405, 1979.
30. Obexer, G., Rumpold, H., and Kraft, D., Target-effector-cell interactions in the human natural killer (NK) system: isolation of target structures, *Immunobiology,* 165, 15, 1983.
31. Phillips, W. H., Ortaldo, J. R., and Herberman, R. B., Selective depletion of human natural killer cells on monolayers of target cells, *J. Immunol.,* 125, 2322, 1980.
32. Jensen, P. J. and Koren, H. S., Depletion of NK by cellular immunoadsorption, *J. Immunol.,* 123, 1127, 1979.
33. Takasugi, M., Akira, D., Takasugi, J., and Mickey, M., Specificities of human cell mediated cytotoxicity, *J. Natl. Cancer Inst.,* 59, 69, 1977.
34. Callewaert, D. M., Lightbody, J. J., Kaplan, J., Jaroszewski, J., Peterson, W. D., and Rosenberg, J. C., Spontaneous cytotoxicity of cultured human cell lines mediated by normal PBL. II. Specificity for target antigens, *Cell Immunol.,* 42, 103, 1979.
35. Hansson, M., Kärre, K., Bakas, T., Kiessling, R., and Klein, G., Intra- and interspecies reactivity of human and mouse natural killer (NK) cells, *J. Immunol.,* 121, 6, 1979.
36. Hansson, M., Kärre, K., Kiessling, R., Roder, J. C., Andersson, B., and Hayry, P., Natural NK cell targets in the mouse thymus: characteristics of the sensitive cell population, *J. Immunol.,* 123, 765, 1979.
37. Hansson, M., Kiessling, R., Anderson, B., Kärre, K., and Roder, J. C., NK-cell sensitive T-cell subpopulation in thymus: inverse correlation to host NK activity, *Nature,* 278, 174, 1979.
38. Mann, M. E., Herberman, R. B., and Holden, H. T., Natural cell-mediated cytotoxicity in mice against non-lymphoid tumor cells and some normal cells, *Int. J. Cancer,* 20, 381, 1977.
39. O'Brien, T., Nendra, J., Stephens, H., Knight, R., and Barrett, A. J., Recognition and regulation of progenitor marrow elements by NK cells in the mouse, *Immunology,* 49, 717, 1983.
40. Saksela, E., Timonen, T., Ranki, A., and Hayry, P., Morphological and functional characterization of isolated effector cells responsible for human natural killer activity to fetal fibroblasts and to cultured cell line targets, *Immunol. Rev.,* 44, 71, 1979.
41. Stern, P., Gidlund, M., Orn, A., and Wigzell, H., Natural killer cells mediate lysis of embryonal carcinoma cells lacking MHC, *Nature,* 285, 341, 1980.
42. Gidlund, M., Orn, A., Pattengale, P. K., Jansson, M., Wigzell, H., and Nilsson, K., Natural killer cells kill tumor cells at a given stage of differentiation, *Nature,* 292, 848, 1981.
43. Werkmeister, J. A., Helfand, S. L., Haliotis, T., Pross, H. F., and Roder, J. C., The effect of target cell differentiation of human natural killer cell activity. A specific defect in target cell binding and early activation events, *J. Immunol.,* 129, 413, 1982.
44. Garson, D., Dokhelar, M. C., Vainchenker, W., and Tursz, T., Protective effects of differentiation inducers on natural killer snesitivity of K562 cells. Analysis at a single-cell level, *Cell Immunol.,* 78, 400, 1983.
45. Dokhelar, M. C. et al., NK cell sensitivity of the leukemic K562 cells: effect of sodium butyrate and hemin inductin, *J. Immunol.,* 128, 211, 1982.
46. Werkmeister, J., Helfand, S., Haliotis, T., Rubin, P., Pross, H., and Roder, J., Tumor cell differentiation modulates susceptibility to natural killer cells, *Cell. Immunol.,* 69, 122, 1982.
47. Gronberg, A., Kiessling, R., Eriksson, E., and Hansson, M., Variants from a MLV-induced lymphoma selected for decreased sensitivity to NK lysis, *J. Immunol.,* 127, 1734, 1981.
48. Durdik, J. M., Beck, B. M., Clark, E. A., and Henney, C. S., Characterization of a lymphoma cell variant selectively resistant to natural killer cells, *J. Immunol.,* 125, 683, 1980.
49. Yogeeswaran, G., Gronberg, A., Hansson, M., Dalianis, T., Kiessling, R., And Welsh, R. M., Correlation of glycosphingolipids and sialic acid in YAC-1 lymphoma variants with their sensitivity to natural killer-cell-mediated lysis, *Int. J. Cancer,* 28, 517, 1981.
50. Young, W. W., Durdik, J. M., Urdal, D., Hakomori, S. I., and Henney, C. S., Glycolipid expression in lymphoma cell variants: chemical quantity, immunologic reactivity, and correlations with susceptibility to NK cells, *J. Immunol.,* 126, 1, 1981.
51. Werkmeister, J. A., Pross, H. F., and Roder, J. C., Modulation of K562 cells with sodium butyrate. Association of impaired NK susceptibility with sialic acid and analysis of other parameters, *Int. J. Cancer,* 32, 71, 1983.
52. Vodinelich, J., Sutherland, R., Schneider, C., Newman, R., and Greaves, M., The transferrin receptor may be a target structure for human natural killer cells, *Proc. Natl. Acad. Sci. U.S.A.,* 80, 835, 1983.

53. Trowbridge, I. S. and Omary, M. B., Human cell surface glycoprotein related to cell proliferation is the receptor for transferrin, *Proc. Natl. Acad. Sci. U.S.A.*, 78, 3039, 1981.
54. Sutherland, R., Delia, D., Schneider, C., Newman, R., Kemshead, J., and Greaves, M., Ubiquitous cell-surface glycoprotein on tumor cells is proliferation associated receptor for transferrin, *Proc. Natl. Acad. Sci. U.S.A.*, 78, 4515, 1981.
55. Abendroth Bishop, G., Gloriose, J. L., and Schwartz, S. A., Relationship between expression of herpes simplex virus glycoproteins and susceptibility of target cells to human natural killer activity, *J. Exp. Med.*, 157, 1544, 1983.
56. Blazar, B. A., Fitzgerald, J., Sutton, L., and Strome, M., Increased sensitivity to natural killing in Raji cells is due to effector recognition of molecules appearing on target cell membranes following EBV cycle induction, *Clin. Exp. Immunol.*, 54, 31, 1983.
57. Blazar, B., Patarroyo, M., Klein, E., and Klein, G., Increased sensitivity of human lymphoid lines to natural killer cells after induction of the Epstein-Barr viral cycle by superinfection on sodium butyrate, *J. Exp. Med.*, 151, 614, 1980.
58. Yasukawa, M. and Zarling, J. M., Autologous herpes simplex virus-infected cells are lysed by human natural killer cells, *J. Immunol.*, 131, 2011, 1983.
59. Ahrlund-Richter, L., Klein, E., and Masucci, C., Somatic hybrids between a high NK-sensitive lymphoid (YACIR) and several low sensitive sarcoma or L-cell-derived mouse lines exhibit low sensitivity, *Somatic Cell Genet.*, 6, 89, 1980.
60. Lin, Y., Collins, J. L., Potek, P. Q., and Cohn, M., An analysis of the sensitivity of somatic cells hybrids to natural killer cell and natural cytotoxic cell-mediated lysis, *J. Immunol.*, 131, 1154, 1983.
61. Roder, J. C., Helfand, S. L., Werkmeister, J., McGarry, R., Beaumont, T. J., and Duwe, A., Oxygen intermediates are triggered early in the cytolytic pathway of human NK cells, *Nature*, 298, 569, 1982.
62. Duwe, A. K., and Roder, J. C., Involvement of hydroxyl free radical, but not superoxide, in the cytolytic pathway of natural killer cells, Revision of an earlier hypothesis, *Medical Biology*, 62, 95, 1984.
63. Pohajdak, B., Gomez, J., Wilkins, J. A., and Greenberg, A. H., Tumor-activated NK cells trigger monocyte oxidative metabolism, *J. Immunol.*, 133, 2430, 1984.
64. Kay, H. D., Smith, D. L., Sullivan, G., Mandell, G. L., and Donovitz, G. R., Evidence for a non-oxidative mechanism of human natural killer (NK) cell cytotoxicity by using mononuclear effector cells from healthy donors and from patients with chronic granulomatous disease, *J. Immunol.*, 131, 1784, 1983.
65. Duwe, A. K., Werkmeister, J., Roder, J. C., Lauzon, R., and Payne, U., Natural killer cell-mediated lysis involves a hydroxyl radical-dependent step, *J. Immunol.*, 134, 2037, 1985.
66. Suthanthiran, M., Solomon, S. D., Williams, P. S., Rubin, A. L., Novogrodsky, A., and Stenzel, K., Hydroxyl radical scavengers inhibit human natural killer cell activity, *Nature*, 307, 276, 1984.
67. Roder, J. C., Arbov, S., Klein, M., Petersson, C., Kiessling, R., Andersson, K., and Hansson, M., Target-effector cell interaction in the natural killer cell system. V. Energy requirements, membrane integrity, and the possible involvement of lysosomal enzymes, *Immunology*, 40, 107, 1980.
68. Kasai, M., Leclerc, J. C., Shen, F. W., and Cantor, H., Identification of Ly5 on the surface of natural killer cells in normal and athymic inbred mouse strains, *Immunogenetics*, 8, 153, 1979.
69. Pollack, S. B., Tam, M. R., Nowinski, R. C., and Emmons, S. L., Presence of T cell-associated surface antigens on murine NK cells, *J. Immunol.*, 123, 1818, 1979.
70. Beaumont, T. J., Roder, J. C., Elliott, B. E., Kerbel, R. S., Dennis, J. W., Kasai, M., and Okumura, K., A comparative analysis of cell surface markers on murine NK cells and CTL target-effector conjugates, *Scand. J. Immunol.*, 16, 123, 1982.
71. Omary, M. B., Trowbridge, I. S., and Scheid, M. P., T200 cell surface glycoprotein of the mouse polymorphism defined by the Ly-5 system of alloantigens, *J. Exp. Med.*, 151, 1311, 1980.
72. Siadak, A. W. and Nowinski, R. C., Identification of Ly-5 and T200 antigens on identical cell surface proteins, *J. Immunol.*, 125, 1400, 1980.
73. Omary, M. B. and Trowbridge, I. S., Disposition of T200 glycoprotein in the plasma membrane of a murine lymphoma cell line, *J. Biol. Chem.*, 255, 1662, 1980.
74. Seaman, W. E., Talal, N., Herzenberg, L. A., Herzenberg, L. A., and Ledbetter, J. A., Surface antigens on mouse natural killer cells: use of monoclonal antibodies to inhibit or to enrich cytotoxic activity, *J. Immunol.*, 127, 982, 1981.
75. Newman, W., Selective blockade of human natural killer cells by a monoclonal antibody, *Proc. Natl. Acad. Sci. U.S.A.*, 79, 3858, 1982.
76. Quan, P. C., Ishizaka, T., and Bloom, B. R., Studies on the mechanism of NK cell lysis, *J. Immunol.*, 128, 1786, 1982.
77. Sparrow, R. L. and McKenzie, I. F. C., A function for human T200 in natural killer cytolysis, *Transplantation*, 36, 166, 1983.
78. Bradley, T. P., Timares Lebow, L., and Bonavida, B., Abst., NK Workshop, Kyoto, Japan, 1983.

79. Hirata, F. and Axelrod, J., Enzymatic methylation of phosphatidylethanolamine increases erythrocyte membrane fluidity, *Nature,* 275, 219, 1978.
80. Hoffman, T., Hirata, F., Bougnoux, P., Fraser, B. A., Goldfarb, R. J., Herberman, R. B., and Axelrod, J., Phospholipid methylation and phospholipase Az activation in cytotoxicity by human natural killer cells, *Proc. Natl. Acad. Sci. U.S.A.,* 78, 3839, 1981.
81. Argov, S., Poros, A., and Klein, E., Cation requirement of natural, in vitro generated and antibody-dependent killing exerted by human lymphocytes, *Immunobiology,* 156, 25, 1979.
82. Goldstein, P. and Smith, E. T., The lethal hit stage of mouse T and non-T cell-mediated cytolysis: difference in cation requirements and characterization of an analytical "cation pulse" method, *Eur. J. Immunol.,* 6, 31, 1976.
83. Strittmatter, W. J., Hirata, F., and Axelrod, J., Increased Ca^{++}-ATPase activity associated with methylation of phospholipids in human erythrocytes, *Biophys. Biochem. Res. Commun.,* 88, 147, 1979.
84. Moon, T. D., Morley, J. E., Vessella, R. L., and Lange, P. H., The role of calmodulin in human natural killer cell activity, *Scand. J. Immunol.,* 18, 255, 1983.
85. Laing, L. P., Boegman, R. J., and Roder, J. C., The inhibitory effect of phenothiazines on NK-mediated cytolysis of tumor cells, *J. Immunopharmacol.,* 8, 1, 1983.
86. Roder, J. C. and Klein, M., Target-effector interaction in the natural killer cell system. IV. Modulation by cyclic nucleotides, *J. Immunol.,* 123, 2785, 1979.
87. Katz, P., Zaytoun, A. M., and Fauci, A. S., Mechanisms of human cell-mediated cytotoxicity. I. Modulation of natural killer cell activity by cyclic nucleotides, *J. Immunol.,* 129, 287, 1982.
88. Orn, A., Hakansson, E. M., Gidlund, M., Ramstedt, U., Axberg, I., Wigzell, H., and Lundin, L. G., Pigment mutations in the mouse which also effect lysosomal functions lead to suppressed natural killer cell activity, *Scand. J. Immunol.,* 15, 305, 1982.
89. Clark, E. A., Shultz, L. D., and Pollack, S. B., Mutations in mice that influence natural killer (NK) cell activity, *Immunogenetics,* 12, 601, 1981.
90. Carpen, O., Virtanen, I., and Saksela, E., The cytotoxic activity of human natural killer cells requires an intact secretory apparatus, *Cell. Immunol.,* 58, 97, 1981.
91. Carpen, O., Virtanen, I., and Saksela, E., Ultrastructure of human natural killer cells: nature of the cytolytic contacts in relation to cellular secretion, *J. Immunol.,* 128, 2691, 1982.
92. Grossi, C. E., Zicca, A., Cadoni, A., Mingari, M. C., Moretta, A., and Moretta, L., Ultrastructural characteristics of human T cell clones with various cytolytic activities, *Eur. J. Immunol.,* 13, 670, 1983.
93. Lagarde, A., Murine cloned cell lines related to the Basophil-Mast Cell lineage and spontaneously cytotoxic towards tumoral cells, *C.R. Acad. Sci. (Paris),* 295, 287, 1982.
94. Neighbour, A. P. and Huberman, H. S., Sr., Sr^{++} induced inhibition of human natural killer (NK) cell mediated cytotoxicity, *J. Immunol.,* 128, 1236, 1982.
95. Hiserodt, J. C., Britvan, L. J., and Targan, S. R., Differential effects of various pharmacologic agents on the cytolytic reaction mechanism of the human natural killer lymphocytes. Further resolution of programming for lysis and KCIL into discrete stages, *J. Immunol.,* 129, 2266, 1982.
96. Weissman, G., Goldstein, F., Hoffstein, S., and Tsung, P. K., Reciprocal effects of cAMP and cGMP on microtubule-dependent release of lysosomal enzymes, *Ann. N. Y. Acad. Sci.,* 253, 1750, 1975.
97. Brandt, E. J., Swank, R. T., and Novack, E. K., in *Immunologic Defects in Laboratory Animals, Vol. 1,* Gershwin, M. E. and Merchant, B., Eds., Plenum Press, New York, 1980, 99.
98. Goldfarb, R. H., Timmonen, T., and Herberman, R. B., Production of plasminogen activator by human natural killer cells (large granular lymphocytes) and the role of neutral serine proteolytic enzymes in the mechanism of NK killing (Abstr.), 1st Int. NK Workshop, 1982.
99. Abo, T., Roder, J. C., Abo, W., Cooper, M. D., and Balch, C. M. NK ($HNK\text{-}1^{+}$) cells in Chediak-Higashi patients are present in normal numbers but are abnormal in function and morphology, *J. Clin. Invest.,* 70, 193, 1982.
100. Hattori, T., Hirata, F., Hoffman, T., Hizuta, A., and Herberman, R. B., Inhibition of human natural killer (NK) activity and antibody dependent cellular cytotoxicity (ADCC) by lipomodulin, a phospholipase inhibition inhibitory protein, *J. Immunol.,* 131, 662, 1983.
101. Roder, J. C., Beaumont, T. J., Kerbel, R. S., Haliotis, T., and Kozbur, D., Selective natural killer resistance in a clone of YAC lymphoma cells, *Proc. Natl. Acad. Sci., U.S.A.,* 78, 6396, 1981.
102. Wright, S. C. and Bonavida, B., Selective lysis of NK-sensitive target cells by a soluble mediator released from murine spleen cells and human peripheral blood lymphocytes, *J. Immunol.,* 126, 1516, 1981.
103. Wright, S. C. and Bonavida, B., Studies on the mechanism of natural killer (NK) cell-mediated cytotoxicity (CMC). I. Release of cytotoxic factors specific for NK-sensitive target cells (NKCF) during co-culture of NK effector cells with NK target cells, *J. Immunol.,* 129, 433, 1982.

104. Blanca, I., Ortaldo, J. R., and Herberman, R. B., Study of soluble natural killer cytotoxic factor(s) released by human peripheral blood lymphocytes (Abstr.), NK Workshop, Kyoto, Japan, 1983.
105. Wright, S. C., Weitzen, M. L., Kahle, R., Granger, G. A., and Bonavida, B., Studies on the mechanism of natural killer cytotoxicity. II. Co-culture of human PBL with NK-sensitive or resistant cell lines stimulates release of natural killer cytotoxic factors (NKCF) selectively cytotoxic to NK-sensitive target cells, *J. Immunol.*, 130, 2479, 1983.
106. Wright, S. C. and Bonavida, B., YAC-1 variant clones selected for resistance to natural killer cytotoxic factors are also resistant to natural killer cell-mediated cytotoxicity, *Proc. Natl. Acad. Sci.*,
107. Wright, S. C. and Bonavida, B., Evidence for the involvement of proteolytic enzymes in the production of natural killer cytotoxic factors (Abstr.), NK Workshop, Kyoto, Japan, 1983.
108. Wright, S. C., Reynolds, C. W., and Bonavida, B., Production of natural killer cytotoxic factors (NKCF) by the RNK rat tumor cell (Abstr.), NK Workshop, Kyoto, Japan, 1983.
109. Wright, S. C., Werkmeister, J., Roder, J. C., and Bonavida, B., Studies on the mechanism of natural killer cell-mediated cytotoxicity. V. The NK resistant YAC-6-28 variant binds NK cells and stimulates release of natural killer cytotoxic factors (NKCF) but is not susceptible to lysis by NKCF, submitted.
110. Podack, E. R. and Dennert, G., Assembly of two types of tubules with putative cytolytic function by cloned natural killer cells, *Nature*, 302, 442, 1983.
111. Podack, E. R. and Dennert, G., Assembly of transmembrane tubules (poly perforins) on target membranes by cloned NK-cells: comparison to poly C9 of complement (Abstr.), NK Workshop, Kyoto, Japan, 1983.
112. Russell, J. H. and Dobos, C. B., Mechanism of immune lysis. II. CTL-induced nuclear disintegration of the target begins within minutes of cell contact, *J. Immunol.*, 125, 1256, 1980.
113. Duke, R. C., Chervenak, R., and Cohen, J. J., Endogenous endonuclease-induced DNA fragmentation: an early event in cell-mediated cytolysis, *Proc. Natl. Acad. Sci., U.S.A.*, 80, 6361, 1983.
114. Ullberg, M. and Jondal, M., Recycling and target binding capacity of human natural killer cells, *J. Exp. Med.*, 153, 615, 1981.
115. Grimm, E. A., Thomas, J. A., and Bonavida, B., Mechanism of cell-mediated cytotoxicity at the single cell level. II. Evidence for first-order kinetics of T cell-mediated cytotoxicity and for heterogeneity of lytic rate, *J. Immunol.*, 123, 2870, 1979.
116. Callewaert, D. M., Johnson, D. F., and Kearney, J., Spontaneous cytotoxicity of cultured human cell lines mediated by normal peripheral blood lymphocytes. III. Kinetic parameters, *J. Immunol.*, 121, 710, 1978.
117. Targan, S. and Dorey, F., Interferon activation of "pre-spontaneous killer (Pre-SK) cells and alteration in kinetics of lysis of both Pre-SK and active SK cells", *J. Immunol.*, 124, 2157, 1980.
118. Hudgin, R. L., Pricer, W. E., and Ashwell, G., The isolation and properties of a rabbit liver binding protein specific for asialoglycoproteins, *J. Biol. Chem.*, 249, 5536, 1974.
119. Baenziger, J. U. and Fiete, D., Recycling of the hepatocyte asialoglycoprotein receptor does not require delivery of ligand to lysosomes, *J. Biol. Chem.*, 257, 6007, 1982.
120. Sando, G. M. and Neufeld, E. F., Recognition and receptor-mediated uptake of a lysosomal enzyme, alpha-L-iduronidase, by cultured human fibroblasts, *Cell*, 12, 619, 1977.
121. Gorczynski, R. M., Kennedy, M., Chang, M.-P., and MacRae, S., Recognition specificities, development, and possible biological function of natural killer cells in the mouse. I. Spleen fragment culture assay for natural killer activity and analysis of lectin-like recognition structures on the surface of murine natural killer cells, *Cell. Immunol.*, 80, 335, 1983.
122. Kahle, R., Hiserodt, J., and Bonavida, B., Characterization of antibody-mediated inhibition of natural killer (NK) cytotoxicity. Evidence for blocking of both recognition and lethal hit stages of cytolysis, *Cell. Immunol.*, 80, 97, 1983.

Chapter 9

NATURAL KILLER CYTOTOXIC FACTORS (NKCF) ROLE IN CELL-MEDIATED CYTOTOXICITY*

Benjamin Bonavida and Susan C. Wright

TABLE OF CONTENTS

* Supported by PHS Grant # CA 35791 awarded by the National Cancer Institute and by a grant from the Margaret E. Early Medical Research Trust.

I. INTRODUCTION

Several cytotoxic effector cells have been described and are considered to play an important role in immune surveillance against infection, cancer, and graft rejection. These effector cells constitute (1) the cytotoxic T lymphocytes (CTL) which can lyse antigen-specific target cells, (2) K cells for antibody-dependent cell-mediated cytotoxicity (ADCC), which can lyse antibody-coated target cells, (3) NK cells present in the peripheral blood which can lyse a variety of NK-sensitive tumor cells, and (4) macrophages and neutrophils which, when activated, can also lyse tumor cells or inhibit tumor growth. While all of these effector cells have in common the destruction of undesired target cells, the mechanisms involved in target cell lysis are not clearly understood. It appears, however, that the various cytotoxic systems have certain features in common, and lysis can be divided into at least three stages: (1) binding of the effector cells to the target cells through specific receptors, (2) activation or triggering of the effector cell in a stage called programming for lysis or the lethal hit, and (3) target cell damage in a killer cell independent stage.[1-4] Numerous studies have examined several characteristics of these cytotoxic systems, such as recognition, specificity, surface phenotype, target structures, and antigens associated with cytotoxicity.[5] The various approaches used in investigating the mechanism of cell-mediated cytotoxicity (CMC) are summarized in Table 1.

The stimulus-secretion model has been proposed for the lytic mechanism of CTL as well as NK cells. According to this model, after the effector cell binds to the target it releases cytotoxic molecules which then lyse the target cell. However, previous attempts to detect soluble cytotoxic factors in the supernatants of CMC reactions were unsuccessful. Cytotoxins can be produced by lymphoid cell populations under different conditions. For instance, it has been well documented that lymphotoxins are released following stimulation of peripheral blood effector cells by antigen or by mitogen.[6] Additional evidence indicates that cell populations containing alloimmune CTL can release forms of LT that retain antigen specificity.[7] Further work is necessary to determine if these molecules may be involved in the CTL lytic mechanism.

These studies prompted us to examine the question of cytotoxic mediators in the NK system. NK cells have been shown to be involved in the first line of defense mechanism and thus are of clinical relevance. Our first objective was to optimize conditions for the generation and assessment of cytotoxic activity mediated by soluble factors. Using these techniques, we have demonstrated that nonimmune effector cells can produce soluble cytotoxic factors that are specific for NK-sensitive target cells. Further studies were undertaken to determine whether NKCF may be the lytic mediators in NK-CMC reactions.

In this review, we will summarize our current knowledge on the role of NKCF in NK-CMC. We will primarily concentrate on our work and propose models when appropriate.

II. THE ROLE OF NKCF IN NK-CMC REACTIONS

A. Generation of NKCF

1. Stimulation by PHA or Con A

Our initial studies employed the miniaturized Marbrook culture system to generate and assay for soluble mediators. This culture system is known to provide optimal conditions for the detection of soluble factors in various immunological cell-mediated reactions.[9] Initially, we used phytohemagglutinin (PHA) and concanavalin A (Con A) as nonspecific stimuli, which have been shown to stimulate the production of various lymphokines, including lymphotoxins.[10,11] Effector cells and PHA were placed in the

Table 1
APPROACHES USED TO STUDY THE MECHANISM OF CMC

Use of chemicals or antibody to define stages and substages of cytotoxic reactions
Use of blocking monoclonal antibodies to assess the functional role of the antigens in CMC
Use of hormones or antibodies to define the role of cell surface receptors
Isolation and characterization of molecules or complexes with cytotoxic activity
Somatic cell hybrids to define chromosomes involved in cytotoxicity
Generation of anti-idiotypic antibodies and characterization of receptors involved in recognition
Definition of cell-cell interaction involved in cytolysis

lower well of the Marbrook vessel and NK-sensitive target cells were added to the upper chamber, which was separated from the lower well by a 0.2 μm nucleopore membrane. After incubation of the chamber for 30 to 40 hr at 37°C, there was significant lysis of the NK-sensitive target achieved, as detected by trypan blue dye exclusion. The NK specificity of these findings was demonstrated using a battery of NK-sensitive and NK-resistant target cells.[12] Similar results were obtained using both human and murine effector cells.

In these initial studies, we ruled out several artifacts that may have resulted in lysis of the NK-sensitive target cells. Target cell lysis was not due to media depletion, since replacement of the 0.2 μm nucleopore membrane by dialysis tubing resulted in no lysis. In addition, the effector cells must be viable to release NKCF. These findings constituted the first evidence of soluble cytotoxic factors with specificity for NK-sensitive target cells.

2. *Stimulation of NKCF by NK-Sensitive Target Cells*

The findings that lectin stimulates release of NKCF were encouraging but did not duplicate the NK-CMC reaction. It was thus necessary to establish conditions to show that coculture of NK cells with NK-sensitive stimulator cells also released NKCF. The Marbrook system was employed, in which NK-sensitive tumor cell lines were used to stimulate effector cells. The results revealed that NKCF are generated upon coculture of human peripheral blood or murine spleen cells with NK target cell.[13,14]

3. *Generation of NKCF in Cell Free Supernatant and Assay for its Cytotoxic Activity*

The previous results in the Marbrook chamber showed that NKCF are produced in the bottom chamber by effector cells stimulated with NK targets and then mediate their cytotoxic activity by diffusion through the nucleopore membrane. Therefore, it was possible to generate NKCF and assay their lytic activity in two separate steps. NKCF in cell free supernatant were produced by coculturing effector cells and stimulators for 24 to 48 hr and then harvesting the cell free supernatant. These supernatants were stored at 20°C until assaying for cytotoxic activity in either the microsupernatant assay or the 16 to 20 hr ^{51}Chromium (^{51}Cr)-release assay.

The microsupernatant assay — This assay employs microtiter plates into which samples of cell free supernatant and target cells were incubated at 37°C for 40 hr and cell viability determined by trypan blue exclusion.[14]

The 16 to 20 hr ^{51}Cr release assay — Cell free supernatant is added to ^{51}Cr-labeled target samples in microtiter plates and allowed to incubate for 16 to 20 hr. Cytotoxicity is measured by assessing radioactivity released above background levels.[15]

B. Correlation Between the Properties of NK-CMC Reaction and the Properties of NKCF

The previous results demonstrated that factors released following stimulation of lymphocytes with either mitogen or NK targets selectively lyse NK-sensitive target cells.

Table 2
CORRELATION BETWEEN NK CMC AND CYTOTOXICITY BY NKCF

NK CMC Reactions	NKCF Properties
Binding to NK-sensitive target	Stimulation by NK-sensitive target
Binding to NK-resistant targets	Stimulation of NKCF by NK resistant
The effector cell is the NK cell	Release by NK effector cells
Defect in bg/bg	Defect in bg/bg
Species specific	Species specific
Activity augmented by IFN-treated NK	Augmentation of NKCF activity by IFN-treated NK
Activity decreased by IFN-treated target cell	Inhibition of NKCF Release by IFN-treated target cell
Variants selected by mutagenesis or by culture in NKCF are resistant in NK-CMC	Variants selected by mutagenesis or by culture in NKCF are resistant to NKCF and NK-CMC

This suggested that NKCF may be involved in the NK-CMC reaction. This hypothesis was further investigated by determining if there is a correlation between the known characteristics of NK CMC and NKCF. Several known features of the NK-CMC reaction have been reported and their relationship to the functional characteristics of NKCF is summarized in Table 2. Each of these correlations will be described separately below.

1. Release of NKCF During Coculture of NK Cells with NK Target Cells

In the NK-CMC reaction, cell-to-cell contact is necessary to initiate the lytic response. We therefore investigated whether NK effector cells stimulated by NK target would release NKCF. Murine spleen cells cocultured with the NK-sensitive target YAC-1 produced NKCF containing supernatants that were selectively cytotoxic to NK target cells. The viability of the stimulator cells was essential since treatment with glutaraldehyde or heating at 56°C for 30 min resulted in no release of NKCF. Similar results were observed using human peripheral blood leukocytes stimulated with the NK-sensitive K562 or Molt-4 target cells. Experiments analyzing the kinetics of production of NKCF indicated that significant levels of cytotoxicity were first detected in supernatants from 20 hr cultures. The cytotoxic activity remained high for up to 50 hr of culture and decreased to low levels thereafter. These results demonstrated that coculture of NK effector cells with NK-sensitive targets induces the release of NKCF, in agreement with the NK-CMC reactions.[13,14]

2. Cells with Surface Phenotype and Characteristics of NK Cells are Involved in Release of NKCF

The nature of the effector cells involved in the release of NKCF was analyzed. Murine spleen cells were treated with anti-Thyl.2 or with antiasialo GM1 antibody plus complement prior to coculture with YAC-1 stimulator cells for the production of NKCF. Treatment with anti-Thy1.2 plus complement did not eliminate NKCF production, while treatment with antiasialo GM1 plus complement inhibited the production of NKCF to the control basal level. These results were valid in both conventional mice and nude spleen cells. Experiments done in parallel with antibody- and complement-treated cells indicated that the NK effector cell that lyses YAC-1 in a 4 hr NK CMC assay is Thy1.2-negative and asialo GM1-positive, in agreement with previous results (Table 3).[13] In man, enrichment of NK in the low density fraction of Percoll gradient resulted in enhanced production of NKCF, and augmentation in NK-CMC reactions.[14] These results demonstrate that cell populations enriched for NK effector cells participate in the production of NKCF.

Table 3
CHARACTERIZATION OF CELLS PRODUCING NKCF

	Activity	
	NK CMC	NKCF production
Mouse spleen cells + anti-Thy1.2 + C¹[a]	+	+
Mouse spleen cells + antiasialo GM1 + C¹	−	−
Mouse spleen cells + C¹	+	+
Mouse thymocytes	−	−
Human LGL[b]	+	+

[a] C¹ complement.
[b] LGL = large granular lymphocytes.

Table 4
CORRELATION BETWEEN STRAIN DISTRIBUTION IN NK-CMC AND PRODUCTION OF NKCF

		NKCF production following stimulation by	
Strains	NK CMC	Mitogen	YAC-1
C57BL/6	Intermediate	+	
Balb/C	Intermediate	+	
Balb/C nude	High	+	+
DBA/2	Intermediate	+	
CBA	High	+	+
bg/bg	Low		−
bg/+	Intermediate		+

3. Correlation Between Strains of Mice with High and Low NK Activity and Their Ability to Generate NKCF

Table 4 summarizes the correlation between strain distribution in NK CMC and production of NKCF. Several strains of mice have been shown to exhibit different levels of NK cytotoxicity. For instance, CBA and nude strains are high NK whereas beige/beige (bg/bg) mice are low NK. This variation may be due to quantitative or qualitative differences in NKCF production or activity. Spleen cells derived from these mice were tested for their ability to produce NKCF following coculture with YAC-1 stimulator cells. The results showed that nude mice produce high levels, whereas the bg/bg mice showed a relative defect in NKCF production as compared to the normal bg/+ littermate.[13] Since bg/bg mice can still form conjugates with YAC-1, we hypothesize that they are unable to synthesize or release NKCF (Figure 1).

4. Correlation Between NK Target Sensitivity to Lysis in NK-CMC and Ability to Stimulate NKCF

The ability of the target cell to stimulate release of NKCF and its sensitivity to lysis by NK cells was investigated. It has been observed that several target cells can bind to the NK effector cells but are not lysed by such cells. This suggests that the resistant cells are defective in either their ability to stimulate release of NKCF or their susceptibility to lysis by NKCF. Accordingly, we tested various stimulator cells of human and rodent origins for NKCF production. The results demonstrate that the majority of

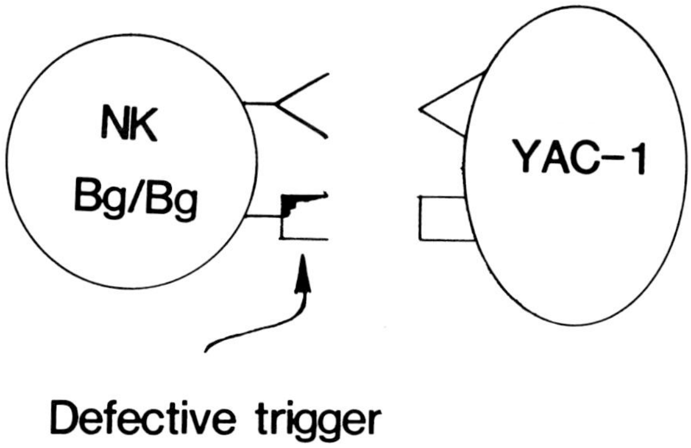

FIGURE 1. Schematic diagram showing that NK cells from bg/bg mice are defective in the trigger for the release of NKCF.

Table 5
CORRELATION BETWEEN ABILITY TO STIMULATE NKCF AND LYSIS BY NK CMC

Species	Stimulator	Lysis in NK CMC	Stimulation of release of NKCF	Sensitivity to NKCF
Mouse	YAC-1	+	+	+
	WEHI-164	+	+	+
	FLD-3	+	+	+
	AKSL-2	−	+	−
	P815	−	+	−
	EL-4	−	−	−
Man	Molt-4	+	+	+
	K562	+	+	+
	RAJI	−	+	−
	WI-L2	−	+	−

target cells stimulate release of NKCF whether they are NK-sensitive or not.[13,14] Thus, many NK-resistant target cells can stimulate the release of NKCF, although they are insensitive to lysis by these factors (Table 5). These data suggest that some tumor cells may escape lysis by NK cells due to a deficiency of NKCF binding sites or else to an inherent insensitivity to the lytic activity of NKCF (Figure 2).

5. Species Specificity of NKCF

It has been shown that lysis of NK-sensitive targets is, in general, species-specific. We tested the species specificity of NKCF using a variety of target cells. The results obtained concur with the NK CMC findings and indicate that NKCF is indeed species-specific even under conditions where the target cell stimulator of NKCF is from a different species.[13]

6. Effect of Interferon (IFN) Treatment of Effector on NKCF Production and Activity

It has been well documented that IFN pretreatment of effector cells results in significantly increased lytic capacity of NK-CMC reactions. Further studies have revealed that the augmented activity is the result of recruitment of pre-NK cells, enhancement of the kinetics of lysis, and enhanced recycling.[16] We proposed that these properties could be due to the augmentation of NKCF production or activity. Experiments were performed in the NKCF system to examine the effect of IFN pretreatment of effector

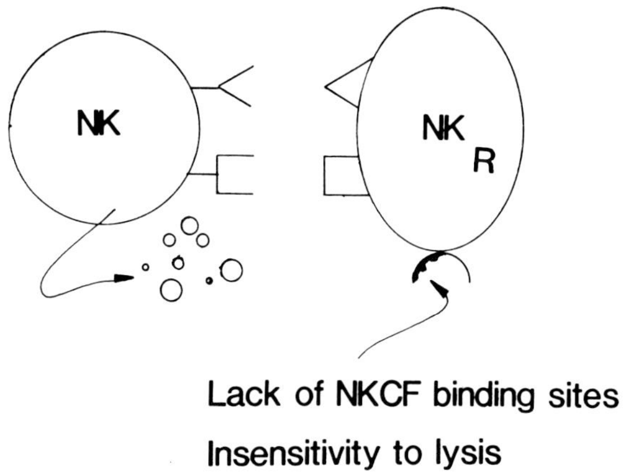

FIGURE 2. Schematic diagram showing that NK-resistant targets (NKR) are deficient in NKCF binding sites or inherently insensitive to NKCF. The NKCF target is still capable of binding to NK and of stimulating the release of NKCF.

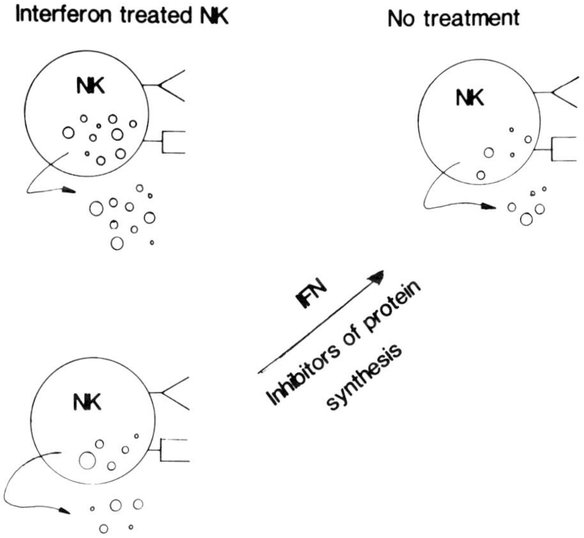

FIGURE 3. Schematic diagram depicting augmentation of NKCF following treatment of NK cell with IFN. However, in the presence of protein synthesis inhibitors there is no augmentation of NKCF but the level returns to normal (equivalent to untreated cells).

cells in the production of NKCF. Murine effector cells were pretreated with either fibroblast IFN or with poly IC, both shown to augment NK-CMC reactions, and co-cultured with YAC-1 stimulator cells. The cell free supernatant was tested for cytotoxic activity against YAC-1 cells. The results indicated that pretreatment of effector cells with IFN augmented the production and activity of NKCF. The mechanism of this augmentation was then investigated. It was found that protein synthesis during the period of IFN treatment was necessary for the augmented activity (Figure 3).[15] These results suggest that the IFN-induced augmentation of NK activity may be due to an increase in the synthesis of NKCF (Table 6).

Table 6
EFFECT OF IFN TREATMENT OF NK EFFECTORS ON NKCF PRODUCTION AND ACTIVITY

Treatment of effector	Activity of NK CMC	Release of NKCF
None	+	+
IFN or PIC	+++	+++
Cycloheximide + IFN	+	+

Table 7
EFFECT OF IFN PRETREATMENT OF TARGET CELLS ON NKCF PRODUCTION

		Cytotoxic activity by	
Treatment	Stimulation of NKCF	NK CMC	NKCF
Target cell alone	++	+	+
Target cell + IFN	±	−	+

7. Effect of IFN Treatment on Target Cell and NKCF Activity

It has been demonstrated that pretreatment of target cells with IFN renders these cells relatively resistant to lysis by NK cells. Nevertheless, target cells are still recognized by the effector cell and form conjugates. It is possible that the NK resistance of such targets is due to an inability to stimulate NKCF release or an insensitivity to lysis by NKCF. Experiments were designed to examine these possibilities. The results showed that IFN-pretreated YAC-1 cells are unable to stimulate the release of NKCF as effectively as normal YAC-1 cells (Table 7). These results suggest that a postbinding event necessary to induce the release of NKCF was defective in IFN-treated YAC-1 cells.[17] Subsequent experiments indicated that IFN-pretreated YAC-1 cells are just as sensitive to NKCF as normal YAC-1. These results ruled out a defect in NKCF receptors or binding sites (Figure 4). Results observed with IFN-treated targets are different from those obtained with the NK-resistant target cells which can stimulate release of NKCF but cannot by lysed by NKCF (see Figure 4). Thus, IFN-treated targets are defective in their ability to stimulate release of NKCF.[17]

8. YAC-1 Variant Resistant to NK CMC are also Resistant to NKCF

Several NK-resistant variants derived from NK-sensitive cell lines have been employed to study the mechanism of NK CMC. As was previously described for IFN-treated YAC cells, such variants may be analyzed in the NKCF system to localize the step at which the NK lytic pathway is blocked. If NKCF are the lytic mediators in NK CMC, then tumor cells selected for variants resistant in NK CMC should also be resistant to NKCF, and inversely, variants selected for resistance to NKCF will also be resistant in NK-CMC reactions. Both of these possibilities were examined.

Variants selected for resistance in NK CMC are also resistant to NKCF — The YAC-6.28 cloned cell lines were derived from the parental YAC-1 NK-sensitive cell line by in vitro mutagenesis and selection for NK resistance.[18] YAC-6-28 continued to express the NK target cell structures and formed conjugates. We hypothesized that NK target cell resistance was due either to failure to simulate release of NKCF, failure to recognize and bind NKCF, or insensitivity to lysis by NKCF. These possibilities were exam-

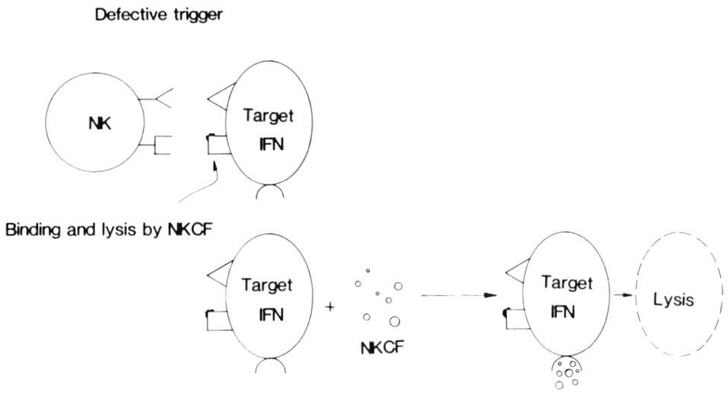

FIGURE 4. This figure shows that IFN-treated target poorly stimulates NK cells to release NKCF. However, the target is susceptible to lysis by NKCF. Thus, it appears as if the defect is localized at the trigger step necessary for stimulation of NKCF production.

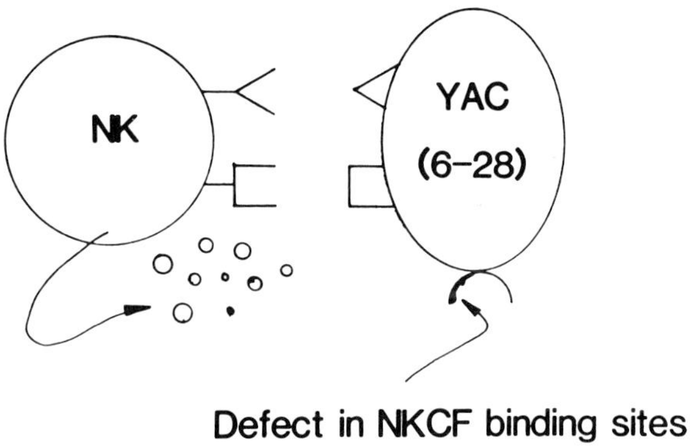

FIGURE 5. This figure shows that the resistant target YAC 6-28 is able to bind to the NK and stimulate release of NKCF but is defective in NKCF binding sites/or insensitive to NKCF.

ined. Coculture of YAC-6-28 target with spleen cells resulted in the production of NKCF. However, the YAC-6-28 was not susceptible to lysis by NKCF (Figure 5). These results suggested that the defect was at the poststimulation level. We then tested for the ability of these cells to adsorb NKCF in order to delineate whether they possess binding sites for NKCF. Our findings indicate that YAC-6-28 resistance to NK CMC is due to a deficiency of NKCF binding sites on the target cells (Figure 6).[19]

Variants selected for resistance to NKCF mediated lysis are also resistant in NK CMC — We predicted that if NKCF is in fact the lytic mediator of NK CMC, variants selected for resistance to NKCF would also be resistant to NK CMC. YAC-R clones were generated by prolonged culture of the initially sensitive YAC-1 cell line in the presence of NKCF. These variants were resistant to NKCF and NK-CMC although they were still able to stimulate release of NKCF (Figure 6).[20] Resistance to lysis by the variants was not a general phenomenon since such cells were lysed by CTL. Table 8 summarizes the various properties of YAC-6-28 and YAC-R resistance targets.

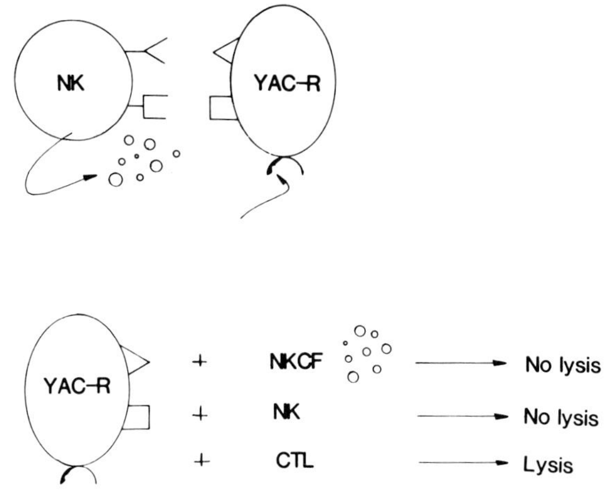

FIGURE 6. This figure shows that the target selected for resistance to NKCF is also resistant to NKCMC. Resistance is due to a defect in NKCF binding sites or insensitivity to NKCF. The target, however, can be lysed by CTL demonstrating that the cell is lysable and is not inherently resistant to lysis.

Table 8
CHARACTERISTICS OF YAC-6-28- AND YAC-R-RESISTANT TARGETS

	YAC-6-28	YA-R
Binding to NK to form conjugates	+	+
Stimulate NKCF	+	+
Bind NKCF		−
Lysis by NKCF	−	−
Lysis by NK CMC	−	−
Lysis by alloimmune CTL	+	+

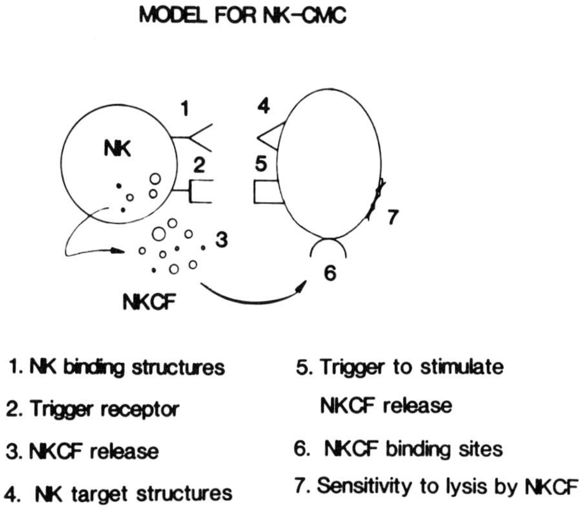

FIGURE 7. This figure schematically diagrams the proposed model of NK-CMC.

III. MODEL PROPOSED FOR THE ROLE OF NKCF IN NK-CMC REACTION

The results of the above experiments and findings led us to propose the following model of NK-CMC reactivity (Figure 7). The first step of the lytic pathway involves the interaction of a receptor on the NK cell which recognizes and binds to the NK target structure on the target cell membrane. The effector cell must then receive a signal from the target to activate the NKCF release mechanism. This is depicted as occurring through the interaction of membrane determinants distinct from those involved in the initial binding step, however it is also possible that the two sets of determinants may be physically linked on the cell surface. The second signal is suggested from the findings that effector cells from low NK strains such as the bg/bg mouse can bind to NK target cells but do not release NKCF (Figure 1).

The NK-sensitive target must be equipped with at least four properties in order to induce lysis by NK cells:

1. The target must bear an NK target structure recognized by the NK cells. This alone is not sufficient, however, since many resistant NK targets can form conjugates with NK cells but are not lysed.
2. The NK target must be able to stimulate the NK cell to release NKCF. This concept is derived from studies which show that IFN-treated target cells cannot stimulate release of NKCF although they are able to bind to NK cells and can be lysed by NKCF (see Figure 4). Stimulation of release is not sufficient to result in lysis of target cells since several NK-resistant target cells can stimulate release of NKCF without being lysed by NKCF or by NK CMC (Figure 2).
3. The NK target cells must express NKCF binding sites. The presence of such sites is revealed in experiments demonstrating that variants derived by mutagenesis or cultured in NKCF do not express NKCF binding sites as measured in absorption assays (see Figures 5 and 6). These cells can bind NK cells to form conjugates and can also stimulate release of NKCF, but are not lysed by NKCF or NK CMC.
4. The target cell must be susceptible to lysis by NKCF. The sensitivity of a target cell to NKCF lytic activity may be due to the ability of the target cell to internalize NKCF, the target cell having a poor repair mechanism, weak inhibitors of NKCF activity in the target cell, or the availability on the target cell of cofactors necessary to activate NKCF.

Our studies are compatible with the above model of NK CMC in which NKCF function as the lytic mediators. This model can be used to dissect CMC into several distinct stages, each of which can be analyzed independently and biochemically. Such analyses should result in the delineation of the molecular basis of CMC by NK cells and also by other cytotoxic cells.

IV. PHYSICAL AND BIOCHEMICAL CHARACTERIZATION OF NKCF

Several physical and biochemical properties of NKCF have been examined using supernatants containing NKCF or semipurified NKCF.

A. Inhibition by Sugars

Recent findings have indicated that certain simple sugars inhibit NK-CMC reactions. We examined the mechanism of this inhibition in the NKCF system. The addition of α-methyl-D-mannoside or *N*-acetyl-D-galactosamine or mannose-6-phosphate to the NKCF assay inhibited lysis at concentrations that had been shown to previously inhibit NK CMC.[21] The blocking activity by simple sugars is consistent with competitive inhibition of the binding of NKCF to the target cells. This could occur by either direct binding of the sugar to NKCF or binding of the sugar to the NKCF receptor on the target cells.

B. Stability of NKCF

The stability of NKCF was examined. It was found that NKCF is stable at −20°C for 1 to 2 months. It is also stable for more than 3 days at 37°C, and unstable at 63°C for 30 min.

C. Effect of Proteolytic Enzymes and Periodate

NKCF activity was found to be sensitive to trypsin or periodate treatment, suggesting that it is a glycoprotein. Furthermore, NKCF was inactivated upon reduction and alkylation. These results suggest that NKCF is a glycoprotein, in which the disulfide bonding may be essential for lytic activity.[22]

D. Effect of Protease Inhibitors

Numerous reports have indicated that proteases are involved in the NK lytic mechanism. This is based on the observation that addition of certain protease inhibitors to an NK-CMC reaction results in inhibition of NK-CMC. These inhibitors do not affect conjugate formation and it has been suggested that they act at a postbinding or lethal hit stage of lysis. According to our model of NKCF, it is possible that proteases are involved in the NKCF release mechanism, inactivating NKCF, or inhibiting NKCF interaction with and lysis of target cells.

Several protease inhibitors which are known to inhibit NK-CMC reactions were examined. No significant effect was seen when the protease inhibitors were added to the NKCF assay. However, pretreatment of effector cells with these inhibitors followed by washing inhibited the production of active NKCF.[23] These results support the hypothesis that a serine-dependent protease is involved in the release and/or activation of NKCF production.

E. Purification of NKCF

Biochemical purification of NKCF was initiated using supernatants derived from murine, rat, and human cultures. Fractionation on HPLC resulted in fractions of 20,000 to 30,000 daltons that retained NKCF activity.[23]

V. RELATIONSHIP OF NKCF TO OTHER CYTOTOXIC MOLECULES

Several cytotoxins have been implicated in CMC reaction. For instance, lymphotoxins have been studied extensively, and have been implicated in several cell-mediated immune reactions. Studies by Hiserodt and Granger[24] have shown that antibodies against human lymphotoxin block xenogenic L cells lysis by mitogen-activated T and B lymphocytes. In addition, the anti-LT serum has been shown to block the lymphocyte independent phase of the reaction, implying that lymphotoxin is transferred from lymphocytes to the target cells.[25] The biochemical nature of the lymphotoxin family of molecules has been extensively analyzed and reviewed by Granger et al.[6] It is not clear whether NKCF is a member of the lymphotoxin family, or is a related one. Granger's studies suggest that the cytotoxic factors lysing NK-sensitive target cells are biochemically distinct from classical lymphotoxin.

Recent studies suggest that the granules present in the LGL fraction are involved in the NK lytic mechanism.[25-27] Cloned NK and T cell killers assemble membrane lesions on target cells during the cytolytic reaction. During this reaction, granules containing the cytolytic percursor molelcules (perforins) are released and the precursors polymerize to form membrane lesions (polyperforins) on the target membranes. Lysis then ensues by channel formation and membrane destruction. Podack has identified the perforins as proteins of 56,000, 38,000, and 22,000 daltons. Likewise, Henkart has shown that granules isolated from rat NK cells are highly cytotoxic to sheep red blood cells. The granules contain major protein bands of 62, 58, 30, 29, and 28 kdaltons and contain hexoses and uric acids.[27] It is not yet clear whether these molecules are involved in NK-CMC reactions and how these findings correlate with our NKCF findings.

A question that is often asked is why different kinetics of lysis are observed with NKCF as compared to NK CMC. If indeed NKCF participates in the lytic reactions, why is lysis not observed in a short term assay, as is expected from the NK-CMC reaction? Though the answer to this question is not yet known, several explanations may be offered. (1) In NK-CMC reactions, in which target cells and effector cells are in direct contact, NKCF release and interaction with target cell is a local phenomenon. NKCF may be focused and easily assembled on target cells to immediately initiate target damage. However, NKCF recovered in the supernatant of a CMC reaction may be much more dilute than the concentrations found in the local microenvironment of effector-target cell conjugates and may also compete with various inhibitors present. Under such conditions, the lytic reaction may take a more prolonged time period to initiate. (2) The repair mechanism may be efficient in the NKCF assay, whereas in the NK CMC reaction, it is at a disadvantage. (3) NKCF alone may not be sufficient to inflict target damage. Cofactors may be required, and these are delivered or activated in the NK-CMC reaction but may be diluted in the NKCF preparations. It is hoped that purifed NKCF studied in detail should resolve the issues raised above.

VI. SUMMARY AND CONCLUSION

A strong correlation was found between the various characteristics attributed to the NK-CMC reaction and the functional characteristics of NKCF. Based on these close relationships, our studies are the first to implicate a role of soluble mediators in a lymphocyte mediated cytotoxicity system.

The demonstration that cytotoxic mediators derived from NK cells participate in the lytic reaction opens new areas of research in the investigation of the complex mechanism of CMC. It also enables us to define several receptor and ligand interactions which can be independently examined. Furthermore, NKCF opens new possibilities to explore the role of soluble mediators in other cytotoxic systems. In addition, the demonstration that low NK strains of mice such as the bg/bg do not generate NKCF upon stimulation provides a good example of the practical application of our findings in clinical setttings, as well as in cases where the NK system is defective. It is also possible that, once purified, and obtained in sufficient quantities, NKCF may be employed therapeutically in vivo.

REFERENCES

1. **Martz, E.**, Mechanism of surface tumor lysis by alloimmune T lymphocytes: resolution and characterization of discrete steps in the cellular interactions, *Contemp. Top. Immunobiol.*, 7, 301, 1977.
2. **Henney, C. S.**, T cell mediated cytolysis: an overview of some current issues, *Contemp. Top. Immunobiol.*, 7, 245, 1977.

3. Goldstein, P. and Smith, E. T., The lethal hit stage of mouse T and non-T cell-mediated cytolysis: differences in cation requirements and characterization of an analytical "cation pulse" method, *Eur. J. Immunol.*, 6, 31, 1976.
4. Goldstein, P. and Smith, E. T., Mechanism of T cell-mediated cytolysis: the lethal hit stage, *Contemp. Top.Immunobiol.*, 7, 273, 1977.
5. Bonavida, B., Mechanism of natural killer cell-mediated cytotoxicity, in *Natural Killer Activity and its Regulation*, Hoshino, T., et al., Eds., Excerpta Medica, Amsterdam, 1984, 97.
6. Granger, G. A., Hiserodt, J. C., and Ware, C. F., Cytotoxic and growth inhibitory lymphokines, in *Biology of the Lymphokines*, Cohen, S., Pick, E., and Opperheim, J. J., Eds., Academic Press, New York, 1979, 141.
7. Hiserodt, J. C., Tiango, G. J., and Granger, G. A., The LT system in experimental animals. IV. Rapid specific lysis of ^{51}Cr-labeled allogeneic target cells by highly unstable high MW lymphotoxin receptor complex(es) in vitro by activated alloimmune murine T lymphocytes, *J. Immunol.*, 123, 332, 1979.
8. Herberman, R. B., *NK Cells and Other Natural Effector Cells*, Academic Press, New York, 1983.
9. Elpert, E. F., Adorini, L., and Couderc, J., A miniaturized in vitro diffusion culture system, *J. Immunol. Methods*, 22, 283, 1978.
10. Ruddle, N. H. and Waksman, B. H., Cytotoxic effect of lymphocyte antigen interaction in delayed hypersensitivity, *Science*, 157, 1060, 1967.
11. Kolb, W. P. and Granger, G. A., Lymphocyte in vitro cytotoxicity: characterization of human lymphotoxin, *Proc. Natl. Acad. Sci. U.S.A.*, 61, 1250, 1968.
12. Wright, S. C. and Bonavida, B., Selective lysis of NK sensitive target cells by a soluble mediator released from murine spleen cells and human peripheral blood lymphocytes, *J. Immunol.*, 126, 1516, 1981.
13. Wright, S. C. and Bonavida, B., Studies on the mechanism of natural killer cytotoxicity. I. Release of cytotoxic factors specific for NK sensitive target cells (NKCF) during co-culture of NK effector cells with NK target cells, *J. Immunol.*, 129, 433, 1982.
14. Wright, S. C., Weitzen, M. L., Kahle, R., Granger, G. A., and Bonavida, B., Studies on the mechanism of natural killer cytotoxicity. II. Co-culture of human PBL with NK-sensitive or resistant cell lines stimulates release of natural killer cytotoxic factors (NKCF) selectively cytotoxic to NK-sensitive target cells, *J. Immunol.*, 130, 2479, 1983.
15. Wright, S. C. and Bonavida, B., Studies on the mechanism of natural killer (NK) cell-mediated cytotoxicity. III. Interferon-pretreatment of effector cell augments the lytic activity of natural killer cytotoxic factors (NKCF), *J. Immunol.*, 130, 2960, 1983.
16. Silva, A., Bonavida, B., and Targan, S., Mode of action of interferon-mediated modulation of natural killer cytotoxic activity: recruitment of pre-NK cells and enhanced kinetics of lysis. *J. Immunol.*, 125, 479, 1980.
17. Wright, S. C. and Bonavida, B. Studies on the mechanism of natural killer (NK) cell-mediated cytotoxicity. IV. Interferon-induced inhibition of NK target cell susceptibility is due to a defect in their ability to stimulate release of natural killer cytotoxic factors (NKCF), *J. Immunol.*, 130, 2965, 1983.
18. Roder, J. C., Beaumont, T. J., Kerbel, R. S., Haliotis, T., and Kozbor, D., Selective natural killer resistance in a clone of YAC lymphoma cells, *Proc. Natl. Acad. Sci. U.S.A.*, 78, 6396, 1981.
19. Wright, S. C., Roder, J. C., Werkmeister, J., and Bonavida, B., Studies on the mechanism of natural killer (NK) cell-mediated cytotoxicity. VI. The NK resistant YAC-6-28 variant binds NK cells and stimulates release of natural killer cytotoxic factors (NK) but is not susceptible to lysis by NKCF, submitted.
20. Wright, S. C. and Bonavida, B., YAC-1 variant clones selected for resistance to natural killer cytotoxic factors are also resistant to natural killer cell-mediated cytotoxicity, *Proc. Natl. Acad. Sci. U.S.A.*, 80, 1688, 1983.
21. Stutman, O., Dien, P., Wisum, R. E., and Latime, C., Natural cytotoxic cells against solid tumors in mice: blocking of cytotoxicity by D-mannose, *Proc. Natl. Acd. Sci. U.S.A.*, 77, 2895, 1980.
22. Wright, S. C. and Bonavida, B., Evidence for the involvement of proteolytic enzymes in the production of natural killer cytotoxic factors, in *Natural Killer Activity and its Regulation*, Hoshino, T., et. al., Eds., Excerpta Medica, Amsterdam, 1984, 145.
23. Wright, S. C., Wilbur, S. M., and Bonavida, B., Biochemical characterization of natural killer cytotoxic factors, in *Mechanism of Cell-Mediated Cytotoxicity II*, Henkart, P. and Martz, E., Eds., Plenum Press, New York, 1985.
24. Hiserodt, J. C. and Granger, G. A., Inhibition of human lymphocyte-mediated mitogen-induced cytotoxicity of murine L-929 cells by heterologous anti-human lymphotoxin antisera in vitro, *J. Immunol.*, 119, 374, 1972.
25. Podack, E. R. and Dennert, G., Assembly of two types of tubules with putative cytolytic function in cloned natural killer cells, *Nature*, 302, 442, 1983.

26. Dennert, G. and Podack, E. R., Cytolysis by H-2 specific T killer cells. Assembly of tubular complexes on target membranes, *J. Exp. Med.*, 157, 1483, 1983.
27. Millard, P. J., Henkart, M. A., Reynolds, C. W., and Henkart, P. A., Purification and properties of cytoplasmic granules from cytotoxic rat LGL tumors, *J. Immunol.*, 132, 3197, 1984.

Chapter 10

CHARACTERISTICS OF CULTURED NK CELLS

Robert C. Burton

TABLE OF CONTENTS

I. INTRODUCTION

The development of the in vitro ^{51}Chromium (^{51}Cr)-release assay by Brunner et al.[1] in 1968 provided a simple technique for measuring target cell lysis by cytotoxic cells. The assay rapidly gained widespread acceptance as the optimal technique for quantitating cytotoxic T (thymus-derived) lymphocyte (T_c)-mediated lysis.[2] Systems were developed to study induction of T_c against alloantigens, autoantigens, and tumor-associated antigens (TAA) in vitro, and in vitro assays of nucleated cells obtained from experimental animals or human patients became major research directions for many laboratories.[2-4] It soon became clear, however, that a significant proportion of the in vitro cytotoxicity observed in many of these systems could not be accounted for by antigen-specific T_c-mediated lysis. This was particularly so when leukocytes obtained from normal or tumor bearing experimental animals or humans were assayed against ^{51}Cr-labeled tumor target cells.[5,6] By 1975, it was recognized that the in vitro "background" lysis of ^{51}Cr-labeled tumor target cells observed in these systems was a phenomenon in its own right: "natural killing".[7,8] The ensuing years have seen numerous and widespread investigations of natural killing, and it is now clear that the phenomenon can be effected by more than one cell type, and that these different cells may be derived from more than one lymphohemapoietic cell lineage.[9,10] The focus of this review is not on these in vivo-derived cytotoxic cells per se, but on the "nonspecific" lysis observed in ^{51}Cr-release assays of cultured lymphohemapoietic mammalian cells and how the effectors of this phenomenon relate to in vivo-derived natural killer (NK) cells.

The observation that cytotoxic cells could be induced in vitro by culturing mouse spleen cells either alone or with irradiated syngeneic normal tissue cells was first made in 1971; the phenomenon was termed autosensitization in vitro.[4] The cytotoxic effector cells were thought to be self-antigen specific T_c.[11,12] My own studies of this phenomenon were stimulated by the need to control for "nonspecific" lysis when assaying for T_c induced to TAA in vitro.[3] In those studies, it was shown that (1) both Thy-1$^+$ and Thy-1$^-$ cytotoxic cells were induced by short-term culture of murine spleen cells alone in fetal calf serum containing media, (2) Thy-1$^+$ cells were absolutely necessary for the in vitro induction of all cytotoxic activity detected, (3) the Thy-1$^-$ NK cell activity of fresh murine spleen cells was rapidly lost in these short term cultures, (4) the specificity of tumor target cell lysis was not restricted by the major histocompatibility complex (MHC), and (5) 10 of 10 lymphoid and solid (carcinoma and fibrosarcoma) tumor target cell lines tested were susceptible to lysis.[13] As part of those studies, cellular competitive inhibition assays[14] were performed which demonstrated that target cell lysis was not blocked by syngeneic normal tissue cells or a wide range of H-2 congenic spleen cells.[13] This led to the conclusion that T_c reactive with self-antigens were not detectable in these cultures.

At that time, the phenomenon of natural killing by uncultured mammalian lymphohemapoietic cells and this culture-induced cytotoxic activity seemed to have little in common. Indeed, the susceptibility of in vivo-derived NK cells to in vitro culture at 37°C and the clear differences in patterns of target cell lysis between fresh and cultured killer cells,[13-15] led us to conclude that the two phenomena were not related.[13] The last 5 years have seen the discovery of specific membrane markers for some NK cell subsets and the development of techniques for long term in vitro culture and cloning of certain cytotoxic cell types.

The work of investigators in these fields has provided new knowledge about the phenomenon of natural killing. The major task of this review is to reappraise the views expressed by the author in 1977.

In the following sections I shall examine the relationships between nonactivated and activated in vivo-derived NK cells, cytotoxic cells induced by short-term culture, and cloned cytotoxic cell lines obtained by long-term culture in interleukin 2 (IL-2)-containing media. I shall concentrate on experimental murine systems, as most of our knowledge about natural killing has been derived from studies in the mouse. Where studies in other mammals provide further insights, and this particularly applied to data obtained from experiments with human peripheral blood leukocytes (PBL), these have been included and compared to the relevant data obtained in murine studies.

II. IN VIVO-DERIVED NK CELLS

A. In Vitro Assay of Killer Cells from "Naive" Donors

It has been clear for a number of years that, given appropriate conditions, all the nucleated lymphohemapoietic cell types obtained from murine spleen, lymph node, or peripheral blood can mediate in vitro lysis of ^{51}Cr-labeled tumor cell lines.[3] This lysis can be spontaneous or nonspecific, antigen-specific, antibody-specific (antibody-dependent cellular cytotoxicity [ADCC]), or lectin-dependent, and can involve direct cell-to-cell lysis of the target or killing through chemical mediators.[3] Indeed, even platelets can mediate ADCC.[16] Therefore, the original definition of natural killing[7,8] might have been expected to encompass a variety of effector cell types.

1. Murine

The discovery of specific alloantigens of murine NK cells which lyse lymphoma targets[17-19] has provided conclusive evidence for heterogeneity of NK cells obtained directly from nonimmunized ("naive") adults of that species.[20] It has been shown that NK cells which express the alloantigens NK-1, NK-2, or NK-3 lyse a certain range of tumor target cells, most of which are lymphomas, while NK cells not expressing these alloantigens kill a nonidentical, but overlapping, range of target cells, most of which are solid tumors.[20-25] The natural killer cells which express these alloantigens have been termed NK or NK_A cells, and those not expressing these alloantigens, NK_B or natural cytotoxic (NC) cells.[20-25]

There is currently some confusion concerning the nomenclature of NK-specific alloantigens, due to incomplete data published to date on the genetic characterization of certain NK-specific alloantisera and lack of definitive studies of the relationships between these sera.[18,19,25] Studies have now been completed which show that CE anti-CBA serum[18] detects the alloantigen NK-2.1[19] and not NK-1.2, an allele of NK-1.1.[17,21,25] Further, genetic studies of C3H anti-St sera have revealed that these sera detect an NK/NK_A cell-specific alloantigen separate to that detected by anti-NK-1.1 or anti-NK-2.1 alloantisera.[21,25] Therefore, I have proposed that the NK/NK_A cell-specific alloantigens be designated thus: NK-1.1, detected by C3H anti-CE or (C3H × BALB/C) F1 anti-CE alloantisera;[17] NK-2.1, detected by CE anti-CBA, NZB anti-BALB/C, (NZB × CE) F1 anti-CBA, or (NZB × CE) F1 anti-BALB/C alloantisera,[18,19,25] and NK-3.1 detected by C3H anti-St alloantisera.[21,25] In this review I have adhered to this nomenclature, adjusting the results reported by investigators using these alloantisera as necessary. It should be noted that my own studies indicate that there are very likely to be additional alloantigenic systems of NK/NK_A cells and NK_B/NC cells.[25]

These two major NK cell subsets can be distinguished on many other grounds apart from the expression of specific membrane markers.[23-25] There is also evidence that there is further heterogeneity within these two classes of effector cells.[21,25] There are, for instance, two subsets of NK cells which lyse the Moloney leukemia cell line YAC and express the NK-specific alloantigen NK-2.1, a Thy-1^+ subset and a Thy-1^- subset.[25,26] These subsets correspond to the NK_I and NK_T subsets of Minato et al.[27] who defined four subsets of murine NK cells on the basis of surface markers, short-term in vitro culture, and responsiveness to interferon (IFN) and IL-2. Further, studies with an EL-4 lymphoma cell line have shown that the NK-2$^+$ NK cells which lyse this target are bone marrow-independent in contrast to the NK-1$^+$, NK-2$^+$, NK-3$^+$ NK cells that lyse YAC, which are bone marrow-dependent.[21,25,28] The NK-1$^-$, NK-2$^-$, NK-3$^-$, NK-$_B$ or NC cells can be divided into at least two subsets: one present in neonatal, cyclophosphamide treated, or lethally irradiated mice, and one absent.[23,25]

Evidence for heterogeneity of NK cells in other experimental animals is much less clear. There is, for example, no evidence that the equivalent of the NK$_B$ or NC cell exists in the rat.[29] However, studies with the monoclonal antibody, (MoAb) OX-8, which reacts with rat cytotoxic/suppressor T cells,[30] have shown that rat splenic NK cells which lyse lymphoma and solid tumor cells are heterogeneous with respect to this marker.[29]

2. Human

Until recently, there was no evidence for heterogeneity of effector cell types of natural killing in the human, where NK cells were usually assayed by in vitro lysis of the erythroleukemic cell line K562.[31] The development of MoAb reactive with cell membrane antigens of human lymphohemapoietic cell subsets and investigations of the in vitro lysis of herpes simplex virus 1 (HSV-1)-infected fibroblasts, have now resulted in evidence which indicates that human NK cells are heterogeneous. Studies with MoAb have shown that there are at least two effectors of natural killing of K562, discernible by their expression of membrane markers.[32-34] One of these is perhaps analogous to the NK$_I$ of Minato et al.[27] as it does not express any mature T cell markers but does express myelomonocytic (M1) and NK cell (HNK-1) markers.[32,33] The second expresses both T and non-T cell markers (T8, T11A, DR, HNK-1) and may be analogous to the NK$_T$ cell.[32-34] This latter subset may contain further heterogeneity, as different groups have found different T cell markers on these cells.[33,34]

Studies in which natural killing of K562 was compared with that of HSV-1 infected or noninfected fibroblast target cells have indicated that there are at least two, and possibly three, subpopulations of human NK cells.[35,36] These studies have shown that NK cells which lyse HSV-1-infected fibroblasts are marrow-dependent, nonlymphoid in origin, reduced in activity in some patients with aplastic anemia who have normal NK cell activity against K562, and are directed against target structures not present on K562.[35,36] When these NK cells were studied with MoAb, it was found that the majority were Ia$^+$ and few reacted with antibodies to the E rosette receptor (Lyt-3, OKT-11A), which suggests that these cells may be analogous to the murine NK$_B$/NC subset. In contrast, the majority of NK cells directed against K562 were T11A$^+$ and did not express Ia antigens. M1, T10, and Leu-7 (HNK-1) were expressed by a portion, but not all of the NK cells which lysed both target types.[35,36]

B. Activated NK Cells: Effects of IFN

In the human and murine systems then, we have a variety of in vivo-derived effector cells which can mediate natural killing. Studies of these cells are, however, further complicated by the effects of IFN. It is now known that NK cells obtained from mammalian species can be activated in vivo by IFN and IFN inducers, or by short-term culture with these agents in vitro.[37] Further, it is possible that activation in vivo by viral infection, an IFN inducer, might not be identical to activation by short term in vitro culture with a particular IFN. Nonetheless, it is clear that NK cells activated in these ways are different from those obtained from nonstimulated mammals. Since these activated NK cells share certain properties with culture-induced killer cells which are not manifested by NK cells obtained from unstimulated mammals, they warrant consideration here.

Table 1
COMPARISON OF NK CELLS FROM NAIVE MICE WITH ACTIVATED NK CELLS

Parameters	NK cells from "naive" mice: NK/NK$_A$: NK$_I$	NK$_T$	NC/NK$_B$	"Activated" NK cells	Ref.
Short-term ^{51}Cr assay					
Lymphoma targets		Lysis	No lysis	Lysis	23,29
"Solid" tumor targets		No lysis	No lysis	Lysis	15,40
Surface markers					
NK-1, NK-2, NK-3	+	+	−	Heterogeneous	21,41,42,48
Asialo Gm1	+	+	−	+	42
Thy-1	−	+	−	Heterogeneous	42,44,46,50
Qa-5	+	+	−	Heterogeneous	43—45
Ly-5	+	+	−	+	38
Other Properties					
Cell size		Small	Large	Large	39,46
F_c receptors		Low	Negative	Increased	24,47
Adherence to nylon wool		Low	Low	Increased	24,46
Lability in culture		Labile	Not labile	Labile	24,46

A number of the differences between activated NK cells and NK cells obtained from "naive" mice are shown in Table 1. In this table, the NK/NK$_A$ cells have been divided into the Thy-1$^-$ NK$_I$ and Thy-1$^+$ NK$_T$ subsets referred to earlier.[25-26,38] Data from my own studies and those of other investigators indicate that "activated" NK cells are also heterogeneous and that this may be related to the mode of activation. Marker studies have revealed that "activated" NK cells can be NK-2-positive or -negative, Thy-1-positive or -negative and Qa-5-positive or -negative depending upon the system under study. Therefore, it is very likely that activated NK cell activity is the sum of the activities of a number of subsets of NK cells. However, to date, there have been no reports which suggest that IFN-activated NK cell activity is mediated by NC/NK$_B$ cell subsets. Indeed, Lattime et al.[49] have shown that IFN-inducing agents do not activate NC/NK$_B$ cells under conditions known to produce NK/NK$_A$ cell activation.[49]

Although there are significant differences between "activated" NK cells and NK/NK$_A$ cells, e.g., "activated" NK cells are large and lyse solid tumor targets, there are also many similarities (Table 1). Therefore, it is likely that NK/NK$_A$ cell subsets contribute to activated NK cell activity. Indeed, Minato and Bloom[38] and Minato et al.[50] have shown that both the Thy-1$^-$ (NK$_I$) and Thy-1$^+$ (NK$_T$) subsets of NK/NK$_A$ cells respond to IFN in vitro and that IFN appears to mediate conversion of NK$_I$ to NK$_T$ cells. This might suggest that activated NK cell activity is largely due to NK$_T$ cells induced by IFN; however, in most systems "activated" NK cells are Thy-1$^-$.[42,44,46] Further, there is evidence that the IFN-responsive cell is Ly-5$^-$, whereas mature NK/NK$_A$ cells are Ly-5$^+$.[38,50]

III. CULTURED NK CELLS

It should be apparent from the foregoing that a consideration of the effects on natural killing of short-term culture, or long-term culture and cloning of lymphohemapoietic cells must take account of the proposition that these measures are acting upon heterogeneous cell populations. Therefore, because these procedures will be both stimulatory and selective for the type of cultured NK cell activity produced, different sys-

Table 2
SUBSETS OF MURINE NK CELLS IN FRESH AND SHORT TERM "UNSTIMULATED" CULTURES OF MURINE LYMPHOHEMAPOIETIC CELLS

Characteristic cell source	1 Fresh spleen	2 Fresh spleen	3 Fresh spleen	4 Fresh spleen	5 Cultured spleen	6 Cultured spleen	6 Cultured bone marrow
Markers							
NK-2	+	+	−	−	−	−	−
Asialo Gm-1	+	+	−	−	−	−	−
Thy-1	+	−	−	−	−	+	−
Lyt-2	−	−	−	−	−	+	−
Qa-5	+	+	−	−	?	−	−
Ly-5	+	+	−	−	?	+	+
Beige activity	−	−	+	+	+	+	+
Nude activity	+	+	+	+	?	−	+
^{89}Sr treatment	Absent	Present	Present	Present	?	Present	?
Neonatal	Absent	Absent	Present	Absent	?	?	?
Radiation	Resistant	Resistant	Resistant	Sensitive	?	?	?
Cyclophosphamide	Sensitive	Sensitive	Resistant	Sensitive	?	?	?
Target preference	YAC	EL-4	WEH1-164	FLD-3	EMT-6	P815	YAC
Nomenclature/ref.							
Burton[20,23,25]	NA_A	NK_A	NK_B	NK_B	"NK_B"	"T_c"	
Minato[27,38]	NK_T	NK_I				TK	NK_M
Stutman[24,49]	NK	NK	NC				

tems, i.e., different species and different mouse strains, or different methods of culture, will probably produce different results.

A. Short-Term "Unstimulated" Cultures

Based on sensitivity to anti-Thy-1.2 and complement treatment and patterns of tumor target cell lysis, the author showed in 1977 that two populations of cytotoxic cells arose in "unstimulated" 7-day cultures of murine spleen cells.[13] Recently, this type of phenomenon has been related to the natural killing observed by uncultured spleen cells. Table 2 summarizes the results of studies from a number of laboratories which now indicate that at least seven different subsets of cells with NK-like activity can be discerned in fresh murine spleen cell suspensions or short term "unstimulated" cultures of murine spleen or bone marrow. It should be noted that uncultured murine bone marrow has virtually no NK cell activity in short-term ^{51}Cr-release assays.[15,27] I have attempted to reconcile the various nomenclatures used by different investigators in this table; however, it is clear that a consensus on a uniform nomenclature for NK cell subsets is needed.

There are three "new" NK-like activities which appear in "unstimulated" short-term (5 to 10 days) cultures of murine spleen or bone marrow. What relation do these cultured NK-like cells bear to the four subpopulations discernible in uncultured murine spleen? All of the NK activity of fresh murine spleen directed against YAC is mediated by NK-1$^+$, NK-2$^+$, NK-3$^+$, NK_A/NK-NK_I/NK_T natural killer cells.[25,27] Studies with NK cell-specific alloantisera have shown that these cells are very labile in "unstimulated" cultures, and by 48 hr less than 20% of the cytotoxicity activity detected in short-term cultures is mediated by NK-2$^+$ cells.[51] Further, removal of NK-2$^+$ cells with antibody and complement prior to short term "unstimulated" culture has no discernible effect on the generation of Thy-1.2$^+$ cytotoxic cells.[51] These results indicate that Thy-1$^+$ and Thy-1$^-$ NK-2$^+$ cells (NK/NK_A-NK_I/NK_T) play no role in the cytotoxicity induced by short-term unstimulated culture. In contrast, the activity of NK_B cells increases in short term "unstimulated" culture and tumor target cells resistant to lysis by fresh NK_B cells become susceptible.[51,52] This indicates that either the effectiveness of killing of target cells with low density of target structures (TS) by NK_B cells is increased by culture, or that new subset(s) of Nk_B-like cells arise in culture. The in vitro generation of this heightened NK_B ("NK_B") activity is not affected by pretreatment of murine spleen cells with anti-NK, antimacrophage or anti-T cell antibodies and complement, nor are "NK_B" cells, themselves, susceptible to this treatment.[51,52]

These results might suggest that "NK_B" cells are similar to NK_M cells which develop in cultures of murine bone marrow.[27,38] However, killer cells derived from bone marrow cultures kill lymphoma targets, such as YAC, whereas "NK_B" cells are directed against nonlymphoma targets and do not kill YAC.[27,38,51,52] In fact, NK_M cells appear to be more closely related to cytotoxic cells obtained from agar-cloned murine bone marrow and promonocytes isolated from liquid bone marrow cultures than to NC/NK_B or "NK_B" cells.[53,54] These granulocyte/monocyte lineage effector cells kill YAC,[53,54] and in the case of the promonocytes isolated from liquid bone marrow cultures, are susceptible to antimacrophage antibodies and complement.[53]

A third cytotoxic cell arises in "unstimulated" cultures which have a peak of activity against P815 about the 6th day of culture. This cytotoxic cell also lyses other lymphoma targets, but does not kill solid tumor targets.[13,51] The identity and target specificity of this cytotoxic effector cell have recently been resolved. It is a mature T_C, which arises from a NK-2$^-$, Thy-1.2$^+$ noncytotoxic precursor in murine spleen, and has the phenotype NK-2$^-$, asialo GM-1$^-$, Thy-1$^+$, Lyt-1$^+$, Lyt-2$^+$, Qa5$^-$, Ly-5$^+$.[27,38,51,52] Bulk cultures of these cells lyse a very wide variety of tumor target cells; however, this is not because the T_C are displaying nonspecific cytotoxicity, as might be implied by some of the terms attached to them, i.e., autoreactive, spontaneous, broadly reactive, or anomalous T_C or "T_C".[4,13,55-57]

In 1977, Ching et al.[58,59] studied Thy-1.2$^+$ cytotoxic cells directed against P815 which arose in "unstimulated" cultures and showed that these T_C could distinguish between syngeneic and allogeneic targets. They interpreted these results to mean that the Thy-1.2$^+$ activity generated by culture was due to activation of individual clones of T_C precursors. A recent study by Good et al.[60] has extended these findings using a limiting dilution split microculture technique to show that this is a clonal phenomenon in which Thy-1$^+$, Lyt-2$^+$ T_C precursors are induced to become T_C with clonally restricted specificity. The induction of multiple clones accounts for the broad range of target cells lysed by bulk cultures.

It should be noted that "unstimulated" is a misnomer, as it is clear that fetal calf and other sera which are absolute requirements for the generation of these in vitro cytotoxic cells contain stimuli to cell proliferation.[61] The recent definition of the effects of IFN and IL-2 on lymphocyte subpopulations provides a means whereby phenomena observed in short term "unstimulated" and stimulated cultures can be understood. It has been shown that IFN acts preferentially on NK_I cells in murine spleen.[27,38,44] T_C precursors, T_C themselves, and NK_M cells are not responsive to IFN.[27] In contrast, IL-2 acts upon the T_C precursors and the NK_T subset of NK/NK_A cells.[27] This is consistent with the proposition that IL-2 acts primarily and perhaps exclusively on Thy-1$^+$ cells.[27] Recent data from Lattime et al.[62] which show that Thy-1$^-$ NC/NK_B cells respond both to IL-2 and IL-3, are not incompatible with this conclusion because the IL-2 source used in their studies was not pure, and could have been contaminated with IL-3.

The data from "unstimulated" cultures of murine spleen are consistent with the proposition that enough IL-2, is generated in such cultures to produce polyclonal activation of T_C precursors, but not sufficient to allow activation of NK-2$^+$, Thy-1$^+$, NK_A/NK-NK_T cells. Further, if IFN is generated, then it is not in amounts sufficient to activate NK-2$^+$, Thy-1$^-$, NK_A/NK-NK_I cells. The heightened NC/NK_B activity ("NK_B")

must result from the activity of factors not yet identified, e.g., IL-3. Since the NK_M cell does not respond to IFN or IL-2,[27] its generation in bone marrow must be the result of other stimuli, such as colony stimulating factor. In summary, these short term "unstimulated" cultures appear equivalent to low-level IL-2 stimulation and thus this phenomenon is quite different to IFN activation of NK cells.

B. Short-Term Stimulated Cultures

I have, for convenience, referred to cultures in which known antigenic or lymphokine stimuli have not been added as "unstimulated" in order to compare them to those cultures in which known stimuli are included, since additional effects are observed in stimulated cultures. For example, mixed lymphocyte cultures (MLC) and mixed lymphocyte tumor cultures (MLTC) are complex in vitro phenomena in which proliferation and differentiation of various nucleated lymphohemapoietic cells takes place and during which lymphokines such as IL-2 and IFN are generated.[63,64] One might predict, therefore, that killer cells generated in MLC and MLTC would include, in addition to alloantigen-specific T_C, T_C, and NK_T responding to IL-2, and NK_I responding to IFN. Where cultures are stimulated by lectins or lymphokines without added antigens, then the types of cytotoxic cells generated might reflect the balance between IFN, IL-2, and other lymphokine stimulation.

Thy-1$^+$, Lyt-2$^+$ T_C derived from Thy-1$^+$, Lyt-2$^+$ T_C precursors, which are not directed against the specific "immunizing" antigens, have been detected in murine MLC, MLTC, F_1 antiparent, and syngeneic antihapten cultures.[55,57,60,65] My own studies in this area, performed in collaboration with a number of colleagues, have indicated that Thy-1$^+$, NK/NK_A-NK_T cells are also induced by MLC, or when the IFN inducer polyinosinic acid is used to stimulate murine spleen cells.[56,66] In addition, Clark and Holley[67] have shown that intraperitoneal injection of allogeniec lymphoid cells rapidly activates NK-1$^+$, asialo $GM_1$$^+$, Thy-1$^+$, NK/$NK_A$-$NK_T$ cells, which show a peak of activity against YAC on the second day after innoculation. These data are all compatible with the proposition that these effects are due to IL-2 production.

Since IFN is generated in mixed lymphocyte cultures,[64] then one might expect that NK-1$^+$, NK-2$^+$, NK-3$^+$, NK/NK_A-NK_I cells might also be detected. Paciucci et al.[68] have detected Thy-1$^-$ cytotoxic cells, which arise from Thy-1$^-$ precursors in MLC. These cytotoxic cells lyse sarcoma targets and require the presence of viable Thy-1$^+$ cells for their activation. Although studies with NK-specific alloantisera have not been reported, it is likely that these are activaed NK cells (Table 1) derived from the NK/NK_A-NK_I subset. Therefore, in these short-term stimulated in vitro murine cultures, there is evidence for activation of NK_T cells and polyclonal activation of T_C by IL-2 and activation of NK_I cells by IFN.

In human studies, Zarling et al.[69,70] have shown that NK-like cells generated in alloantigen-stimulated and autologous lymphoblastoid cell line-stimulated cultures can be distinguished from T_C, because they do no express the human T cell markers T3 or T8. Further, this group have also shown that the NK-like cells generated in such MLC are derived from cells which express the phenotype of one subset of fresh human NK cells (M-1$^+$, B-73.1$^+$.)[71] The data of Lopez-Botet et al.[72] support these findings, because they have shown that T3$^+$, T8$^+$ T cell blasts and T8$^-$ NK-like cells develop in MLC, or cultures of human PBL with IL-2. These findings, and those of others[73] indicate that polyclonally activated T_C, which express mature human T cell markers, and NK-like cells with a phenotype found on fresh human NK cells, develop in stimulated human cultures. The first of these cytotoxic cells is probably equivalent to the polyclonally activated murine T_C, while the second almost certainly corresponds to either or both of the NK/NK_A subpopulations of murine spleen, i.e., NK_T and/or NK_I.

IV. NK CELL LINES

From the foregoing, it can be predicted that cloned cytotoxic cell lines derived from long-term cultures will consist of T_C and various subsets of NK cells, depending upon the conditions of culture. In particular, the balance between IL-2, IL-3, and IFN activities and the presence or absence of strong stimulating antigens will have a major effect on the cell lines obtained. Further, there will be the possibility that these long-term lines might undergo malignant transformation, either spontaneously, or in response to continued stimulation by lymphokines. This might well result in unexpected changes in in vitro function and/or the expression of surface markers not normally present on that cell type. Such transformed cells might well have no corresponding in vivo cell type.

A. Murine NK Cell Lines

Since most of the systems used to derive NK cell lines employ stimulation with IL-2, it is not unexpected that Thy-1^+ cytotoxic cell lines with NK-like activity would be the most common cloned lines obtained. This is in fact the case, and where appropriate marker studies have been performed, it has been shown that Thy-1^+, asialo GM_1^+, NK-1^+ and/or NK-2^+, Lyt-1^-, Lyt-2^- uncloned or cloned NK cell lines can be readily established in IL-2-containing media.[74-77] These lines have a phenotype identical to that of the NK/NK_A-NK_T subset (Table 2), as might have been predicted. Although IL-2 has been shown to be an absolute requirement for proliferation of these NK_T cells in vitro and for the derivation of cloned lines, IFN does have a modulating effect on both the proliferation and the cytotoxicity of the cultured cells.[76,78] Very recently, uncloned Thy-1^- NC/NK_B-like cell lines have been obtained by use of IL-3 conditioned media,[79] which further emphasizes the differential effects of different lymphokines on different NK cell subsets.

Cloned Thy-1^+ NK-like cell lines not expressing the typical NK_T phenotype have been obtained. Brooks et al.[80] found dense Lyt-2 expression on two Thy-1^+, Lyt-1^-, NK-2^+ cloned cytolytic cell lines with NK-like activity. To date, no corresponding Lyt-2^+, NK-2^+ cell has been demonstrated in fresh murine spleen (Table 2). Suzuki et al.[77] found that only 7 to 15% of the cells in 11 cloned NK lines, in which more than 85% of the cells expressed asialo GM_1 or Ly-5, expressed Thy-1.2. Are these NK_T lines with low Thy-1 expression, or are they mixtures of Thy-1^+ and Thy-1^- lines? Do these lines represent a new NK phenotype? This current confusion concerning the expression of T cell markers, and in particular Lyt-2, on NK cell lines has not been resolved.

It has recently been shown that cloned MCH-restricted male antigen-specific T_C kept in culture in the presence of IL-2 for over 2 years lost their antigenic specificity and acquired high NK-like activity.[81] These lines maintained their typical T_C phenotype, i.e., Thy-1^+, Lyt-2^+. Further, cytotoxicity of one of these lines was not inhibitied by monoclonal anti-Lyt-2 antibodies which do inhibit specific T_C mediated lysis.[81] We have recently shown that 3 alloantigen-specific cytotoxic T cell cloned lines express NK-1 and/or NK-2.[82] On two of these lines, the expression of NK-2 was 20 to 50% that of the expression of this antigen on cloned NK cell lines, however, the third C57BL/6 anti-DBA/2 cloned cytotoxic T cell line expressed as much NK-1 and NK-2 as any NK-like line.[82] These results have been interpreted to mean that NK cells and T cells are closely related.[80,82] Since these lines most closely resemble NK_T cells, it is possible that there is a close relationship between this subset of NK cells and T_C. A more trivial explanation would be that the expression fo T cell-specific markers on cloned NK cell lines and vice versa are "artefacts" due to malignant transformation.

B. Human NK Cell Lines

In human systems, cloned lines with NK cell-like activity, but with mature T lymphocyte phenotypes have been obtained by a number of investigators.[83,85] It is possible that these are, in fact, typical T_C with a clonally restricted receptor directed against a widely shared or cross-reacting TS. On the other hand, they may represent clones similar to the Lyt-2^+ NK lines described in murine systems. Uncloned and cloned NK cell lines with a non-T_C phenotype have also been obtained by a number of investiagors.[86-89] These lines lack the mature T cell markers T3, T4, and T8, and fall into two groups. There are those which express the E-rosette receptor[86-88] and one cloned NK cell line derived from the null cell fraction of human PBL, which did not.[89] Flomenberg et al.[88] derived three cloned NK cell lines from patients with primary T cell immunodeficiencies and found that they expressed the E rosette receptor and reacted with the MoAb 3A-1, which detects an antigen on all T cells and LGL. They compared these cell lines to the NK_T cells of mice. In contrast, the NK cell line derived from the null cell fraction of PBL by Hercend et al.[89] responded to IFN and had a phenotype which would make it analogous to the murine NK_I cell.

V. COMMENTS AND CONCLUSIONS

In vitro culture is a powerful tool for studying certain properties of lymphohemapoietic cells. The use of "unstimulated" and stimulated culture conditions for the study of mammalian NK cells has produced new insights into the types of lymphohemapoietic cells which mediate natural killing and their response to biological regulatory lymphokines, in particular IFN, IL-2, and IL-3. In fact, it appears that the results obtained in a particular culture system will depend upon the balance between IL-2, IL-3, and IFN stimulation, although long-term continuous and cloned cell lines have only been obtained to date with IL-2 or IL-3 stimulation.

These findings emphasize the limitations of in vitro culture as an investigatory tool in the study of mammalian lymphohemapoietic cells. The technique exerts both selective and stimulatory pressures on lymphohemapoietic cells. Thus, major lymphohemapoietic cell subsets may not survive under in vitro conditions, while the stimulation of other subsets might result in the emergence of very minor in vivo subsets with in vitro properties quite dissimilar to their in vivo role. Further, partial or complete malignant transformation may occur with the appearance of in vitro cell types which have no in vivo counterpart. Nonetheless, it should be clear from the foregoing that study of the characteristics of cultured NK cells has, within a very short space of time, added significantly to our knowledge of natural killing.

ACKNOWLEDGMENTS

Dr. Noel Warner, Dr. Stanley Chism, Dr. Henry Winn, and Dr. Scott Barlett were major collaborators in my studies in this area over the last 10 years. I have been supported by the National Health and Medical Research Council of Australia throughout this period, with additional support from the National Cancer Institute and the National Institutes of Health of the U.S. I wish to thank Ms. Elinor Couper for her care and patience in typing this manuscript.

REFERENCES

1. Brunner, K. T., Mauel, J., Cerottini, J. C., and Chapius, B., Quantitative assay of the lytic action of immune cells on ^{51}Cr labelled allogeneic target cells, *Immunology,* 14, 181, 1968.
2. Cerottini, J. C. and Brunner, K. T., Cell mediated cytotoxicity allograft rejection and tumor immunity, *Adv. Immunol.,* 18, 67, 1974.
3. Burton, R. C., Chism, S. E., and Warner, N. L., *In Vitro* induction and expression of T cell immunity to tumour associated antigens, in *Contemporary Topics in Immunobiology,* Vol. 8, Warner, N. L. and Cooper, M. D., Eds., Plenum Press, New York, 1978, 69.
4. Cohen, I. R., Globerson, A., and Feldman, M., Autosensitisation *in vitro, J. Exp. Med.,* 133, 834, 1971.
5. Takasugi, M., Mickey, M. R., and Terasaki, P. I., Reactivity of lymphocytes from normal persons on cultured tumour cells, *Cancer Res.,* 33, 2898, 1973.
6. Herberman, R. B., Aoki, T., Nunn, M., Lavrin, D. H., Soares, N., Gazdar, A., Holden, H., and Chang, K. S. S., Specificity of ^{51}Cr release cytotoxicity of lymphocytes immune to murine sarcoma virus, *J. Natl. Cancer Inst.,* 53, 1103, 1974.
7. Kiessling, R., Klein, E., and Wigzell, H., "Natural" killer cells in the mouse. I. Cytotoxic cells with specificity for mouse Moloney leukemia cells. Specificity and distribution according to genotpye, *Eur. J. Immunol.,* 5, 112, 1975.
8. Herberman, R. B., Nunn, M. E., and Lavrin, D. H., Natural cytotoxic reactivity of mouse lymphoid cells against syngeneic and allogeneic tumours. I. Distribution of reactivity and specificity, *Int. J. Cancer,* 16, 216, 1975.
9. Herberman, R. B., Ed., *Natural Cell Mediated Immunity Against Tumours,* Academic Press, New York, 1980.
10. Herberman, R. B., Ed., *NK Cells and Other Natural Effector Cells,* Academic Press, New York, 1982.
11. Cohen, I. R. and Wekerle, H., Regulation of autosensitisation: the immune activation and specific inhibition of self-recognising thymus-derived lymphocytes, *J. Exp. Med.,* 137, 224, 1973.
12. Ilfield, D., Carnoud, C., and Klein, E., Cytotoxicity of autosensitised lymphocytes restricted to the H-2K end of targets, *Immunogenetics,* 2, 231, 1975.
13. Burton, R. C., Chism., S. E., and Warner, N. L., *In vitro* induction of tumour specific immunity. VII. Does autosensitisation occur with *in vitro* culture of T lymphocytes?, *J. Immunol.,* 119, 1329, 1977.
14. Chism, S. E., Burton, R. C., Grail, D. L., Bell, P. M., and Warner, N. L., *In vitro* induction of tumour specific immunity. VI. Analysis of immune response by cellular competitive inhibition. Limitations and advantages of the technique, *J. Immunol. Methods,* 16, 245, 1977.
15. Burton, R. C., Grail, D., and Warner, N. L., Natural cytotoxicity of hemapoietic cell populations against murine lymphoid tumors, *Cancer,* 37, 806, 1978.
16. Winn, H. J., personal communication.
17. Glimcher, L., Shen, F. W., and Cantor, H., Identification of a cell surface antigen selectively expressed on the natural killer cell, *J. Exp. Med.,* 145, 1, 1977.
18. Burton, R. C., and Winn, H. J., Studies on natural killer (NK) cells. I. NK cell specific antibodies in CE anti-CBA serum, *J. Immunol.,* 126, 1985, 1981.
19. Pollack, S. B. and Emmons, S. L., NK-2.1: an NK associated antigen detected with NZB anti-BALB/c serum, *J. Immunol.,* 129, 2277, 1982.
20. Burton, R. C., Barlett, S. P., Kumar, V., and Winn, H. J., Studies on natural killer (NK) cells. II. Serological evidence for heterogeneity of NK cells, *J. Immunol.,* 127, 1864, 1981.
21. Burton, R. C., Barlett, S. P., and Winn, H. J., Alloantigens on natural killer cells, in *International Review of Cytology,* Bourne, G., Ed., Academic Press, in press.
22. Stutman, O., Paige, C. J., and Figarella, E. F., Natural cytotoxic cells against solid tumours in mice. I. Strain and age distribution and target cell susceptibility, *J. Immunol.,* 21, 1819, 1978.
23. Lust, J. A., Kumar, V., Burton, R. C., Bartlett, S. P., and Bennett, M., Heterogeneity of natural killer (NK) cells in the mouse, *J. Exp. Med.,* 154, 306, 1981.
24. Stutman, O., Lattime, E. C., and Figarella, E. F., Natural cytotoxic cells against solid tumors in mice: a comparison with natural killer cells, *Fed. Proc., Fed. Am. Soc. Exp. Biol.,* 40, 2699, 1981.
25. Burton, R. C., Scott, S. P., Lust, J. A., and Kumar, V., Natural killer cell subsets, in *NK Cells and Other Natural Effector Cells,* Herberman, R. B., ED., Academic Press, New York, 1982, 173.
26. Mattes, M. J., Sharrow, S. O., Herberman, R. B., and Holden, H. T., Identification and separation of Thy-1 positive mouse spleen cells active in natural cytotoxicity and antibody dependent cell-mediated cytotoxicity, *J. Immunol.,* 123, 2851, 1979.
27. Minato, N., Reid, L., and Bloom, B. R., On the heterogeneity of murine natural killer cells, *J. Exp. Med.,* 154, 750, 1981.

28. Kumar, V., Luevano, E., and Bennett, M., Hybrid resistance to EL-4 lymphoma cells. I. Characterisation of natural killer cells that lyse EL-4 cells and their distinction from marrow dependent natural killer cells, *J. Exp. Med.*, 150, 531, 1979.
29. Brooks, C. G., Flannery, G. R., Cantrell, D. A., Gray, J. D., Robins, R. A., and Baldwin, R. W., Rat NK cells active against lymphoma and sarcoma tumor cells are probably identical, *J. Immunol.*, 128, 913, 1982.
30. Brideau, R. J., Carter, P. B., McMaster, W. R., Mason, D. W., and Williams, A. F., Two subsets of rat T lymphocytes defined with monoclonal antibodies, *Eur. J. Immunol.*, 10, 609, 1980.
31. Pross, H. F. and Baines, M. G., Spontaneous human lymphocyte mediated cytotoxicity against tumor target cells. I. The effect of malignant disease, *Int. J. Cancer*, 18, 593, 1976.
32. Zarling, J. M., Clouse, K. A., Biddison, W. E., and Kung, P. C., Phenotypes of human natural killer cell populations detected with monoclonal antibodies, *J. Immunol.* 127, 2575, 1981.
33. Abo, T., Cooper, M. D., and Balch, C. M., Characterisation of HNK-1^+ (Leu-7) human lymphocytes. I. Two distinct phenotypes of human NK cells with different cytotoxic capability, *J. Immunol.*, 129, 1752, 1982.
34. Perussia, B., Fanning, V., and Trinchieri, G., A human NK and K cell subset shares with cytotoxic T cells expression of the antigen recognized by antibody OKT-8, *J. Immunol.*, 131, 223, 1983.
35. Fitzgerald, P. A., Evans, R., Kirkpatrick, D., and Lopez, C., Heterogeneity of human NK cells: comparison of effectors that lyse HSV-1-infected fibroblasts and K562 erothryoleukaemia targets, *J. Immunol.*, 130, 1663, 1983.
36. Lopez, C., Kirkpatrick, D., Fitzgerald, P. A., Ching, C. Y., Pahwa, R. N., Good, R. A., and Smithwick, E. M., Studies of the cell lineage of the effector cells that spontaneously lyse HSV-1-infected fibroblasts (NK HSV-1), *J. Immunol.*, 129, 824, 1982.
37. Djeu, J. Y., Heinbaugh, J. A., Holden, H. T., and Herberman, R. B., Augmentation of mouse natural killer cell activity by interferon and interferon inducers, *J. Immunol.*, 122, 175, 1979.
38. Minato, N. and Bloom, B. R., Heterogeneity and regulation of the natural killer cell system, in *NK Cells and Other Natural Effector Cells*, Herberman, R. B., Ed., Academic Press, New York, 1982, 131.
39. Tai, A., Burton, R. C., and Warner, N. L., Differential natural killer cell reactivity against T cell lymphomas by cells from normal or stimulated mice, *J. Immunol.*, 124, 1705, 1980.
40. MacFarlan, R. I., Ceredig, R., and White, D. O., Comparison of natural killer cells induced by Kunjin virus and Corynebacterium parvum with those occurring naturally in nude mice, *Infect. Immun.*, 26, 832, 1979.
41. Kumar, V., Barnes, M. C., Bennett, M., and Burton, R. C., Differential lysis of endogenous and activated natural killer cells by anti-NK-1.2 antibody and complement, *J. Immunol.*, 128, 1482, 1982.
42. Bukowski, J. F., Biron, C. A., and Welsh, R. M., Elevated natural killer cell mediated cytotoxicity, plasma interferon, and tumor cell rejection in mice persistently infected with lymphocytic choriomeningitis virus, *J. Immunol.*, 131, 991, 1983.
43. Chun, M., Pasanen, V., Hammerling, U., Hammerling, G., and Hoffman, M. K., Tumor necrosis serum induces a serologically distinct population of NK cells, *J. Exp. Med.*, 150, 426, 1979.
44. Chun, M., Fernandes, G., and Hoffman, M. K., Mechanism of NK cell activation: relationship between $Qa5^+$ NK cells and lymphocytes, *J. Immunol.*, 126, 331, 1981.
45. Clark, E. A., Engel, D., and Windsor, N. T., Immune responsiveness of SM/J mice: hyper-NK cell activity mediated by NK-1^+ Qa5-cells, *J. Immunol.*, 127, 2391, 1981.
46. Kiessling, R., Eriksson, E., Hallenbeck, L. A., and Welsh, R. M., A comparative analysis of the cell surface properties of activated versus endogenous mouse natural killer cells, *J. Immunol.*, 125, 1551, 1980.
47. Welsh, R. M., Cytotoxic cells induced during lymphocytic choriomeningitis virus infection of mice. I. Characterisation of natural killer cell induction, *J. Exp. Med.*, 148, 163, 1978.
48. McKinnon, K. P., Hail, A. H., and Ruebush, M. J., Elicitation of natural killer cells in beige mice by infection with vesicular stomatitis virus, *Infect. Immun.*, 32, 204, 1981.
49. Lattime, E. C., Pecoraro, G. A. Cuttito, M., and Stutmann, O., Solid tumors are killed by NK and NC populations: interferon inducing agents do not augment NC cell activity under NK activating conditions, in *NK Cells and Other Natural Effector Cells*, Herberman, R. B., Ed., Academic Press, New York, 1982, 179.
50. Minato, N., Reid, L., Cantor, H., Lengyel, P., and Bloom, B. R., Mode of regulation of natural killer cell activity by interferon, *J. Exp. Med.*, 152, 124, 1980.
51. Bartlett, S. P. and Burton, R. C., Studies on natural killer (NK) cells. III. Effects of *in vitro* culture on spontaneous cytotoxicity of murine spleen cells, *J. Immunol.*, 128, 1070, 1982.
52. Bartlett, S. P. and Burton, R. C., Cultured natural killer cells, in *NK Cells and Other Natural Effector Cells*, Herberman, R. B., Ed., Academic Press, New York, 1982, 807.

53. Lohmann-Matthes, M. L., Domzig, W., and Roder, J., Promonocytes have the functional characteristics of natural killer cells, *J. Immunol.*, 123, 1883, 1979.
54. Claesson, M. H. and Olsson, L., Autoreactive natural killer like cells from agar cloned murine bone marrow cells, *Nature*, 283, 578, 1980.
55. Ishikawa, H. and Dutton, R. W., Spontaneous and induced *in vitro* F_1 antiparental cytotoxic T lymphocyte responses: target specificities of cytotoxic effectors, *J. Immunol.*, 123, 2741, 1979.
56. Dorfman, N., Winkler, D., Burton, R. C., Kossayda, N., Sabia, P., and Wunderlich, J., Broadly reactive murine cytotoxic cells induced *in vitro* under syngeneic conditions, *J. Immunol.*, 129, 1762, 1982.
57. Shain, B., Holt, C. A., and Lilly, F., Lack of specificity for viral and H-2 antigens by anomalous T killer cells generated in murine leukocyte cultures, *J. Immunol.*, 129, 722, 1982.
58. Ching, L. M., Marbrook, J., and Walker, K. Z., Spontaneous clones of cytotoxic T cells in culture. I. Characteristics of the response, *Cell Immunol.*, 31, 284, 1977.
59. Ching, L. M., Marbrook, J., and Walker, K. Z., Spontaneous clones of cytotoxic T cells in culture. II. Specificity of the response, *Cell. Immunol.*, 31, 293.
60. Good, M. F., Boyd, A. W., and Nossal, G. J. V., Analysis of true antihapten cytotoxic clones in limit dilution microcultures after correction for "anti-self" activity: precursor frequencies, Ly-2 and Thy-1 phenotype, specificity and statistical methods, *J. Immunol.*, 130, 2046, 1983.
61. Golub, S. H. and Zielske, J., Induction of cell mediated cytotoxic responses against human tumor cells and fibroblasts, *Proc. Am. Assoc. Cancer Res.*, 16, 170, 1975.
62. Lattime, E. C., Pecoraro, G. A., and Stutman, O., The activity of natural cytotoxic cells is augmented by interleukin 2 and interleukin 3, *J. Exp. Med.*, 157, 1070, 1983.
63. Gillis, S., Ferm, M. M., Ou, W., and Smith, K. A., T cell growth factor: parameters of production and a quantitative microassay for activity, *J. Immunol.*, 120, 2027, 1978.
64. Virelizier, J. L., Allison, A. C., and DeMayer, E., Production by mixed lymphocyte cultures of type II interferon able to protect macrophages against virus infections, *Infect. Immun.*, 17, 282, 1977.
65. Kärre, K. and Seeley, J. K., Cytotoxic Thy-1.2^+ blasts with NK-like target cell activity in murine mixed lymphocyte cultures, *J. Immunol.*, 123, 1511, 1979.
66. Kärre, K., Seeley, J. K., Eriksson, E., Burton, R. C., and Kiessling, R., "Anomalous" Thy-1^+ killer cells in allogeneic and F_1-anti-parental mixed leukocyte culture: relation to natural killer cells and allospecific cytotoxic T lymphocytes, *J. Exp. Med.*, 157, 385, 1983.
67. Clark, E. A. and Holly, R. D., Activation of natural killer (NK) cells *in vivo* with H-2 and non-H-2 alloantigens, *Immunogenetics*, 12, 221, 1981.
68. Paciucci, P. O., MacPhail, S., Bach, F. H., and Zarling, J. M., Requirements for T cells in alloantigen induced generation of non-T cell mediated cytotoxicity against syngeneic mouse sarcoma cells, *J. Immunol.*, 125, 36, 1980.
69. Zarling, J. M., Dierckins, M. S., Sevenich, E. A., and Clouse, K. A., Stimulation with autologous lymphoblastoid cell lines: lysis of Epstein-Barr virus positive and negative cell lines by two phenotypically distinguishable effector cell populations, *J. Immunol.*, 127, 2118, 1981.
70. Zarling, J. M., Bach, F. H., and Kung, P. C., Sensitisation of lymphocytes against pooled allogeneic cells. II. Characterisation of effector cells cytotoxic for autologous lymphoblastoid cell lines, *J. Immunol.*, 126, 376, 1981.
71. Strassmann, G., Bach, F. H., and Zarling, J. M., Depletion of human NK cells with monoclonal antibodies allows the generation of cytotoxic T lymphocytes without NK-like cells in mixed cultures, *J. Immunol.*, 130, 1556, 1983.
72. Lopez-Botet, M., Silva, A., Rodriguez, J., and De-Landazuri, M. O., Generation of T cell blasts with NK-like activity in human MLC: cellular precursoes, IL2 responsiveness and phenotype expression, *J. Immunol.*, 129, 1109, 1982.
73. Masucci, M. A., Klein, E., and Argov, S., Disappearance of the NK effect after expantation of lymphocytes and generation of similar non-specific cytotoxicity correlated to the level of blastogenesis in activated cultures, *J. Immunol.*, 124, 2458, 1980.
74. Dennert, G., Yogeeswaran, G., and Yamagata, S., Cloned cell lines with natural killer activity: specificity, function and cell surface markers, *J. Exp. Med.*, 153, 545, 1981.
75. Nabel, G. Bucalo, L. R., Allard, J., Wigzell, H., and Cantor, H., Multiple activities of a cloned cell line mediating natural killer cell function, *J. Exp. Med.*, 153, 1582, 1981.
76. Kuribayashi, K., Gillis, St., Kern, D. E., and Henney, C. S., Murine NK cell cultures: effects of interleukin-2 and interferon on cell growth and cytotoxic reactivity, *J. Immunol.*, 126, 2321, 1981.
77. Suzuki, R., Handa, K., Itoh, K., and Kumagai, K., Natural killer (NK) cells as a responder to interleukin 2 (IL 2). I. Proliferative response and establishment of cloned cells, *J. Immunol.*, 130, 981, 1983.
78. Riccardi, C., Vose, B. M., and Herberman, R. B., Modulation of IL 2-dependent growth of mouse NK cells by interferon and T lymphocytes, *J. Immunol.*, 130, 228, 1983.

79. Djeu, J. Y., Lanza, E., Pastore, S., and Hapel, A. J., Selective growth of natural cytotoxic cells but not natural killer cells in interleukin-3, *Nature,* 306, 788, 1983.
80. Brooks, C. G., Kuribayashi, K., Sale, G. E. and Henney, C. S., Characterisation of five cloned murine cell lines showing high cytolytic activity against YAC-1 cells, *J. Immunol.,* 128, 2326, 1982.
81. Acha-Orbea, H., Groscurth, P., Lang, R., Stitz, L., and Hengartner, H., Characterization of cloned cytotoxic lymphocytes with NK-like activity, *J. Immunol.,* 130, 2952, 1983.
82. Brooks, C. G., Burton, R. C., Pollack, S. B., and Henney, C. S., The presence of NK alloantigens on cloned cytotoxic T lymphocytes, *J. Immunol.,* 131, 1391, 1983.
83. Pawelec, G. P., Hadam, M. R., Ziegler, A., Lohmeyer, J., Rehbein, A., Kumbier, I., and Wernet, P., Long-term culture, cloning, and surface markers of mixed leukocyte culture-derived human T lymphocytes with natural killer-like cytotoxicity, *J. Immunol.,* 126, 1892, 1982.
84. Sugamura, K., Tanaka, Y., and Hinuma, Y., Two distinct human cloned T cell lines that exhibit natural killer-like and anti-human effector activities, *J. Immunol.,* 128, 1749, 1982.
85. Sheehy, M. J., Quintieri, F. B., Leung, D. Y. M., Geha, R. S., Dubey, D. P., Limmer, C. E., and Yunis, E. J., A human large granular lymphoctye clone with natural killer-like activity and T cell-like surface markers, *J. Immunol.,* 130, 524, 1983.
86. Kornbluth, J., Flomenberg, N., and Dupont, B., Cell surface phenotype of a cloned line of human natural killer cells, *J. Immunol.,* 129, 2831, 1982.
87. Krensky, A. M., Ault, K. A., Reiss, C. S., Strominger, J. L., and Burakoff, S. J., Generation of long-term human cytolytic cell lines with persistent natural killer activity, *J. Immunol.,* 129, 1748, 1982.
88. Flomenberg, N., Welte, K., Mertelsmann, R., O'Reilly, R., and Dupont, B., Interleukin 2-dependent natural killer (NK) cell lines from patients with primary T cell immunodeficiencies, *J. Immunol.,* 130, 2635, 1983.
89. Hercend, T., Meuer, S., Reinherz, E. L., Schlossman, S. F., and Ritz, J., Generation of a cloned NK cell line derived from the "null cell" fraction of human peripheral blood, *J. Immunol.,* 129, 1299, 1982.

Chapter 11

LECTIN-DEPENDENT KILLER CELLS*

Benjamin Bonavida

TABLE OF CONTENTS

* Supported in part by CA 35791 for the National Cancer Institute and in part from the Cancer Research Coordinating Committee.

I. INTRODUCTION

Several effector cells, both of lymphoid and nonlymphoid origin, have been shown to be involved in cell-mediated cytotoxicity (CMC). Some of these effector cells are antigen-specific, such as those mediated by the cytotoxic T lymphocytes (CTL), and others appear to be antigen-nonspecific such as the natural killer (NK) and killer cells for antibody-dependent cell-mediated cytotoxicity (ADCC), macrophages, and neutrophils (Table 1). These cytotoxic effector mechanisms are operative in vivo and can be readily demonstrated and maintained in vitro. Many of these cells have been shown to play an important role in immune surveillance against infection and malignant disease.

Cytotoxic T cells develop following sensitization with virally infected cells, tumor cells, and allogeneic graft. These T cells have been shown in the syngeneic system to be H-2-restricted. Killer (K) cells for ADCC are cytotoxic cells which can mediate their cytotoxic function against antibody-coated target cells. They bear Fc receptors which bind to the Fc fragment of the antibody and this interaction appears to initiate the events which lead to cytotoxicity. NK cells are present in the peripheral blood, and without active sensitization express cytotoxicity against a variety of sensitive tumor targets and virally infected cells. There are also recent demonstrations of the possible importance of NK cells in hemopoietic regulation.[1] Activated macrophages and neutrophils are rendered cytotoxic against a variety of tumor and nontumor target cells. Also recently described are lymphokine-activated killer (LAK) cells that kill tumor cells.[2]

Clearly, there are several effector cell mechanisms by which the body can defend itself against foreign invaders. However, there may be other effector cells which have yet to be discovered. It is also possible that there are other pathways or systems by which the same effector cells can be triggered and exhibit their cytotoxic potential. In the latter category, cells exist that express cytotoxicity against a variety of target cells in the presence of lectin or following enzymatic or chemical modification of the target cell (Table 2).

The lectin-dependent cellular cytotoxicity (LDCC) system is observed in the presence of lectin such as phytohemagglutinin (PHA) or concanavalin A (Con A), and the oxidative-dependent cellular cytotoxicity (ODCC) systems are observed following enzymatic treatment by neuraminidase and galactose oxidase (NAGO) or by periodate (IO_4) modification of the target cells.[3-7] Both CTL[8] and normal human peripheral blood cells[9] exert these various cytotoxic activities. More recent, however, is the observation of a lectin-dependent cytotoxic system in which normal murine spleen cells kill NK-sensitive targets in the presence of lectins.[10] These NK-LDCC cells differ from the CTL-LDCC system in mice in that the effector cells are not sensitized and the target specificity is restricted to the NK-sensitive targets.

The exact biological and physiological function of the LDCC, ODCC, or NK-LDCC systems is not clear. It is possible that lectin-like molecules are expressed on certain types of target cells and that such lectins mimic plant lectins and become targets for LDCC, ODCC, or NK-LDCC. In such a case, these systems add a new dimension to the natural cytotoxic systems discussed above and amplify the effector mechanisms in favor of the immune surveillance. Under certain circumstances, however, it is possible that such highly cytotoxic systems attack normal host tissue leading to clinical manifestations.

In this review article, I will summarize our data and, briefly, the data of others in the lectin-dependent cytotoxic effector mechanisms.

Table 1
CYTOTOXIC EFFECTOR CELLS

Effector	Specificity
CTL	Antigen-specific — MHC-restricted
NK	NK-sensitive targets
ADCC	Antibody-coated target cells
Macrophages	Tumor targets; infected targets
Neutrophils	Tumor targets; infected targets
LAK	Tumor targets

Table 2
LDCC AND ODCC

Effector	Target
CTL	Lectin-coated; IO_4 or NAGO-modified
Human peripheral blood	Lectin-coated; IO_4 or NAGO-modified
Macrophages	Lectin-coated red blood cells
Murine pre NK or T cells	Con A + NK-sensitive targets

Table 3
CTL-MEDIATED LDCC IN MICE

Effector[a]	Target (^{51}Cr)	Lectin[b]	%Lysis (E:T=20:1)
C57BL/6 anti-G.35	G-35	None	45
($H\text{-}2^b$ anti-$H\text{-}2^d$)	($H\text{-}2^d$)	PHA	44
		Con A	42
C57BL/6 anti-G.35	EL-4	None	0
($H\text{-}2^b$ anti$H\text{-}2^d$)	($H\text{-}2^b$)	PHA	56
		Con A	55
C57BL/6 anti-G.35	SJL/J blasts	None	0
($H\text{-}2^b$ anti-$H\text{-}2^d$)	($H\text{-}2^s$)	PHA	13.0
	C58NT/D rat tumor	None	2
		PHA	19
Normal Balb/c	EL-4	None	4
		PHA	5
		Con A	4

[a] The effector cells were prepared by immunizing C57BL/6 mice with allogeneic G.35 targets and 9 days later the peritoneal exudate cells were obtained and used in the ^{51}Cr release assay.

[b] 10 $\mu\ell$ PHA and 10 μg Con A were used.

II. T CELL-MEDIATED LDCC AND ODCC

A. Differences Between Man and Animal Systems

T lymphocytes have been shown to exhibit nonspecific cytotoxicity in a variety of systems, both in humans and in animals. In the animal systems, this phenomenon has been observed with lymphocytes sensitized in vitro with PHA or Con A,[11] in lymph nodes of mice sensitized with oxazolone or picrylchloride,[12] with lymphocytes sensitized against allogeneic stimulator cells,[5,13] and in spleen cells of mice sensitized in vivo with Con A.[14] In all of these systems, cytotoxicity was mediated by activated T cells, while untreated lymphocytes from normal mice were not found to be cytotoxic (Table 3). These results suggest that LDCC detects the presence of activated T cells present in a mixed cell population.

Table 4
LDCC IN NORMAL HUMAN PERIPHERAL BLOOD

Sample Number[a]	Target[b]	Lectin	% Lysis (E:T=20:1)
1	EL-4	PHA	14
2	EL-4	PHA	16
3	EL-4	PHA	23
4	EL-4	PHA	31
5	T-24	PHA	19
6	HCV/29	PHA	36
7	Raji	Con A	34

[a] Human peripheral blood was separated over a Ficoll-hypaque gradient and macromolecular cells used as effectors.

[b] Various targets of murine or human origin were used. EL-4 is a chemically induced lymphoma in C57BL/6 mice. T-24 and HCV/29 human cell lines were derived from a transitional cell carcinoma of the bladder. Raji is a B cell derived from a patient with Burkitt's lymphoma.

In man, however, mitogen-induced cellular cytotoxicity (MICC) by normal peripheral blood has been observed against chicken red blood cells and tumor target cells.[15,16] The effector cells mediating these cytotoxic activities were initially comprised of T cells and required long periods of incubation (more than 18 hr), in contrast to the LDCC assay which is obtained in less than 4 hr of incubation. Thus, the presence of LDCC and ODCC in the peripheral blood of man was investigated in order to demonstrate whether such effector cells might exist in the nonactivated or sensitized state as required for the murine system. Indeed, T-dependent LDCC was observed with normal peripheral blood with a variety of target cells including syngeneic, allogeneic, and even xenogeneic target cells (Table 4).[9,17] Thus, unlike the mouse, and like the NK cells, LDCC effector cells were shown to be present naturally in the peripheral blood.

B. Characterization of the Effector Cells in LDCC

1. In the Mouse

The effector cells mediating LDCC in mice have been reported to be T-dependent but it is not clear whether the LDCC is mediated by an antigen-specific CTL or polyclonally activated CTL. Preliminary studies in our laboratory suggested that specific CMC and LDCC are mediated by the same CTL population.[3] This premise has been supported by some reports, but not by others. In all studies, the ^{51}Chromium (^{51}Cr)-release assay has been used to elucidate the identity of the LDCC effector cells. With the ^{51}Cr-release assay, whole effector populations have been employed so that only circumstantial evidence can be obtained. We reexamined the question, with the introduction of the single-cell assay for cytotoxicity[18] using two target conjugates in which both specific and lectin-coated targets were bound to single CTL.

These studies resulted in unequivocal evidence that single CTL is capable of mediating both specific cell-mediated cytotoxicity (SCMC) and LDCC.[8] The evidence supports the notion that antigen-specific CTL is endowed with the capacity to bypass antigen recognition and to lyse target cells nonspecifically. This evidence consists pri-

Table 5
SCMC AND LDCC ARE MEDIATED BY THE SAME CTL

	% Target cells killed[b]	
Two target conjugates[a]	Both targets	One target
EL-4 (Con A) and P815	26 ± 6.7	49.6 ± 10.0
EL-4 (PHA) and P815	23.3 ± 2.9	46.7 ± 13.8
EL-4 ($NaIO_4$) and P815	27.7 ± 7.3	43.2 ± 3.4

[a] Two target conjugates are formed between a single C57BL/6 anti-P815 PEL and two targets. The destruction of each target was made possible by labeling one of the target and the two target conjugates relocated in a microlocator.

[b] Mean value ± SD of three experiments.

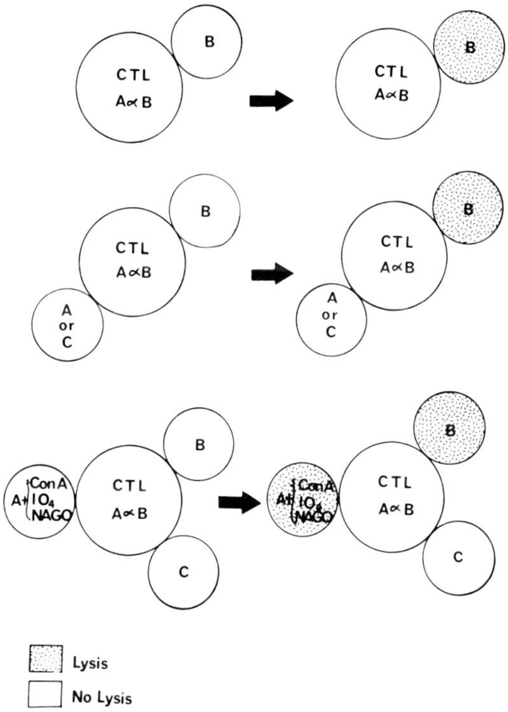

FIGURE 1. This figure schematically represents the ability of CTL to bind and kill target cells. Target B is recognized and killed specifically by A anti-B CTL. Target A and C are not killed unless the cell is modified by Con A, IO_4, or NAGO.

marily of (1) the frequency of lymphocytes target conjugates is the same for both SCMC and LDCC and (2) the frequency of binders and killers of tumor target conjugates is the same for autologous targets and heterotargets. The same results are true for LDCC, whereby the target cells are oxidized by periodate, ruling out artifacts that may be introduced by the addition of exogenous lectins (Table 5). The cytotoxic potential of CTL is schematically diagrammed in Figure 1.

Table 6
LDCC AND NK/K CYTOTOXICITY ARE MEDIATED BY DISTINCT SUBPOPULATIONS OF HUMAN PBL

	% Target cells killed	
Two target conjugates[a]	Both targets	One target
K562-LGL-Raji (Con A)	0	58.7
K562-LGL-Raji (PHA)	0	47.6
MOLT-4-LGL-Raji (Ab)	31.3	35.9

[a] The two target conjugates were performed according to procedures previously described in Reference 20. The target K562 and MOLT-4 are NK-sensitive targets and Raji (Ab) serves as ADCC target.

2. In Man

In the peripheral blood, significant LDCC has been observed with a variety of target cells. Preliminary findings have demonstrated that T cells and Fc-bearing cells mediate the LDCC phenomenon.[9,19] Since normal human peripheral blood lymphocytes (PBL) express several cytotoxic functions, among which are NK, ADCC, and LDCC, the relationship of these various cytotoxic mechanisms, and the identity of the cells involved, has been the subject of controversy. We have reported the NK and K cell subpopulation with multiple cytotoxic functions.[20] The relationship of NK/K to LDCC was examined using the two target conjugates and employing the same rationale as used for the CTL-LDCC. The results revealed that LDCC and NK/K are mediated by distinct subpopulations of effector cells even though they both copurify in the large granular lymphocyte (LGL) fraction (Table 6).[17] The results also demonstrate that lectins cannot trigger NK/K cells to mediated LDCC, even under conditions whereby the target is already bound to the NK effector cells (see below for details). The surface phenotype of the LDCC effector cells is characteristic of T cells using monoclonal fluorescent antibody markers. The cytotoxic potential of PBL in man is schematically shown in Figure 2.

C. Mechanism of T-LDCC

1. Requirements for Mitogenicity

The various lectins that were tested and found effective in mediating LDCC were also shown to exhibit mitogenic activity. Lectins that do not exhibit mitogenic activity were found to be noneffective in LDCC even though they were able to lead to the formation of stable lymphocyte-target conjugates. It was postulated, then, that lectin serves as a "glue" bringing cells in close proximity and leading to lysis. However, the demonstration that several nonmitogenic lectins (which form stable conjugates) do not mediate LDCC suggests that lectin plays a dual role, i.e., binding and activation (Table 7). The requirements for mitogenic lectins in LDCC were corroborated in studies using chemical and enzymatic modification of target cells for ODCC. Thus, periodate modification or NAGO treatment result in target cells which induce mitogenic stimulation in culture. Using these modifications, it was possible to obtain nonspecific lysis in ODCC. Under conditions where mitogenesis is blocked, as in reduction with borohydride, the modification is effective in inhibiting the ODCC phenomenon.[8,21] Another example of the importance of mitogenicity is the demonstration that lectins such as peanut agglutinin (PNA) and soybean agglutinin (SBA), which are not mitogenic in mice, are also noneffective in LDCC, even though they provide adequate binding.[22]

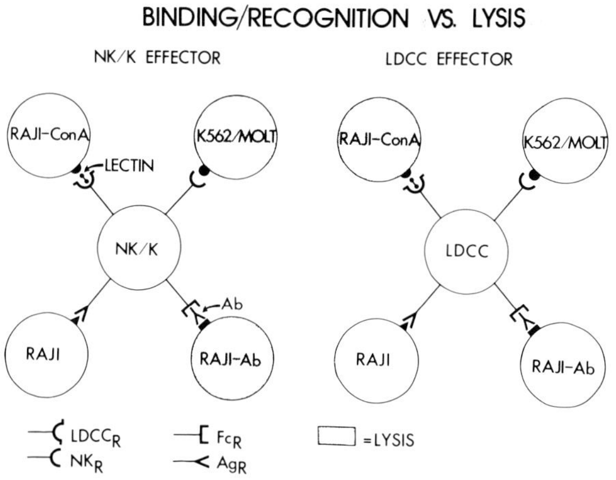

FIGURE 2. The cytotoxic potential of human PBL is represented. Effector cells for NK and K for ADCC are mediated by one subpopulation while the effector for LDCC is mediated by another subpopulation. Binding of various targets (NK, ADCC, LDCC, and NK resistant) can take place with the effector cell. However, killing is only seen with the corresponding target.

Table 7
REQUIREMENT FOR MITOGENIC LECTIN FOR LDCC[a]

Agent	Conjugate formation	Lysis	Mitogenicity
PHA, Con A, LNA	+	+	+
PNA, SBA (mouse)	+	−	−
NASE + PNA/SBA	+	+	+
WGA	+	−	−
PLL	+	−	−
$NaIO_4$, NAGO	+	+	+
$NaIO_4$ or NAGO + $NaHB_4$	−	−	−

[a] This table summarizes findings obtained in both the ^{51}Cr release assay and the single cell assay in which the various agents were tested for binding, lysis, and mitogenicity.

However, treatment of the target cells using neuraminidase followed with PNA or SBA resulted in mitogenic properties which were also effective in LDCC (Table 7). The mechanisms involved are not clear, but some possible explanations will be described in Section 2 below. From the physiological point of view, it would be of interest to assess the role of natural lectins isolated from cells which have been shown to induce mitogenic activity.[23] These naturally developed lectins should be tested for LDCC. If LDCC is achieved, then LDCC may play a very important role in vivo in immunosurveillance and in other regulatory functions as well.

2. Role of Target Cell Structures in LDCC and ODCC: The Effect of Pretreatment of Target or Effector Cells with Lectin and Wash

It has been shown that the addition of lectin to effector and target cells leads to LDCC. In our laboratory, experiments were performed to delineate whether pretreatment of the target cells or effector cells, or both, with lectin followed by wash leads to lysis. Varying results were obtained, depending on the lectin used. Whereas with Con

Table 8
SUMMARY OF LDCC REACTIONS BY PNA AND SBA[a]

Treatment	Single cell assay (LDCC) Binding	Lysis
Target cell — lectin (PNA or SBA)	+	−
Target cell — n'ase[b] + lectin	+	+
CTL — lectin	−	−
CTL — n'ase — lectin	−	−

[a] This table summarizes results obtained in the dissociation between binding and lysis.[22]
[b] N'ase, neuraminidase.

A, SBA, and PNA, only target cell pretreatment was effective,[13,24] pretreatment of the effector cells did not lead to any significant binding or lysis. In other systems, however, such as PHA, lentil lectin (LNA), or IO_4 modification, both effector cell and target cell modification led to lysis.[13,24] ODCC was always better when the target cells were modified.[21] Since lectins are multivalent, they may interact with both the effector and target cells, even when pretreatment and wash are performed. Thus dissociation of binding and the lysis events in cytotoxicity have not easily been achieved.

Initially, experiments were devised to dissociate the phenomenon of binding from that which leads to lysis. Lectins such as SBA an PNA were shown to induce binding with an equal frequency to that observed in the SCMC by the CTL.[22] These results indicated that only the CTL were able to bind target cells in the presence of those lectins. However, no binding was obtained unless the target cells were previously treated with lectin. The advantage of this system is that it allows for the importance of the modification to be examined separately, on either the effector cells or the target cells. These results indicated that lysis occurs only when the target cells are treated with neuraminidase and SBA but not when the effector cells are treated with neuraminidase and SBA. This was corroborated in the single cell assay, in which pretreatment of target cells with SBA led to lymphocyte-target cell binding, but pretreatment of the effector cells did not lead to binding. However, when neuraminidase and SBA were used to treat target cells, both binding and lysis took place. Interestingly, in the pretreatment of effector cells with SBA and neuraminidase, no binding or lysis was observed, even though the effector cells were coated with lectin (Table 8).[22] It appears, then, that the CTL-SBA is unable to interact with appropriate ligands present on the target cells. A schematic diagram depicting these experiments is illustrated in Figure 3.

These experiments demonstrated that target cell structures are important for LDCC, but it is not clear how these structures are involved in lysis and binding. It is possible that following modification of the target cell with neuraminidase and lectin, cell membrane perturbation takes place, which allows these target cells to become recognized by CTL and thus leads to lysis. Alternatively, it has been suggested by Berke et al.[24] that lectin modification of target cells results in the modification of H-2 antigens, and the modified antigen is recognized by the antigen receptor on the CTL. Below, we will describe experiments which are pertinent to Model I without ruling out Model II.

3. Lectin may Induce Target Cell Membrane Modifications Which are Necessary for Lysis

Pretreatment of target cells with lectin and/or chemical or enzymatic modification (ODCC) which leads to lysis is abolished by sugar inhibitors and/or reduction by bo-

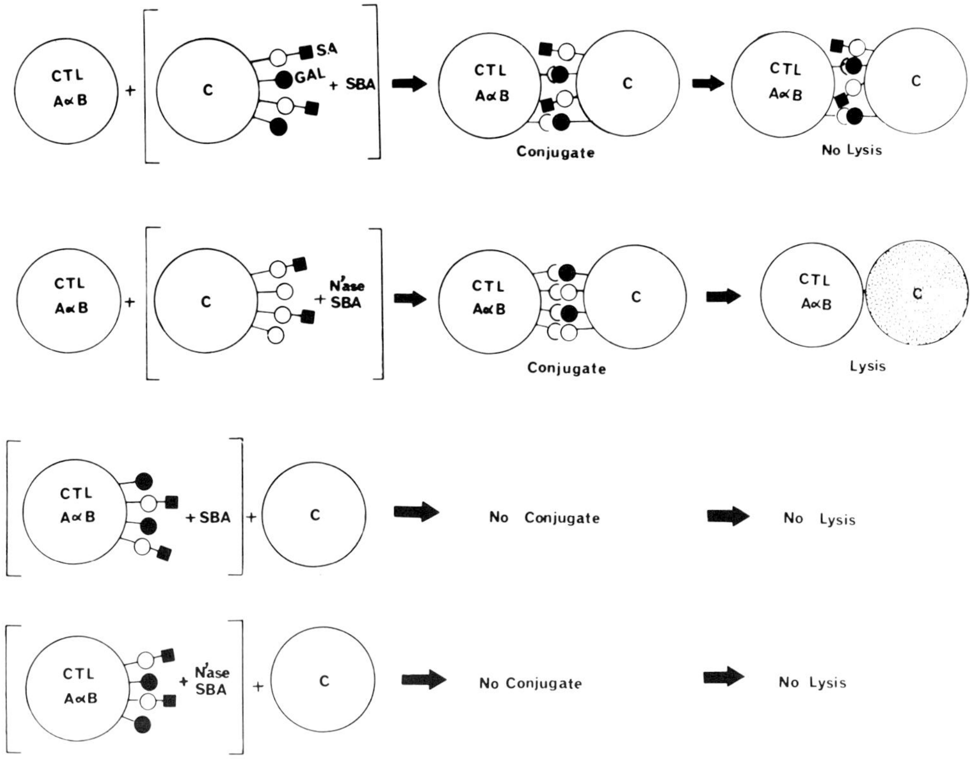

FIGURE 3. The ability of antigen-specific CTL (A anti-B) to bind and kill target cells under different conditions is shown. In the presence of SBA, binding takes place but no killing. Modification of target cells with neuraminidase and SBA leads to lysis. However, pretreatment of CTL with SBA in the presence or absence of neuraminidase modification does not lead to binding or lysis.

rohydride. This suggests that intercross-linking may be required between the effector cells and target cells to achieve lysis. Alternatively, intracross-linking may take place and the target cells may undergo structural changes which make them susceptible to lysis while losing their ability to bind to the lymphocytes. It is possible, then, that lectin plays a dual role, i.e., to modify the target cells and also provide the binding.

In order to test this hypothesis, we performed a series of experiments which enabled us to differentiate between these two models. We made use of two modifications which, taken alone, were not sufficient to initiate LDCC or ODCC. It was reasoned that if one signal were to be involved in the membrane target modification and the other were to provide for binding, lysis would thus be achieved. Following this rationale, target cells were treated with IO_4 and then treated with the reducing agent borohydride. These modifications rendered the cells insusceptible to binding or lysis. The modified and reduced target cells were then used in the presence of SBA, which does not mediate LDCC. Under these conditions, target cell lysis was achieved (Table 9).[26] Other lectins, such as wheat germ agglutinin (WGA) and PNA, were also effective in the same system, but addition of the agglutinating agent poly-L-lysine (PLL) was not effective (Table 10). These results suggest that the second signal provided by the SBA is also important for LDCC and cannot be substituted by non-LDCC agglutinating agents. Shown schematically in Figure 4, the data indicates that target cell membrane perturbations are probably the result of lectin interaction with the target cells, and this perturbation, in conjunction with binding of the target cells to the lymphocyte, results in lysis. These experiments also provide further evidence of the dissociation between

Table 9
LDCC IN IO_4 + BH_4-TREATED TARGETS[a]

Lectin	(IO_4) mM	% ^{51}Cr Release[b] 0	KBH$_4$ 25 mM	5 mM
None	0	0.2 ± 2	0.8 ± 1	1.8 ± 2
	5	19.7 ± 2	8.9 ± 3	4.1 ± 2
SBA (20 μg/mℓ)	0	4.1 ± 2	4.9 ± 2	4.6 ± 2
	5	19.5 ± 1	18.3 ± 3	19.7 ± 1
Con A (20 μg/mℓ)	0	21.0 ± 3	19.7 ± 1	18.9 ± 3
	5	14.9 ± 1	16.9 ± 1	15.7 ± 1

Note: In these experiments, the effector cell was treated with IO_4, incubated at 37°C for 1 hr, and then treated with KBH_4. At this point, SBA or Con A was added to the effector and target cell mixtures.

[a] CTL = C57BL/6 αP815; TC = EL4; the CMC was performed in a 3 hr ^{51}Cr release at E:T = 20:1
[b] E:T ratio was 20:1

Table 10
LDCC IN IO_4 + BH_4-TREATED TARGET CELLS: REQUIREMENTS OF LDCC LECTINS[a]

Lectin	(IO_4^-) mM	% ^{51}Cr Release KBH$_4$ 0	KBH$_4$ 5 mM	KBH$_4$ 10 mM
None	0	3.0 ± 1	1.3 ± 2	2.9 ± 1
	5	17.5 ± 3.1	1.0 ± 0	0.7 ± 3
SBA (20 μg/mℓ)	0	2.4 ± 1	2.5 ± 0	2.1 ± 0.7
	5	18.8 ± 3	27.9 ± 5	16.3 ± 3
PNA (20 μg/mℓ)	0	2.6 ± 0	4.4 ± 1.7	6.3 ± 2
	5	17.2 ± 3.4	18.9 ± 4	16.1 ± 1
WGA (20 μg/mℓ)	0	5.3 ± 1	8.6 ± 4	9.8 ± 0
	5	19.6 ± 2	27.8 ± 3	16.4 ± 3

[a] The same protocol was used as for Table 9.

binding and lysis in LDCC and ODCC. The exact nature of the membrane perturbation event is not understood at present. It is postulated that a target antigen for cytotoxicity (TAC) plays a role in ODCC, as shown in Figure 4.

D. Role of Class I Antigens in LDCC

It has been suggested that Class I antigens play a role in the mechanism of T-dependent CMC.[24] This has led to the proposition that lectin, in conjunction with Class I antigens, modifies target cells and becomes recognized by the antigen-specific CTL. This has been corroborated by the demonstration that (1) cells which lack Class I antigens are poor target cells for LDCC, (2) the treatment of target cells with papain, which removes Class I antigens, renders the cells resistant to lysis by CTL in the presence of lectin, and (3) anti-H-2 antibodies can block LDCC. However, these experiments do not rule out the possibility that Class I antigens may not always be required for cytolysis and papain treatment, a nonspecific protease, may in addition to removing Class I antigens, remove important surface membrane antigens involved in cytotoxicity.

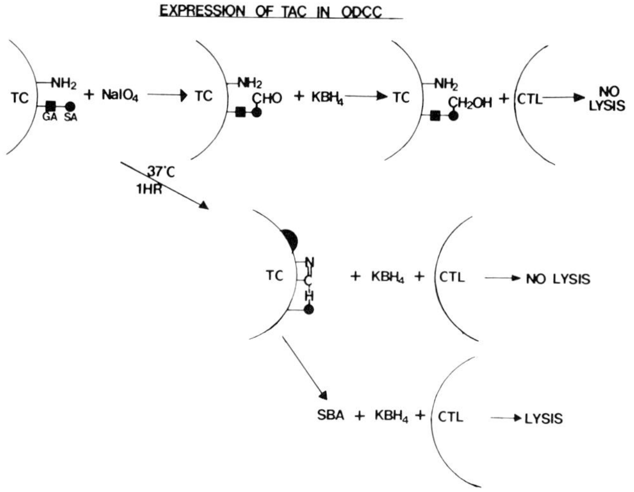

FIGURE 4. Target cells modified with $NaIO_4$ (oxidation of sialic acid [SA]) and reduced with KBH_4 are not lysed. However, following incubation at 37°C for one hour of the oxidized and reduced target, followed by addition of SBA, lysis is obtained.

Table 11
EFFECT OF PAPAIN PRETREATMENT ON LDCC ON HUMAN CULTURE CELL LINES

Target cell line[a]	Papain (mg/mℓ)	Background[b] % cytotoxicity (SD)	LDCC[c] % cytotoxicity (SD)
RAJI (HLA^+)	0.0	4.51 ± 0.78	35.54 ± 2.37
	0.5	1.93 ± 1.27	31.74 ± 0.46
	1.0	0.06 ± 1.11	28.92 ± 2.71
	2.5	0.71 ± 0.81	17.52 ± 0.16
DAUDI (HLA^-)	0.0	2.82 ± 0.78	66.69 ± 2.06
	0.5	2.58 ± 0.38	35.28 ± 0.32
	1.0	0.87 ± 0.94	28.91 ± 0.17
	2.5	0.88 ± 0.03	30.33 ± 0.71

[a] ^{51}Cr-labeled targets (2×10^5 cells/mℓ) cocultured with PBL (8×10^6 cells/mℓ) at 40:1 E/T ratio. The cells were treated with papain for 1 hr at 37°, washed and used in the assay.
[b] Targets cultured in medium and 10% FCS.
[c] For LDCC: 40 μg/mℓ of Con A in medium and 10% FCS was used.

We examined these possibilities in LDCC in man.[27] PBL were used as effector cells with both HLA^- and HLA^+ as target cells. The genetically deficient Class I HLA^- target cell Daudi was used. The LDCC system was performed in the presence of Con A. Our first experiments were designed to delineate whether HLA^- Daudi cells would serve as target cells in LDCC. Indeed, it was demonstrated that Daudi, in the presence of Con A, served as a good target cell in LDCC. The cytotoxic activity obtained was comparable to that obtained with HLA^+ target cells such as Raji (Table 11). Thus, it appears as though Class I HLA antigens are not necessary for lysis.The effect of papain treatment of target cells was examined using both HLA^+ and HLA^- target cells, as shown in Table 12. Increased concentrations of papain resulted in a decrease in the LDCC for

Table 12
RECOVERY OF LDCC FOLLOWING TREATMENT OF DAUDI WITH PAPAIN[a]

Target	Papain (mg/mℓ)	% Control following preincubation 0 hr	1 hr	2 hr
Daudi	0	100	100	100
	0.5	52.6	71.0	100
	1.0	38.8	52.6	88.7
	2.5	37.1	48.9	81.3
Raji	0	100	100	100
	0.5	83.8	100	100
	1.0	68.8	78.0	100
	2.5	48.8	70.9	89.8

[a] Cells were treated with various concentrations of papain and then incubated at 37°C for 1 hr or 2 hr prior to addition of radiolabeled target cells. The assays were completed after 3 hr of incubation. The results are calculated as percent of control in the absence of any treatment.

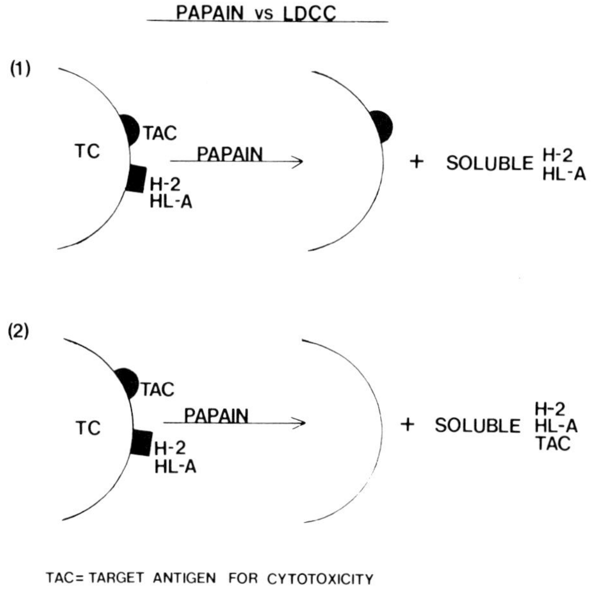

FIGURE 5. This figure represents the effect of papain on target cells. Papain treatment solubilizes Class I H2 or HL-A antigens and in addition, it also digests antigens associated with cytotoxicity.

both Raji and Daudi. This indicated that papain removes from HLA⁻ target cells surface structures important for lysis (Figure 5). However, the reduction in cytotoxicity following papain treatment was never complete. Thus, an effort was made to delineate whether the residual activity obtained following papain treatment was due to target cell-resistant antigens and/or the rapid recovery of papain-sensitive molecules during

Table 13
FREQUENCY OF BINDERS AND KILLERS BY HLA-DAUDI TARGET CELL[a]

Target	Con A	% Binding	% Target cell death
Daudi	−	18.0 ± 1.7	6.5 ± 4.7
	+	31.8 ± 0.6	40.0 ± 3.1
Raji	−	24.6 ± 4.5	17.5 ± 3.5
	+	27.9 ± 2.1	35.3 ± 1.2

[a] The single cell assay was performed with LGL as described in Reference 8.

the cytotoxic assay. At different times after papain treatment, treated cells were examined for their susceptibility to lysis. The cells were incubated at 37° and then used in the test. It was demonstrated that LDCC recovers within a short period of time and this explains the failure to achieve complete inhibition following papain treatment (Table 12).

The results of these studies suggested that papain treatment of target cells, such as HLA-Daudi, results in the release or removal of sensitive target antigens that are important for LDCC. In addition, papain-sensitive molecules recover fairly rapidly within the incubation period for cytotoxicity in a manner similar to the recovery of HLA antigens. This observation is reminiscent of our studies with the Lyt-2 molecules on CTL and their removal by trypsin.[28]

The question remained, however, as to whether the LDCC phenomenon observed with Raji and Daudi was mediated by the same or different effector cells. To answer this question, we examined the frequency of binders and killers using the single cell assay, and also examined the frequency of conjugates formed by OKT4 fluorescent lymphocyte bound to targets. We found that the frequency was the same for both Raji and Daudi target cells and the frequency of binders and killers for Daudi was within the range observed with HLA^+ Raji target cells (Table 13). These results are consistent with the same population of effector cells as those involved in the mediating LDCC with HLA^+ and HLA^- target cells. Although recent experiments were performed with human PBL and not with mouse-generated CTL, we would like to extrapolate the present findings to the other effector cells involved in LDCC. Indeed, mouse CTL lyse HLA^- Daudi targets in the presence of Con A, therefore extrapolation seems valid.

In conclusion, our results demonstrate that Class I HLA antigens are not crucial in LDCC. Since HLA^- target cells serve as targets, the use of papain as an indicator for the involvement of Class I antigens on a membrane is not conclusive.Other papain-sensitive molecules which are removed are also important.

III. NK LECTIN-DEPENDENT CELL CYTOTOXICITY (NK-LDCC)

The effect of lectin on CMC has been well documented in the CTL system in which an antigen-specific CTL becomes nonspecific when mitogenic lectins such as Con A and PHA are added to the cytotoxic mixture. However, the effect of lectins on NK cells has not been thoroughly examined. Previous studies have shown that the addition of the lectin Helix Pomatia to a mixture of B6 nude spleen cells and the NK-resistant K562 target cells results in enhancement of cytotoxicity.[29] This enhancement has been correlated with the levels of NK activity against the sensitive YAC-1 target cells. However, these studies do not clarify the exact nature of the effector cells that mediate this particular cytotoxic activity or whether the activity is due to NK or non-NK effector cells.

Table 14
SUSCEPTIBILITY OF NK-LDCC TO αThy1.2+c′[a]

Effector	% ^{51}Cr release (100:1)
SJL/J	7.1
SJL/J + Con A	24.2
SJL/J + αThy1.2+c′	3.4
SJL/J + αThy1.2+c′ + Con A	4.1
SJL/J + c′ + Con A	26.0
SJL + A-GMI + C′	23.5
CBA	69
CBA + Con A	64.7
CBA + αThy1.2+c′	57
CBA + αThy1.2+c′ + Con A	55
CBA + c′ + Con A	58
CBA + A-GMI + C′	24

[a] In these experiments, the effector cells were derived from spleen cells passaged through a nylon wool column. The cells were treated with antibody for 30′ at 4°C and complement for 30′ at 37°C. The cells were recounted for viability and used in the cytotoxic assay.

We examined this question to explore whether NK cells can mediate a LDCC against NK-sensitive target cells and also whether other effector cells are involved in this system. Our previous studies did not clearly indicate that normal spleen cells or normal T cells from mice do mediate LDCC. Activation of such cells (antigenic stimulation) was required for LDCC.[13] By examining the effect of various lectins on normal spleen cells, both from high NK- and low NK-sensitive mice, and using NK-sensitive target cells, we obesrved a significant cytotoxic activity in the low NK strain of mice.[10] We then examined the specificity of the lectin and found that the same requirements which apply to the classical T cell-dependent LDCC (i.e., Con A, PHA, and wheat germ agglutinins) were all effective in mediating NK-LDCC. However, PLL and nonmitogenic lectins were not effective. This phenomenon, labeled NK-LDCC, was examined in various strains of mice. A high NK-LDCC activity was obtained in the low NK strains, such as the SJL/J and the beige-beige mice. This effect was also noticeable in the C57BL/6. However, there was no noticeable effect in the Balb/c nude mice and the effect was seldom seen with a high NK strain such as CBA. These results suggest that NK-LDCC activity is seen in strains of mice that have low, or no, NK activity.

The specificity of the cytotoxic activity was then tested with NK-sensitive and NK-resistant targets and it became clear that the activity was restricted to the the NK-sensitive target cells. The surface phenotype of the effector cells involved in NK-LDCC was examined using antibodies directed against the Thy-1.2 antigen and against the asialo Gm-1 antigen on the effector cells. The results demonstrate that the cytotoxic activity is sensitive following the treatment with anti-Thy-1.2 antibody and complement, and is resistant to the effect of antiasialo Gm-1 (Table 14). As expected in controls, however, NK activity was found insensitive to Thy-1.2+C and sensitive to asialo Gm-1. This suggests that the effector cell in NK-LDCC is Thy-1.2^{+} asialo Gm-1^{-}. We further examined the susceptibility of the derived NK-resistant target cells in NK-LDCC,[30] using YAC-R resistant subclones derived following culture of YAC-1 in NKCF.[30] YAC-R15 was not effectively lysed in the presence of Con A and YAC-R1.1 showed intermediate lysis (Table 15). This suggests that the mechanism of recognition and lysis is consistent with a NK-like cell.

Table 15
SUSCEPTIBILITY OF NK-RESISTANT TARGET IN NK-LDCC

Effector target[a]	% ^{51}Cr release (0:1)
SJL/J	
YAC-1 + Con A	32
YAC-1	13
YAC-R1.1 + Con A	21.6
YAC-R1.1	2.5
YAC-R15 + Con A	10.5
YAC-R15	3.5
CBA	
YAC-1	53.0
YAC-R15	11.8

[a] The variant YAC targets have been derived as described in Reference 30.

Table 16
EFFECT OF PRETREATMENT OF EFFECTOR OR TARGET WITH CON A ON NK-LDCC[a]

Effector	Target	% ^{51}Cr release (200:1)
SJL	YAC-1	3.8
SJL/J + Con A	YAC-1	25.8
SJL/J pretreated with Con A	YAC-1	23.5
SJL/J	YAC pretreated with Con A	22.08
CBA	YAC-1	21
CBA + Con A		33
CBA pretreated with Con A		36
CBA+	YAC pretreated with Con A	22

[a] The cells were pretreated with Con A for 1 hr at 37°C, washed and used in the assay.

The effect of pretreatment of the effector cells or target cells with Con A was then examined (Table 16). In the T cell-dependent LDCC, pretreatment of the effector cells with Con A did not mediate LDCC, whereas pretreatment of the target cells with Con A did mediate LDCC. Similar experiments were performed in the NK-LDCC system. It was found that both pretreatment of effector cells, or of target cells and wash, resulted in cytotoxic activity. The addition of α-methyl mannoside (α-MM) in the wells inhibited both NK cells and the NK-LDCC system. Pretreatment of the target cells with Con A and wash with excess α-MM, which should presumably remove the Con A, resulted in no loss of cytotoxic activity. In the CTL system, however, this cytotoxic activity was reduced extensively. This suggests that the mechanism by which Con A mediates LDCC by CTL and by the putative NK-LDCC effector cells is distinct. It also suggests that the Con A may not be directly involved in the cytotoxic reaction, but may serve as an activator. It is possible that Con A may be activating a precursor of NK cells which become activated by the lectin in the low NK strains of mice. In the high NK, this population is probably differentiated to mature NK cells and therefore cannot interact with the lectin for cytotoxicity.

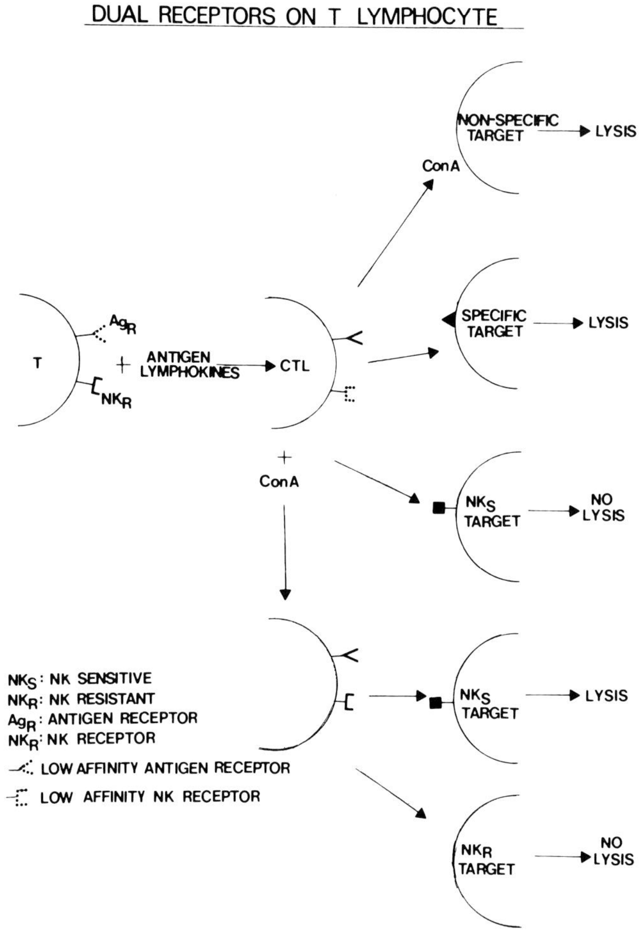

FIGURE 6. The T lymphocyte is shown to carry on its membrane two receptors, one for specific antigen and one for NK target recognition. In the presence of antigen or lymphokine, the antigen specific receptor is fully functional while the NK receptor is of weak affinity. Following addition of Con A both receptors become functional and the cell lyses both antigen-specific and NK-sensitive targets.

Alternatively, we postulate that the effector cell which mediates this phenomenon is not classical NK cell or pre-NK cell. It may be a cell that expresses the Thy-1 antigen and does not express the asialo Gm-1. However, it remains to be shown whether surface Lyt antigens are present on these cells in order to further confirm the T cell nature of these cytotoxic effector cells.

We hypothesize that this particular NK-LDCC expresses two receptors, one for specific antigen and one for an NK target antigen. As shown in Figure 6, the cell differentiates into a cytotoxic lymphocyte following activation by antigen or in the presence of lymphokines. The CTL then have a functional receptor for antigen and a weak receptor for NK cells. In the presence of Con A, the CTL may mediate nonspecific target cell lysis and the CTL may then interact with an NK-sensitive target cell and mediate lysis. Thus, it seems that Con A may play a role in either the activation of the NK receptor, or in allowing the NK-sensitive target cell to be recognized by the effector cell. The dual role receptor hypothesis on the T lymphocytes would thus hold true.

This suggestion, that a cell can express two receptors, is in agreement with recent studies from the laboratory of Binz et al.[31] which demonstrated that CTL clones that have an idiotype-specific receptor may indeed lyse NK-sensitive target cells through different receptors. We have also shown that both NK and ADCC effector cells are mediated by the same cell.[20] This suggests that different receptors on the lymphocytes may function as stimuli for cytotoxicity.

IV. GENERAL COMMENTS

The studies described in this review are primarily related to the phenomenon of lectin-dependent K cells. This review has covered the phenomenon mediated by various effector cell populations in both man and in animals. The studies, in general, encompass work done in the author's laboratory with a few references to other investigators' work. The studies presented are slanted towards the author's bias and should be viewed as such.

The phenomenon of lectin-dependent K cells is described in various systems and is used as a probe to investigate the mechanism of CMC. This phenomenon provides additional tools to investigate the complex mechanism of CMC. The findings have been primarily directed at the cellular and functional levels and very little has been focused on the biochemical nature underlying this phenomenon. For example, it is possible to generate antibodies directed against surface membrane antigens involved in lysis, which would hopefully lead to characterization of the functional molecules involved. A major drawback of any biochemical study is that the lectins are nonspecific and interact with various molecules on the surface of cells. Likewise, the enyzmatic or chemical modification seen in ODCC is also nonspecific but appears to be more restricted than the lectins, and fewer molecules are modified. Future studies on ODCC may provide better means to delineate the nature of the target molecules involved in binding, activation, and sites of lysis. Nevertheless, the studies here have proposed several working models and hypotheses which can be experimentally verified (Figure 7).

Even though the studies with lectins have provided new insights to the mechanism of CMC, one may question the physiological role of such systems in vivo. Interestingly, it has been shown that mammalian cells bear surface lectins, and that such lectins can be isolated and shown to be mitogenic in vitro.[23] It is therefore conceivable that under special circumstances, target cells that express such lectins may be rendered susceptible to lysis by the PBL. Thus, LDCC and ODCC may play important regulatory and surveillance roles. Such a possibility deserves serious consideration and investigation.

Regardless of whether the LDCC or ODCC phenomena play a role in vivo, it is possible to apply these systems to assess the cytotoxic potential of specific subpopulations of cells as well as the frequency of K cells present in the blood. Such evaluations may have important implications in cases of immunodeficiency, immunosuppression, and the effect of biological response modifiers.

ACKNOWLEDGMENT

The following investigators in my laboratory who contributed to the research presented in this review are acknowledged: Drs. T. P. Bradley and John Fan, Mr. J. Katz, Ms. L. Lebow, and Ms. H. Ostergaard. I also thank Kirman Ridd for editing and James Jun for typing the manuscript.

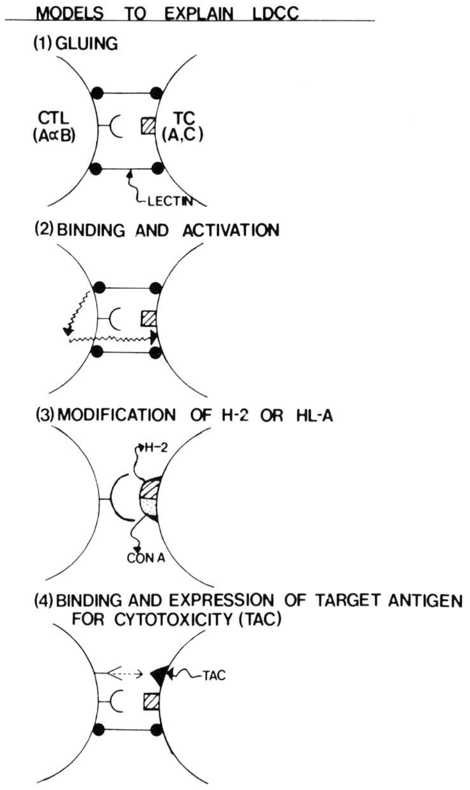

FIGURE 7. Four models for LDCC are represented. The first model suggests that the lectin acts as a gluing agent to make contact between the effector and target. The second model proposes that the lectin plays a dual role of binding and activation. The third model proposes that the lectin modifies Class I antigens (H2 or HL-A) and the resulting modification is recognized by the antigen specific receptor. This interaction leads to binding and lysis. The fourth model suggests that following modification of the target cell by lectin there follows a modulation or perturbation that leads to the expression of TAC. TAC can then bind to the effector cell in the presence of the lectin.

REFERENCES

1. Herberman, R. B., Ed., *NK Cells and Other Natural Effector Cells,* Academic Press, New York, 1982.
2. Grimm, E. A., Mazumder, A., Zhang, H. Z., and Rosenberg, S. A., Lymphokine activated killer cell phenomenon. Lysis of natural killer-resistant fresh solid tumors by interleukin 2 activated autologous human peripheral blood lymphocytes, *J. Exp. Med.,* 155, 1825, 1982.
3. Bonavida, B. and Bradley, T. P., Studies on the induction and expression of T-cell mediated immunity. V. Lectin-induced nonspecific cell-mediated cytotoxicity by alloimmune lymphocytes, *Transplantation,* 21, 94, 1976.
4. Forman, J. and Moller, G., Generation of cytotoxic lymphocytes in mixed lymphocyte reaction. I. Specificity of the effector cells, *J. Exp. Med.,* 138, 672, 1973.
5. Bevan, M. J. and Cohn, M., Cytotoxic effects of antigen- and mitogen-induced T cells on various targets, *J. Immunol.,* 114, 559, 1975.
6. Novogrodsky, A., Induction of lymphocyte cytotoxicity by modification of the effector or target cells with periodate or with neuraminidase and galactose oxidase, *J. Immunol.,* 116, 1089, 1975.

7. Schmitt-Verhulst, A. and Shearer, G. M., Effects of sodium periodate modification of lymphocytes on the sensitization and lytic phases of T cell-mediated lympholysis, *J. Immunol.*, 116, 947, 1976.
8. Bradley, T. P. and Bonavida, B., Mechanism of cell-mediated cytotoxicity at the single cell level. III. Evidence that cytotoxic T lymphocytes lyse both antigen-specific and nonspecific targets pretreated with lectins or periodate, *J. Immunol.*, 126, 208, 1981.
9. Bonavida, B., Robins, A., and Saxon, A., Lectin-dependent cellular cytotoxicity in man, *Transplantation*, 23, 261, 1977.
10. Bonavida, B., Lectin-dependent natural killer cellular cytotoxicity in mice (NK-LDCC): a new subpopulation of NK-like cytotoxic cells, in *NK Cells and Other Natural Effector Cells*, Herberman, R. B., Ed., Academic Press, New York, 1982, 483.
11. Anderson, J., Sjoberg O., and Moller, G., Contact sensitivity in the mouse. X. Non-specific cytotoxicity of T blasts in the draining lymph nodes. *Transplant. Rev.*, 11, 131, 1972.
12. Asherson, G. L. and Ferluga, J. X., Non-specific cytotoxicity of T blasts in the draining lymph nodes, *Immunol. Today*, 25, 471, 1972.
13. Bonavida, B. and Bradley, T. P., Studies on the induction and expression of T cell-mediated immunity. V. Lectin-induced non-specific cell-mediated cytotoxicity by alloimmune lymphocytes, *Transplantation*, 21, 94, 1976.
14. De Bracco, M. M., Isturiz, M. A., and Manni, J. A., Cell-mediated cytotoxicity characterization of effector cells, *Immunol. Today*, 30, 325, 1976.
15. Holm, G. and Perlmann, P., Cytotoxic potential of stimulated human lymphocytes, *J. Exp. Med.*, 125, 721, 1967.
16. Nelson, D. L., Bundy, B. M., West, T. D., et al., The nature of the effector cells mediating mitogen-induced cellular cytotoxicity (MICC) and antibody-dependent cellular cytotoxicity (ADCC), *Cell Immunol.*, 23, 89, 1976.
17. Bradley, T. P. and Bonavida, B., Mechanism of cell-mediated cytotoxicity at the single cell level. VII. Trigger of the lethal hit event is distinct for NK/K and LDCC effector cells as measured in the two target conjugate assay, *Cell. Immunol.*, 83, 199, 1984.
18. Bonavida, B., Bradley, T. P., and Grimm, E. A., The single cell assay in cell-mediated cytotoxicity, *Immunol. Today*, 4, 196, 1983.
19. Lang, N. P., Ortaldo, J. R., Bonmard, G. D., and Herberman, R., Interferon and prostaglandins: effects on human natural and lectin-induced cytotoxicity, *J. Natl. Cancer Inst.*, 69, 229, 1982.
20. Bradley, T. P. and Bonavida, B., Mechanism of cell-mediated cytotoxicity at the single cell level. IV. Natural killing and antibody dependent cellular cytotoxicity can be mediated by the same human effector cell as determined by the two target conjugate assay, *J. Immunol.*, 129, 2260, 1982.
21. Fan, J. and Bonavida, B., Studies on the induction and expression of T-cell mediated immunity. XIV. Role of Lyt-2 antigens of CTL and H-2 antigens of target cells on antigen non-specific oxidation dependent cellular cytotoxicity (ODCC) mediated by sodium periodate oxidation of either effector or target cells, *J. Immunol.*, 131, 1426, 1983.
22. Bradley, T. P. and Bonavida, B., Mechanism of cell-mediated cytotoxicity at the single cell level. V. The importance of target cell structures in cytotoxic T-lymphocyte mediated antigen non-specific lectin-dependent cellular cytotoxicity, *J. Immunol.*, 129, 2352, 1982.
23. Novogrodsky, A. and Ashwell, G., Lymphocyte mitogenesis induced by a mammalian liver protein that specifically binds desialylated gycoproteins, *Proc. Natl. Acad. Sci. U.S.A.*, 74, 676, 1977.
24. Berke, G., McVey, H. E., and Clark, W. R., T-lymphocyte mediated cytolysis. I. One common mechanism for target recognition in specific and lectin-dependent cytolysis, *J. Immunol.*, 127, 776, 1982.
25. Green, W. R., Ballas, Z. K., and Henney, C. S., Studies on the mechanism of lymphocyte mediated cytolysis. XI. The role of lectin in lectin dependent cell-mediated cytotoxicity, *J. Immunol.*, 121, 1566, 1978.
26. Bonavida, B. and Ostergaard, H., Role of target cell structure on CMC. I. Expression of target cell antigen for cytotoxicity (TAC) following modification by IO_4 borohydride, in preparation.
27. Bonavida, B. and Katz, J., Role of target cell structure on CMC. II. Involvement of papain sensitive membrane structure in HL-A- target cell in LDCC, in preparation.
28. Fan, J. and Bonavida, B., Studies on the induction and expression of T-mediated immunity. XII. The concommitant loss and recovery of membrane associated non-specific cytotoxic activity of alloimmune T lymphocytes following treatment with trypsin, *J. Immunol.*, 127, 18, 1981.
29. Brunda, M. J., Herberman, R. B., and Holden, H. J., in *Natural Cell-Mediated Immunity Against Tumors* Herberman, R. B., Ed., Academic Press, New York, 1980, 525.
30. Wright, S. C. and Bonavida, B., YAC-1 resistant clones selected for resistance to natural killer cytotoxic factors are also resistant to natural killer cell mediated cytotoxicity, *Proc. Natl. Acad. Sci. U.S.A.*, 80, 1688, 1983.
31. Binz, H., Fenner, M., Frei, D., and Wigzell, H., Two independent receptors allow selective target lysis by T cell clones, *J. Exp. Med.*, 157, 1252, 1983.

Chapter 12

MLC-INDUCED CYTOTOXICITY AS A MODEL FOR THE DEVELOPMENT AND REGULATION OF NK CYTOTOXICITY

Paula J. D'Amore and Sidney H. Golub

TABLE OF CONTENTS

I. INTRODUCTION

Evidence is accumulating which indicates that natural killer (NK) activity is of some importance in human malignant disease and that NK cell function can be affected by tumor cells and their products. For example, NK activity is depressed in patients with large tumor burdens,[1,2] including cancer patients whose ability to produce interferon (IFN) is normal.[3] Hershey et al.[4] correlated NK activity to certain histopathological features in melanoma patients. Recent animal studies indicate that NK cells can inhibit metastasis formation.[5] Therefore, NK cells may be of biological significance as antitumor effectors and a thorough understanding of these cells and their activity is essential.

A useful means for studying NK cells and their activity is to induce NK cytotoxicity in vitro. Several systems have been used to generate NK or NK-like cytotoxicity in vitro, including simply culturing lymphocytes in the presence of fetal calf serum,[6,7] stimulating lymphocytes with antigen or the supernatants of antigen-stimulated cultures,[8,9] stimulation of lymphocytes with autochthonous or allogeneic lymphoblastoid cell lines (LCL),[10,11] and most recently, the lymphokine-activated killer cell system (LAK)[12] which generates cells bearing a resemblance to mixed lymphocyte culture (MLC)-generated NK cells.

We have chosen as our model system the MLC which generates NK-like cells as well as allospecific cytotoxic T lymphocytes (CTL) in vitro. There are several attractive features of MLC as a model of NK development and regulation. First, it is a system which allows for the generation of cytotoxic cells which have NK-like specificity from precursor cells that are NK-inactive. Therefore, this presents the possibility of studying the development of NK cytotoxicity and the regulation of such development. Second, the simultaneous development of allospecific and NK cytotoxic cells allows for comparisons of the target specificity of these cells. Is there a relationship between the antigenic determinants involved in recognition by the CTL and NK-like cells? Is allospecific killing and NK-like cytotoxicity mediated by the same cell population or two different populations? Another area of interest in the MLC-generated NK system is the phenotype of the effector cells. A remarkably heterogeneous group of cells appear to mediate this type of cytotoxicity and these cells are phenotypically quite different from fresh NK cells.

An area that warrants considerable attention is the regulation of NK cells. Although many studies have focused on soluble mediators such as IFN, prostaglandins, and interleukin 2 (IL-2) as regulators of NK activity, much less is known about the cellular interactions which affect the development and cytotoxic activity of NK cells. Defining the type of cells that can activate or suppress NK activity and when such cells can exert their regulatory influence is of considerable importance. An MLC provides an excellent model for such studies because it allows for analysis of the induction of NK activity and its subsequent decline.

This review will attempt to provide an overview of our work and that of others in the various areas outlined. We shall attempt to critically review the nature of MLC-induced NK-like cells including a discussion of the precursors of these cells, their phenotypes, the specificity of the cytotoxicity they mediate, and the mode of regulation of their function. Although the opinions expressed are those of the authors, this report is also a product of the diligent work of two former graduate students in this laboratory, Janet Seeley, Ph.D. and Marc Golightly, Ph.D., whose initial contributions to the MLC studies made our subsequent investigations possible.

II. DEVELOPMENT OF NK-LIKE EFFECTOR CELLS IN VITRO

Some of the experimental data on the development of cytotoxic NK cells from their precursors and some of the data on the cell lineage to which NK cells belong are rather difficult to reconcile. Some human NK cells have been shown to express T cell-associated antigens[13-15] whereas murine NK cells develop as an autonomous function of the bone marrow[16] and are found in the spleens of congenitally athymic mice.[17] Some investigators have suggested that NK cells represent a heterogeneous population composed of more than one cell type derived from different cell lineages.[18,19] A model system for studying NK development in vitro might allow analysis of this problem in that studies of NK cells induced in MLC allow for the generation of these cells from NK inactive precursors. Therefore, it is possible to determine what precursor cells are essential for NK (or NK-like) maturation as well as the regulatory events involved in NK development and the kinetics of development. Because an MLC generates NK-like cells and allospecific CTL, it provides an excellent means of studying the development of both types of cells in concert in order to determine if NK-like cells are of the T lineage or if there is any relationship between NK and T cells. One apparent difference between NK-like cytotoxicity and allospecific killing is in the kinetics of development. In our initial MLC studies[20] a 13-day time course study was performed to compare the development of NK-like and allospecific killing. Differences in the time of appearance and the duration of the NK-like and allospecific response became apparent. Alloreactivity to the original stimulator cell was evident on day 5 of MLC, peaked on days 6 to 7, and retained considerable activity through day 13. In contrast, the NK-like cytotoxicity against K562 peaked on days 4 to 5 and declined thereafter, returning to baseline levels on day 9. A similar pattern of cytotoxicity was found directed towards the EBV-transformed lymphoblastoid cell line derived from peripheral blood lymphocytes (PBL) of the original responder type. These studies clearly showed that two distinct cytotoxicities are generated in a MLC with different times of appearance. We have further analyzed the kinetics of NK-like and allospecific killing generated in MLC using single cell analysis.[21] A number of MLC were maintained in culture for a period of 1 to 7 days. The effector cells generated were assayed for their NK-like activity against K562. The maximum response to K562 was found on day 3 with an increase in both the number of cells able to bind K562 and the number of cytotoxic cells. Thereafter, the number of binders and killers declined and returned to baseline on days 6 and 7. Allospecific killing appeared later than the NK-like response with a maximum number of binders and killers of the alloantigen target appearing on days 6 and 7. The increased number of cells binding and killing the allospecific target correlates with the well-known proliferation of allospecific cells activated in MLC. Callewaert et al.[22] have shown that elimination of dividing cells in MLC by treatment with BUDR and light completely abrogates the CTL response but does not affect the NK-like cytotoxicity. In addition to providing further evidence for the generation of two distinct cytotoxicities generated in MLC, these results indicate that proliferation is not required for the cytotoxic response of MLC NK-like cells. The increased number of NK target binders and killers that we have found in single cell analysis may simply reflect the differentiation of nonbinding, noncytotoxic NK precursors into cells that can bind the target and their subsequent development into mature NK cells capable of lysing target cells. It is interesting that a similar increase in the number of cells that can bind and kill K562 was observed from in vivo IFN-treated patients.[23] This suggests that IFN may be one factor involved in the conversion of nonbinding precursors into NK cells. Similar kinetic experiments have also shown that MLC induces two cytotoxic activities (NK-like and allospecific) which appear at different times.[24-26] Seeley and Karre[25] have demonstrated that mouse cells kept in MLC exhibit the same pattern of induction with maximum NK-like activity on days 3 to 4 and allospecific killing peaking on day 6.

Further differences in patterns of development between NK-like cells and allospecific CTL have been shown in secondary MLC.[27] MLC cells were restimulated on day 14 with the original stimulator cells. Allospecific killing displayed a classical memory response resulting in 100% lysis of the alloantigen-bearing target. In contrast, cytotoxicity against K562 was only slightly activated in secondary MLC, especially when compared to the substantial increase induced in primary MLC. Seeley and Kärre[25] have confirmed these results in both the mouse and human systems.

Although it is apparent that an allogeneic MLC induces both allospecific and NK cytotoxicity, an obvious question is whether the NK-like activity is merely due to fresh NK cells present at the initiation of the culture which are maintained in MLC or is there *de novo* generation of NK-like effector cells? Our approach to this question was to deplete fresh PBL to be used as responders in MLC of NK cells prior to sensitization.[27] It is generally accepted that the NK activity of fresh PBL is mediated by a population of cells which express an Fc receptor (FcR). Therefore, lymphocytes to be used as responders were separated into Fcγ+ and Fcγ− fractions by absorption to immune complex monolayers. As expected, the anti-K562 cytotoxic activity was enriched in the Fcγ+ fraction and depleted in the Fcγ− fraction. When the Fcγ+-enriched cell population was used as responders in MLC, the NK-like activity of day 5 MLC cells was negligible. This would indicate that the cytotoxic activity of the NK-enriched population was not maintained in culture and no new NK cells were generated. In contrast, the Fcγ− cell population, depleted of NK activity, responded well in MLC and developed NK-like activity by day 5 of MLC. These results clearly demonstrate that the NK-like cytotoxicity characteristic of MLC cells represents *de novo* generation from an NK inactive precursor cell and is not the result of fresh NK cells maintained from the initiation of the MLC. Similar experiments by other investigators have shown that NK-like cells are derived from noncytotoxic precursor cells.[24,25,28-30] However, conflicting results have recently been reported by Strassman et al.[31] They have found that when fresh PBL, depleted of OKM1+ or B73.1+ cells, were used as responders in an allogeneic MLC, minimal NK-like activity was generated. Therefore, the authors suggested that NK-like activity generated in MLC is derived in part from residual fresh NK cells expressing the OKM1 or B73.1 phenotypic markers which are activated in MLC by IFN. Major differences in our system and the one described by Strassman et al. are in the culture conditions and the days in which the cultures were tested. We used a single allogeneic stimulus instead of a pool of allogeneic cells and we tested on day 3 as opposed to day 7. By day 7 in our system, the NK-like activity of MLC cells had returned to baseline level. Therefore, testing only on day 7 and not before might fail to reveal all cytotoxic cells that had developed. We agree with Strassman et al. that elimination of Fcγ+ cells by treatment with the monoclonal antibody (MoAb) B73.1 may be different than absorption of lymphocytes to immune complexes. Recently, we have removed B73.1+ or OKM-1+ cells from fresh PBL using a panning technique and depleted Fcγ+ cells by adherence to EAγ monolayers. When any of these cell populations (OKM-1−, B.73.1−, or EAγ−) were cultured in MLC, NK-like activity was generated.[31a] We have seen a substantial increase in NK cytotoxicity on day 3 in all cases. Therefore, we believe these results confirm our previous data that the NK-like activity of MLC effector cells is not due to residual NK cells but is due to newly developed effector cells generated from NK inactive precursors.

One of the precursors necessary for the development of NK-like activity in MLC is T cells. Populations rich in E rosette-forming cells with no NK activity respond in MLC producing strong anti-K562 cytotoxicity.[27] A weak NK response and minimal blastogenesis is produced when E rosette-depleted, Fcγ+ cells are used as responders in

MLC.[29] The activation of T cells appears to be a requirement for in vitro development of NK activity in other systems also.[29,32,33] These results indicate that NK cells may be part of the T cell lineage or that NK cells are under T cell regulation. To investigate the relationship between NK cells and T cell activity, we have studied the presence of FcR for IgM and IgG on the precursors of in vitro-generated NK activity using MLC or the T cell stimulus.[34] Depleting Fcγ+ cells on EAγ monolayers prior to MLC resulted in post-MLC NK-like effectors. The precursor in this case was presumed not only to be Fcγ− but also Fcμ−, as we could detect few Fcμ+ cells prior to incubation. Furthermore, pre-MLC Fcμ depletion confirmed the absence of precursors bearing the Fcμ receptor, as no change in post-MLC activity occurred. The participation of Fcγ+ receptor cells in the generation of cytotoxic effectors was further examined by enrichment of Fcγ+ cells by EAγ rosette formation. Fcγ+ cells were able to generate NK-like cytotoxic cells in MLC. Therefore, there appears to be great heterogeneity with respect to the precursors of MLC-induced NK activity. E+, Fcμ-γ− and Fcμ-γ+ cells are all capable of giving rise to MLC cells with NK-like cytotoxic activity.

Further heterogeneity is indicated by the recent studies of Abo and Balch.[35] They have demonstrated that fresh PBL, expressing the HNK-1 differentiation antigen, do not proliferate in an allogeneic MLC whereas HNK-1 depleted cells do respond in MLC generating a cell population with NK-like cytotoxic activity. HNK-1 is a differentiation antigen expressed on a large portion of fresh NK cells. These results also indicate that MLC-generated NK-like cells can be derived from noncytotoxic precursors.

The newest approach that we have taken to the question of the precursor of MLC-generated NK activity is described in Torten et al.[36] In this study, we explored the use of thymocytes to generate NK-like cytotoxicity. We found that thymocytes could be used to generate cytotoxic effectors against K562 as long as the MLC was supplemented with IL-2. The most interesting feature of the thymocyte system is the finding that the anti-K562 effectors generated from thymocytes are almost exclusively Fcγ-positive. In this sense, they are very similar to standard peripheral blood NK cells and distinct from the predominantly Fcμ-positive effectors generated in MLC from PBL. Separation of thymocytes into Fcμ+ and Fcμ− fractions prior to MLC resulted in development of anti-K562 cytotoxicity only from the Fcμ+ cells. These results suggest that there is a population of thymus-derived human T cells that can contribute to NK cytotoxicity. The thymocyte that develops into the NK-like effector cell has the Fcμ receptor in common with the PBL-derived, MLC-induced, NK-like effector cell. One means of explaining this concurrence is the possibility that these two cells represent the same stage in a common pathway.

III. CHARACTERISTICS OF EFFECTORS

The effector cells generated in MLC that mediate NK-like cytotoxicity represent a heterogeneous population with regard to the surface markers. Furthermore, there are some clear phenotypic differences between fresh NK cells and MLC-generated NK-like effector cells. Although the precursors of MLC NK-like cells are noncytotoxic and for the most part do not express the Fcγ receptor, alloactivation may stimulate NK precursors and their expression of the Fcγ receptors. In the initial studies of Seeley et al.,[27] MLC-generated cells were found to contain a much lower proportion of Fcγ+ cells as compared to fresh PBL. In order to determine whether Fcγ+ cells were responsible for the NK-like cytotoxic activity, MLC cells were separated into Fcγ+ and Fcγ− populations by absorption to immune complex monolayers. The anti-K562 activity of the Fcγ− cells was comparable to the NK activity of unfractionated MLC cells. Although the adherent cell population containing the Fcγ+ cells was greatly enriched for cytotoxic activity against K562, it represented only a small percentage of the total population of MLC cells. Therefore, MLC-induced NK-like activity is mediated by a heterogeneous population of cells which, unlike fresh NK cytotoxicity, is not exclusively mediated by Fcγ receptor bearing cells. Other investigators have obtained similar results.[24,25,28,30,37]

We have further investigated the nature of the NK-active Fcγ− cell population generated in MLC. While it is generally accepted that fresh NK activity is mediated by a population of lymphocytes bearing the Fcγ receptor, other reports have indicated that Fcμ+ cells contribute to the cytotoxic activity of fresh NK cells.[38,39] Therefore, we tested the hypothesis that Fcμ receptor cells, in addition to Fcγ+ cells, were involved in MLC-generated NK-like activity.[32] MLC cells were fractionated into Fcμ+ and Fcμ− populations using a EAμ rosette separation technique. The unfractionated Fcμ+ and Fcμ− cells were tested for cytotoxicity against K562. Fcμ+ cells displayed substantial cytotoxicity against K562. NK activity was also detected in the Fcμ− MLC population. Thus it appears that MLC-induced anti-K562 effectors are a heterogeneous population containing both Fcμ+ and Fcμ− cells. However, the net gain in NK-like activity found in MLC appears to be due primarily to the increase in activity of the Fcμ receptor-bearing cells. This became evident in comparing nonstimulated control cultures with MLC-cultured cells. The majority of the NK activity against K562 in the nonstimulated control cultures was in the Fcμ− fraction, while Fcμ+ cells had very little cytotoxic activity. In contrast, the majority of the NK activity in MLC was in the Fcμ+ cell population. To confirm our findings that MLC Fcμ+ cells were cytotoxic against K562, we utilized a combined rosetting and single cell cytotoxicity test. This allowed us to identify at the single-cell level what cell was actually binding to and killing the NK target. Fresh PBL, prior to stimulation in MLC, contained less than 1% EAμ+ cells that could bind K562 and no EAμ+ cells that were cytotoxic. With time in MLC, the proportion of both EAμ+ binders and killers increased, with peak binding found on day 3 and the maximum number of killers found on days 5 to 7. The number of EAγ+ target binding cells showed a slight increase from 7.3% on day 0 to 10.3% on day 3. The number of EAγ+ cytotoxic cells remained around 3% at all times. Therefore, it became apparent by single-cell analysis that the proportion of Fcγ+ cytotoxic effector cells generated in MLC appears to be stable or declining during MLC, while the proportion of Fcμ+ killer cells increases. The fact that the total number of Fcμ+ cytotoxic cells increases post-MLC clearly indicates that a new type of cytotoxic cell is emerging rather than an indirect augmentation of the existing NK cells by the MLC. If the latter possibility were the case, one would expect the increase in NK activity to be confined to the Fcγ+ cells.

In addition to the expression of Fcμ and Fcγ receptors on NK-like cells, variability in T cell markers had also been established. We have found NK-like activity associated with both E rosette-forming cells and cells that fail to form high-affinity E rosettes.[27] A stronger anti-K562 response is usually associated with the cells not expressing the E receptor. Poros and Klein[40,41] have also found NK-like activity associated with the E rosette-forming population as well as the cells that do not form E rosettes. The strongest NK-like activity was found in the population depleted of T cells with E receptors. It should be noted that the Fcμ+ effector cells generated in MLC that we demonstrated were also E rosette-bearing cells and that the cytotoxic activity of the Fcμ− cells appeared in both the E rosetting and non-E rosetting cell populations.[34] Ausiello et al.[42] have done extensive cell separation experiments to characterize the MLC-generated NK-like effector cells. They have also found that cytotoxic activity against NK-sensitive target cells is found among Fcγ+ and Fcγ− cells. In addition, when the Fcγ+ and Fcγ− populations were separated into E rosette and non-E rosette fractions, NK-like activity was found in all the subsets. The authors concluded that NK-like cytotoxic activity is mediated by a population of Fcγ+ and Fcγ− effector cells that may or may not express T cell markers. Santoli et al.[30] compared the NK-like effector cells generated when either unfractionated PBL or E+ Fcγ− cells were used as responders in MLC. In either case, NK-like activity was associated with both E receptor and non-E receptor cells. Further characterization of the NK-like effector cells generated from E+ Fcγ− responder cells led those investigators to conclude that NK-like cytotoxicity is mediated by a population of newly generated effector cells that have maintained T cell markers. This was based on the fact that all of the NK-like effectors generated from Fcγ− E+ cells reacted with two MoAb reactive with T cells, OKT3, and B36.1. In contrast, when unfractionated PBL were used as responders, anti-K562 activity was associated with the non-T cell population as well as the E+ OKT3+ population. As suggested by Santoli et al., these results might explain the work of Zarling and colleagues.[43,45] Zarling has found that treatment of MLC-effector cells with OKT3 or OKT8 and complement eliminated the cytotoxicity against the allogeneic stimulator cells and autochthonous LCL without affecting NK-like activity against K562. In these studies, unfractionated PBL were used as the responders in MLC. Therefore, it is possible that the NK-like activity of the OKT3− MLC effector cell population was the result of preexisting NK cells not expressing T cell markers that were maintained in MLC. Alternatively, the cytotoxicity against K562 and the cytotoxicity against the LCL may be mediated by different cell types. Our binding studies[21] would be consistent with separate anti-K562 and anti-LCL effectors. Zarling and Kung[43] have also reported that OKM1 and complement eliminated the cytotoxic activity of fresh and poly I:C activated NK cells but did not affect the cytotoxicity of MLC cells against K562. The OKT3 results are worth noting, as fresh NK cells do not generally express the OKT3 marker even if they are E+. Thus, the OKT3 and the E receptor markers have to be considered to be quite distinct in these systems, as MLC-induced NK-like cells may be positive or negative for either marker while fresh NK cells appear to be heterogeneous only for the E marker.

From the results presented in this section, it is obvious that MLC-generated NK-like cells represent an extremely heterogeneous population that is phenotypically quite different from fresh NK cells. However, it is unlikely that the disparity in surface marker expression indicates no functional relationship between MLC-NK and peripheral blood NK. Differences in the activation event leading to NK activity and the precursor cells from which these cells are derived may result in NK cells with different phenotypes. Whether these cells are all of the same lineage at different stages of differentiation or whether they are cells of different lineage cannot be fully answered at this time.

IV. SPECIFICITY

MLC results in the development of a cytotoxic specificity in addition to, and distinct from, the allospecific specificity mediated by CTL. The distinction of NK specificity from allospecificity can be made by answering the following questions.

(1) Are the MLC-generated effector cells able to kill a spectrum of targets similar to that of fresh NK cells?
(2) Are different recognition sites involved in the killing of the allospecific target by the CTL and the lysis of NK-sensitive targets by NK-like cells?
(3) If different recognition sites are involved in allospecific and NK-like cytotoxicity, are they executed by the same effector cell population or is MLC-induced NK a separate cytotoxic activity mediated by a subpopulation of cells distinct from alloreactive T cells?
(4) If NK-like cytotoxicity is mediated by a separate population of cells, do the effector cells recognize a structure common to all NK targets or are the MLC NK-

like cells a heterogeneous population composed of clonally distributed subpopulations, each recognizing different target specificities?

Our initial studies were aimed at determining whether effector cells generated in MLC were cytotoxic against a spectrum of targets quite different from the allospecific target recognized by the CTL. NK-like activity was found against a broad range of targets including LCL targets derived from the same individual as the PBL of the original MLC responder.[20] The cytotoxicity against autochthonous LCL targets was called "anomolous killing" (AK). However, cytotoxicity could not be detected against mitogen-activated lymphocyte targets autochthonous to the responder cells. To rule out the possibility that an EBV-associated antigen was the target antigen for NK-like activity, other targets were tested. EBV-negative T cell lines, HSBII and MOLT-4, were as sensitive to lysis as three EBV-transformed LCL (the autochtonous LCL, Daudi, and SB). Cytotoxicity did not appear to be related to HLA determinants as HLA-negative targets such as Daudi and K562 were sensitive to NK-like activity. This broad range of cytotoxicity resembles the pattern of fresh NK cell activity reported by Takasugi and colleagues,[46] who observed that normal PBL are cytotoxic for a wide spectrum of cell lines. Our data was consistent with the concept that in vitro allostimulation in MLC leads to an augmented cytotoxic response against a variety of target cell lines in addition to the CTL response to the original stimulator cells. Other investigators have also shown that MLC-activated NK cells are able to lyse a large number of target cells, including those that are only slightly susceptible to lysis by fresh NK cells.[24,25,48] Thus, AK appears to have a somewhat broader target spectrum than NK cytotoxicity although it does resemble the specificity IFN-activated NK cells.

These results, however, did not provide evidence as to whether different recognition sites are involved in NK-like and allospecific killing. Our approach to this question was to determine by cold target inhibition analysis whether NK targets would inhibit the cytotoxicity developed in MLC against the alloantigen-bearing target and whether the allospecific target would inhibit anti-K562 activity.[27] When unlabeled allotargets were added to a mixture of MLC-effector cells and ^{51}Cr-labeled allospecific targets, efficient homologous inhibition occurred. Unlabeled K562 targets were also able to inhibit the killing of ^{51}Cr-labeled K562 by MLC effector cells. However, alloantigen-bearing targets would not inhibit the cytotoxicity developed in MLC against K562 nor would K562 inhibit the cytotoxicity against the allospecific targets. These results demonstrated that different recognition sites are involved on the NK-like target and allospecific target. The CTL-mediated allospecific killing is directed against the histocompatibility antigens present on the original stimulator cells and the NK-like response is directed toward antigens distinct from the alloantigen present on the tumor cell lines. When K562 and the autochthonous LCL were tested in cold target analysis, some partial cross-reactivity was observed, indicating that K562 and the autochthonous LCL may share some common target determinant. Bolhuis[24] and Bolhuis and Ronteltap[28] have done similar cold target competition studies to distinguish the CTL and NK recognition sites. They also found that alloblasts could not inhibit the cytotoxicity against K562. However, the authors demonstrated that K562 and T24, a bladder cancer cell line, could sometimes inhibit the lysis of PHA lymphoblast target cells. This would occur only when the killing of autochthonous PHA lymphoblasts was observed. Bolhuis and colleagues[24,28,37] also used a monolayer absorption technique to analyse NK and CTL specificity. MLC-generated NK-like cytotoxic activity could only be absorbed out by monolayers of NK-sensitive targets and not by lymphoblasts of the original MLC stimulator cell. Using this technique, the CTL response was depleted only on monolayers of the original stimulator cells and not on monolayers of K562 or T24. This provides further evidence that distinguishes AK from allospecific cytotoxicity.

Seeley and Kärre[25,26] have found a similar lack of cross-reactivity between NK and allospecific killing using mouse MLC-generated effector cells. NK-sensitive targets, YAC-1 and MPC-11, could inhibit cytotoxicity against YAC-1 but not the CTL response to the allospecific target. Conversely, the allospecific target did not cross-compete with the killing of YAC-1 targets.

Taken together, the cold target inhibition data and the monolayer absorption results indicate that the NK-like and allospecific reactivities are directed against different specificities with distinct recognition sites.

Although the previous data supports the concept that different recognition sites are involved in NK-like and allospecific killing, it was still not clear whether the two cytotoxic activities were mediated by the same population of effector cells. We turned to single-cell analysis to investigate this.[21,49] We felt it was important to use this type of analysis since cold target competition can show substantial differences in compatibility with different effectors despite the fact that the effectors may have similar levels of cytotoxic activity against the same target. Single-cell analysis also allows for a quantitative analysis of the numbers of effector cells reacting with various targets. This technique offers an additional dimension in evaluating the specificity of NK-like cells and CTL, in that one can directly visualize what type of target an effector cell is binding and determine if any one effector cell can bind more than one type of target. Klein[48] has proposed that NK represents a stage in the development and/or differentiation of a CTL. As discussed above, this concept is clearly correct in that the NK-like cells develop from T cells and are cytotoxic. However, the CTL has the connotation of allospecificity. The data from competition and absorption analyses would argue against allospecificity of NK-like cytotoxicity. Our objective was to directly test if one population of MLC effector cells could mediate NK and allospecific killing or whether these two cytotoxic responses were executed by two separate subpopulations. We felt that if NK is a function of the developing alloreactive T lymphocytes, there should be a point in time when a cell changes from NK reactivity to alloreactivity. Therefore, the MLC-generated cells were tested daily in single cell analysis with both NK and allospecific targets simultaneously. Accordingly, we could determine if there was a time when an effector cell could bind the NK-sensitive and allospecific targets simultaneously. Relatively few effector cells were found which could bind both targets during a 7-day interval. Therefore, we feel this is quite conclusive evidence that the NK-like cytotoxic activity developed in MLC is distinct from alloreactivity and is mediated by a separate subpopulation of cells. Zarling and colleagues[43-45,50] have also found that NK-like and allospecific killing are not executed by the same cell population. By treating MLC-generated effector cells with OKT3 or OKT8 MoAb and complement, the cytotoxic activity against the allospecific target cells as well as the autochthonous EBV-transformed LCL was depleted. However, reactivity against the NK-sensitive target, K562, was unaffected. Using single-cell analysis with both the allospecific target and autochthonous LCL, we have found that MLC-generated effector cells can bind both targets simultaneously. However, a small number of double target binders of the autochthonous LCL and K562 were found, suggesting that in addition to CTL, AK cells may also have some activity against the NK-sensitive targets. These results confirm our original data in which there was a partial cross-reactivity in cold target competition between autochthonous LCL and K562.[27] Thus, there appear to be distinct cytotoxic activities developed in MLC. The allospecific CTL are cytotoxic for the alloantigen-bearing targets and also for the autochthonous LCL (AK). The NK-like effectors do not kill alloantigen targets but can kill NK-sensitive targets and perhaps mediate AK as well. Other features that distinguish NK-like and AK cytotoxicity remain undefined.

If the NK-like response is mediated by a separate subpopulation of MLC-generated cells, do NK-like cells recognize a structure common to all NK-sensitive targets or is the NK population composed of clonally distributed subpopulations, each recognizing a limited set of target antigens? Using several different NK target combinations in single-cell analysis with MLC effector cells, relatively few double target binders were found. This would imply considerable heterogeneity among NK cells and would indicate clonal distribution of receptors for the various target structures unique to each NK-sensitive target. The question of specificity can also be addressed by cloning the MLC-activated cells in IL-2. This approach would have the advantage of providing separate clonal populations for analysis of specificity. However, IL-2 is clearly a regulatory molecule for NK cytotoxicity and might well affect the specificity and function of the cloned cells. Even with this limitation, indications from IL-2 cloning studies are that MLC-generated NK-like cells are heterogeneous with regard to specificities recognized.[51]

In summary, MLC clearly results in two separate cytotoxicities, NK-like and alloreactivity, which are mediated by different cell populations. The target specificites recognized by the MLC-generated NK-like effector cells are quite distinct from those found on the allospecific target. We are proposing that the NK-like population is heterogeneous in nature, comprised of clonally distributed subpopulations, each recognizing different target specificities. However, it seems unlikely that each and every NK-like effector cell can only recognize one target specificity. There may be a limited number of target receptors and each population of cells might express more than one receptor, with the receptor specificities being randomly distributed. In this case, only an occasional cell would express receptors for any two preselected targets under test. Thus, with either single or multiple specificities, cytotoxicity would appear to be polyclonal.

VI. REGULATION

It has become increasingly apparent that NK cells are subject to regulatory controls including both activating and inhibitory signals. Soluble mediators of NK function have been identified and cellular regulation of NK function and development, perhaps via mediators, has also been observed. MLC allows for the generation of cytotoxic cells which have NK-like specificity from noncytotoxic precursors thereby allowing the examination of the development of cytotoxicity. Establishing an in vitro model of NK regulation may provide useful information for determining the relevant in vivo regulatory events.

Several investigators have focused on the contributions of soluble mediators such as IFN and IL-2 to the augmented NK response found in early MLC. Lymphocytes in response to the allogeneic stimulus in MLC have been shown to produce IFN.[52,53] Maximum IFN-γ production has been found on days 4 to 6 in human MLC and days 5 to 8 in mouse MLC.[53] Trinchieri et al.[52] have characterized the cells responsible for the IFN production as E+ and E+ Fcγ− cells. The kinetics of IFN production are similar to that of NK-like activity generated in MLC. Therefore, the conditions for the development of NK-like cytotoxicity and for IFN production coincide. However, enthusiasm for the MLC system would be limited if it simply reflected the in vitro production of IFN producing the augmented NK response. While the participation of IFN or other soluble mediators cannot be completely dismissed, it seems unlikely that IFN is the sole regulator of NK-like activity. For example, IFN appears to augment NK cytotoxicity primarily by activating Fcγ receptor cells.[54,55] while the MLC system generates primarily Fcμ-bearing NK effectors. Furthermore, cyclosporin A allows development of MLC-generated NK cytotoxicity despite decreased IFN production and allospecific cytotoxicity.[56] MLCs in which additional IFN was added during the development of the cytotoxic effectors give rise to a lower NK response than cells cultured in MLC without added IFN.[57] Pretreatment of MLC-generated effector cells with IFN for 1 hr results in an increased NK response. This is another characteristic shared by NK and MLC-derived NK-like cells which is not shared by CTL. In contrast, MLCs in which IFN was added at the initiation of the culture yield cells unable to respond to a second exposure to IFN.[57,58] Whisler et la.[59] described a similar system for in vitro induction of NK cytotoxicity which was not inhibited by anti-IFN serum. Therefore, it would appear that NK genertion can be independent of IFN production in the MLC.

IL-2 has also been shown to generate natural cytotoxicity in vitro. An LAK cell system has recently been described by Grimm et al.[12] in which nonadherent PBL are kept in culture for a minimum of 3 days in lectin-free IL-2 supernatants. Both LAK cells and MLC cells have been shown to lyse autochthonous fresh tumor cells, allogeneic tumor cells, and cultured tumor cell lines. The LAK cells bear a resemblance to MLC-generated NK cells in relation to kinetics of development and generation of effector cells from noncytotoxic precursors. In addition, IFN does not appear to be the sole stimulus needed for LAK cell induction. It remains to be determined if IL-2 is the sole T cell product governing the development of NK-like cells or if allostimulation in MLC provides other signals. The fact that MLC induction of NK-like cytotoxicity is resistant to cyclosporin A[56] argues that IL-2 is not the sole factor involved.

Very little is known as to why NK-like activity declines in late MLC. Our findings that NK-like activity generated in MLC returns to baseline by day 9 and that secondary MLC was ineffective in generating NK-like cytotoxicity[22,29] suggested to us the possibility of MLC-developed suppressor cells for NK function or development. Our first question was whether a suppressor cell was activated in late MLC.[60,61] This putative suppressor cell would be expected to inhibit both MLC-induced and fresh NK activity. To test this hypothesis, mixing experiments were performed in which effector cells kept in MLC for various time periods were mixed with fresh PBL of the original responder type. The NK activity of the cell mixture was compared to that obtained by the fresh PBL alone. Late MLC cells, especially day 12 cells, could inhibit the cytotoxic activity of autochthonous fresh NK cells. Suppression of MLC-generated NK-like activity was also seen when the day 12 MLC cells were mixed with day 3 MLC effector cells. To determine what portion of the cytotoxic reaction was affected by the suppression, the single-cell cytotoxicity assay was used. We established that suppression is manifested at the level of target recognition which was reflected in the decreased number of target-binding conjugates (TBC) found when day 12 MLC cells were added to fresh NK cells or day 3 MLC cells. Therefore, suppression is directed towards functionally active NK cells, preventing them from binding to target cells and thereby decreasing the number of available cytotoxic effector cells. A soluble suppressive factor did not appear to be causing the suppression, since the addition of the supernatant from the 12-day MLC had no effect on the binding and killing activity of the fresh PBL. Studies were conducted to evaluate the phenotype of the suppressor cell. The suppressor cells generated in the day 12 MLC, in addition to being nonadherent, express the Fcμ receptor but not the Fcγ receptor. The most interesting marker was the HNK-1 antigen, as suppression of fresh NK activity was alleviated when HNK 1+ cells were removed from the 12-day MLC. Our results also indicate that the suppressor cell is HLA-DR−, Leu 4−, and Leu 2a−. This would imply that the suppressor cell is not an activated T cell nor a typical T suppressor cell. Therefore, the suppressor cell population within the 12-day MLC is an Fcμ+, HNK 1+ cell.

Although we established that suppression is manifested at the level of target recognition, we were interested in the mechanism underlying the suppression. How were fresh NK cells prevented from binding to the NK-sensitive target, K562? Throughout the mixing experiments we consistently found a small number of day 12 MLC cells and fresh PBL bound to each other. The removal of various subpopulations from the day

12 MLC such as Leu 4+, Leu 2a+, HLA-DR+, or B73.1+ cells did not alleviate the suppression of fresh NK activity and had no effect on the number of fresh PBL-day 12 MLC cell conjugates. However, when HNK-1-depleted day 12 MLC cells were mixed with fresh PBL, there was no suppression of fresh NK activity and a marked reduction in the number of day 12 MLC cell-fresh PBL conjugates was found. Our hypothesis was that the suppressor cell was binding to fresh NK cells. Therefore, HNK-1+, B73.1+, or EAγ+ cells were removed from the fresh PBL and the remaining cells were mixed with the day 12 suppressor cells. In all three circumstances the number of fresh PBL-day 12 MLC cell conjugates was markedly reduced. It would appear that late MLC generates a cell population expressing the Fcμ receptor and HNK-1 differentiation antigen. These cells are capable of mediating suppression by binding to HNK-1+, Fcγ+ NK cells within the fresh PBL. In turn, HNK-1+, Fcγ+ NK cells are rendered incapable of binding to target cells.

As will be discussed in the last section, we are proposing a model of NK suppression of feedback inhibition in which cells generated in late MLC expressing NK surface markers function as immunoregulators, inhibiting the cytotoxic activity of fresh NK cells.

We have shown that a suppressor cell activated in late MLC can inhibit the activity of fresh NK cells. Perhaps a suppressor function exists for the generation of NK-like cells and this is the reason for the decline in NK-like activity found in late MLC. Therefore, we wanted to see if the removal of various subpopulations at the beginning of MLC on day 0 would affect the kinetics of NK development. To address this question, different cell populations such as unfractionated fresh PBL, B73.1-depleted, or HNK-1-negative cells, were used as responders in MLC. As expected, maximum NK-like activity was found on day 3 and declined thereafter when either unfractionated or B73.1-depleted PBL were the responder cell population. However, when HNK-1 negative cells were used as responders, NK-like activity did not decline after 3 days in MLC and remained as high or higher by day 7. These results clearly indicate that in addition to soluble mediators such as IFN and IL-2, cellular regulation of NK cytotoxicity exists.

In summary, the regulatory events which affect NK activity appear to be quite complex. It is evident that a number of factors including soluble mediators and regulatory cells can augment or inhibit NK activity. In addition, NK cells themselves may function as immunoregulators controlling their own cytotoxic activity. A thorough understanding of the mechanisms underlying these regulatory events and the in vivo relevance of these interactions is needed.

VI. CONCLUSIONS

Considerable information has now accumulated on MLC-induced NK cytotoxicity and the current state of the art is summarized in Table I. Enough data has now been assembled to permit some speculations on the implications of this phenomenon. There are two general interpretations possible concerning this type of cytotoxicity. The first, or "null" hypothesis, would hold that MLC-induced NK cytotoxicity has no relationship whatsoever to standard NK activity. The alternative view would be that MLC-induced NK is an accurate, albeit limited, model for the actual events involved in the in vivo development of NK cytotoxicity.

The null interpretation, if correct, would also be quite informative as to the nature of NK cell. If true, it would indicate that a variety of mechanisms must exist to achieve the same end result. Standard NK cells and in vitro-generated NK-like cells have cytotoxic activities against a similar spectrum of targets. This would imply that there is either a strong evolutionary pressure to develop such broadly reactive cytotoxic cells

Table 1
CHARACTERISTICS OF MLC-GENERATED NK-LIKE CELLS

I. Kinetics of development
- 1 MLC: Maximum cytotoxic activity on day 3
  - Increased number of TBC
  - Increased number of cytotoxic effector cells
- 2 MLC: Minimal activation

II. Precursors
- Fcγ−
- B73.1−
- OKM.1−
- E rosette +
- Fcμ-γ−, Fcμ-γ+
- HNK-1−
- Fcμ+ thymocytes

III. Effector cell characteristics

High activity	Low activity
Fcγ−	Fcγ+
Fcμ+ (E+)	Fcμ- (E+ and E−)
E−	
OKM1−	
OKT3−, OKT8−	

IV. Cytotoxic specificity
- Cytotoxic towards a broad spectrum of targets. Different recognition site from that found on allospecific target
- Mediated by separate population of cells — not allospecific CTL
- Subpopulations — each recognizing a limited set of target structures

V. Regulation
- Augmentation
  - IFN (?)
  - IL-2 (?)
- Suppression
  - HNK-1+ cells

or that this cytotoxicity is an epiphenomenon and simply mirrors some other important event. Suppressor cell functions or hematopoietic regulation would be candidate functions for both types of cells. At present, there is no absolutely convincing evidence to disprove the contention that in vitro-induced NK and standard NK are unrelated activities. However, there are a number of lines of evidence that are more easily interpreted if one assumes that these two types of cytotoxicity are related.

The most convincing similarities between NK cells and MLC-induced NK-like cells are (1) the similarities in target spectrum including the lack of activity of both cell types against alloantigens; (2) the similar influences of IFN and IL-2 on both cell types; and (3) the finding that both are susceptible to suppression by one suppressor cell type. In fact, the only obvious distinction between NK cells and NK-like cells is in surface marker phenotype. Even in this feature there are some interesting overlapping markers such as T cell markers and the Fcμ receptor. Therefore, it is likely that NK-like cells are the same cell type as NK cells but are at a different stage of development or activation.

The various cell types that have been identified as NK-like can be arranged in a tentative sequence for the development of NK cells, as shown in Figure 1. The precursor would be a T cell which when activated by alloantigen and possibly by IL-2 would then express the Fcμ receptor followed by acquisition of cytotoxic function. Further differentiation would yield a typical Fcγ+ NK cell. Finally, this cell would mature into a post-NK cell with suppressor functions and would limit the entry of new cells into this pathway. In summary, this postulated pathway would be a Fcμ-γ− T cell (noncy-

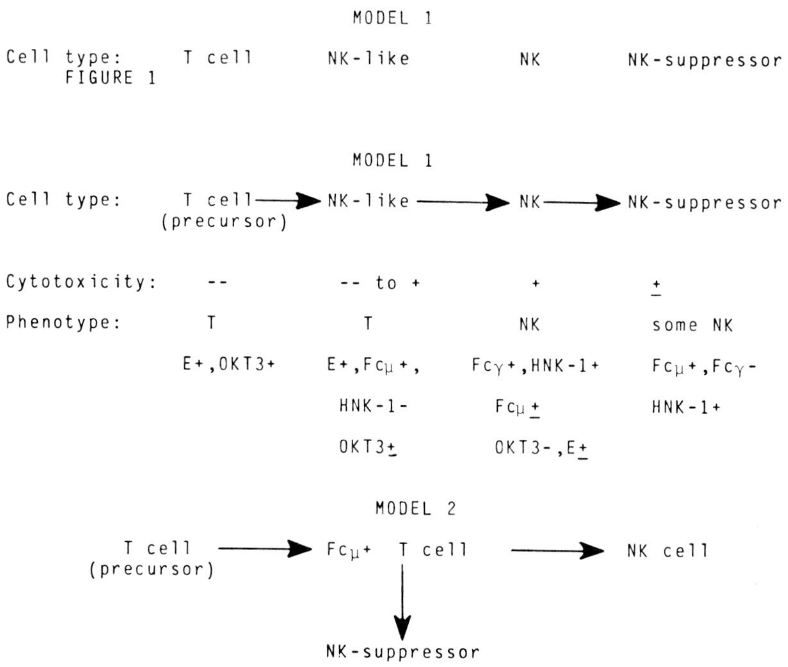

FIGURE 1. Two possible models for the relationship of MLC-induced NK-like cytotoxicity to the standard NK activity seen in PBL without culture.

totoxic) to a noncytotoxic Fcμ+ cell to a cytotoxic Fcμ+ cell to cytotoxic Fcγ+ NK cell to the Fcγ− NK suppressor cell.

The problem with this model is that we have not yet seen mature typical NK cells as a product of in vitro culture of peripheral blood T cells. However, when we start with the relatively mature thymocyte population that bears the Fcμ receptor, we have observed the development of HNK-1+, Fcγ+ effector cells. It is possible that it is difficult to stabilize PBL T cells at the mature NK stage as the agents promoting their further differentiation are still present.

Alternatively, the Fcμ+ cell may reflect a branch point in the developmental sequence. This possibility is shown as Model 2 in Figure 1. With one set of signals, the Fcμ+ cell may become an NK cell. With different signals it might differentiate into an NK suppressor cell. At present, we cannot distinguish between these two models. The clonal expansion at each of these phenotypes may allow for a more comprehensive analysis of their functions.

In summary, MLC-induced NK-like cells bear enough similarities to NK cells that the possibility that they represent a stage in NK maturation should be considered. These cells have also provided an insight into the self-regulating nature of cytotoxic cells.

ACKNOWLEDGMENTS

The work reported here was supported in part by NIH Grant CA 12582, by NIH Fellowship CA 09120, and by the CCCI. The authors thank Ms. Cynthia McGruder for preparation of the manuscript.

REFERENCES

1. Pross, H. F. and Baines, M. G., Spontaneous human lymphocyte-mediated cytotoxicity against tumor target cells. I. The effect of malignant disease, *Int. J. Cancer,* 18, 593, 1976.
2. Takasugi, M., Ramseyer, A., and Takasugi, J., Decline of natural nonselective cell-mediated cytotoxicity in patients with tumor progression, *Cancer Res.,* 37, 413, 1977.
3. Kadish, A. S., Doyle, A. T., Steinhauser, E. H., and Ghossein, N. A., Natural cytotoxicity and interferon production in human cancer: deficient natural killer activity and normal interferon production in patients with advanced disease, *J. Immunol.,* 127, 1817, 1981.
4. Hershey, T., Hobbs, A., Edwards, A., McCarthy, W. H., and McGovern, V. J., Relationship between natural killer cell activity and histological features of lymphocyte infiltration and partial regression of the primary tumor in melanoma patients, *Cancer Res.,* 42, 363, 1982.
5. Hanna, N. and Fidler, I. J., Role of natural killer cells in the destruction of circulating tumors emboli, *J. Natl. Cancer Inst.,* 65, 801, 1980.
6. Zielske, J. V. and Golub, S. H., Fetal calf serum-induced blastogenic and cytotoxic responses of human lymphocytes, *Cancer Res.,* 36, 3842, 1976.
7. Ortaldo, J. R., Bonnard, G. D., and Herberman, R. B., Cytotoxic reactivity of human lymphocytes cultured in vitro, *J. Immunol.,* 119, 1351, 1977.
8. Koide, Y. and Takasugi, M., Augmentation of human natural cell-mediated cytotoxicity by a soluble factor. I. Production of N-cell-activating factor (NAF), *J. Immunol.,* 121, 872, 1978.
9. Lazda, V. A. and Baram, P., In vitro stimulation of natural killer (NK) cells by soluble factor(s) generated in antigen-stimulated rhesus monkey peripheral blood lymphocyte cultures, *J. Immunol.,* 122, 2068, 1979.
10. Svedmyr, E. A., Deinhardt, F., and Klein, G., Sensitivity of different target cells to the killing action of peripheral lymphocytes stimulated by autologous lymphoblastoid cell lines, *Int. J. Cancer,* 13, 891, 1974.
11. Jondal, M. and Targan, S., In vitro induction of cytotoxic effector cells with spontaneous killer cell specificity, *J. Exp. Med.,* 147, 1621, 1978.
12. Grimm, E., Mazumder, A., Zhang, H., and Rosenberg, S., Lymphokine-activated killer cell phenomenon. Lysis of natural killer-resistant fresh solid tumor cells by interleukin 2-activated autologous human peripheral blood lymphocytes, *J. Exp. Med.,* 155, 1823, 1982.
13. Kaplan, J., Callewaert, D., and Peterson, W. D., Expression of human T lymphocyte antigens by killer cells, *J. Immunol.,* 121, 1366, 1978.
14. Fast, L., Hansen, J., and Newman, W., Evidence for T cell nature and heterogeneity within natural killer (NK) and antibody-dependent cellular cytotoxicity (ADCC) effectors: a comparison with cytolytic T lymphocytes (CTL), *J. Immunol.,* 127, 448, 1981.
15. Masucci, G., Masucci, M. G., and Klein, E., Human blood lymphocyte subsets separated on the basis of nylon adherence, SRBC and EA rosetting: natural cytotoxicity and characterization with monoclonal reagents, *Cell. Immunol.,* 69, 166, 1982.
16. Haller, O., Kiessling, R., Ozu, A., and Wigzell, H., Generation of natural killer cells: an autonomous function of the bone marrow, *J. Exp. Med.,* 145, 1411, 1977.
17. Kiessling, R., Klein, E., and Wigzell, H., Natural killer cells in the mouse. I. Cytotoxic cells with specificity for mouse moloney leukemia cells. Specificity and distribution according to genotype, *Eur. J. Immunol.,* 5, 221, 1975.
18. Minato, N., Reid, L., and Bloom, B., On the heterogeneity of murine natural killer cells, *J. Exp. Med.,* 154, 750, 1981.
19. Burton, R. G., Alloantisera selectively reactive with NK cells: characterization and use in defining NK cell classes, in *Natural Cell Mediated Immunity against Tumors,* Herberman, R. B., Ed., Academic Press, New York, 1980, 19.
20. Seeley, J. K. and Golub, S. H., Studies on cytotoxicity generated in human mixed lymphocyte cultures. I. Time course and target spectrum of several distinct concomitant cytotoxic activities, *J. Immunol.,* 120, 1415, 1978.
21. D'Amore, P. J. and Golub, S. H., Detection of double target binders at the single cell level: an evaluation of the specificity of NK and MLC-induced NK-like cells, *Cell. Immunol.,* 71, 66, 1982.
22. Callewaert, D. M., Lightbody, J. J., Kaplan, J., Jaroszewski, J., Peterson, W. D., and Rosenberg, J. C., Cytotoxicity of human peripheral lymphocytes in cell-mediated lympholysis; antibody-dependent cell-mediated lympholysis and natural cytotoxicity assays after mixed lymphocyte cultures, *J. Immunol.,* 121, 81, 1978.
23. Golub, S. H., D'Amore, P. J., and Rainey, M., Systemic administration of human leukocyte interferon to melanoma patients. II. Cellular events associated with changes in NK cytotoxicity, *J. Natl. Cancer Inst.,* 68, 711, 1982.
24. Bolhuis, R., Development of NK activity during in vitro culture, in *Natural Cell Mediated Immunity against Tumors,* Herberman, R. B., Ed., Academic Press, New York, 1980, 449.

25. Seeley, J. K. and Kärre, K., MLC-induced cytotoxicity against NK-sensitive targets, in *Natural Cell Mediated Immunity against Tumors*, Herberman, R. B., Ed., Academic Press, New York, 1980, 477.
26. Kärre, K. and Seeley, J. K., Cytotoxic THY 1.2-positive blasts with NK-like target selectivity in murine mixed lymphocyte cultures, *J. Immunol.*, 123, 1511, 1979.
27. Seeley, J. K., Masucci, G., Poros, A., Klein, E., and Golub, S. H., Studies on cytotoxicity generated in human mixed lymphocyte cultures. II. Anti-K562 effectors are distinct from the allospecific CTL and can be generated from NK-depleted T-cells, *J. Immunol.*, 123, 1303, 1979.
28. Bolhuis, R. and Ronteltap, C., Generation of natural killer (NK) cell activity after mixed lymphocyte culture (MLC): activation of effector cells in NK cell-depleted cell populations, *Immunol. Lett.*, 1, 191, 1980.
29. Masucci, G., Poros, A., Selley, J. K., and Klein, E., In vitro generation of K562 killers in human T-lymphocyte subsets, *Cell. Immunol.*, 52, 247, 1980.
30. Santoli, D., Francis, M. K., and Trucco, M., Phenotypic and functional characterization of allospecific and non-specific (NK- and K-like) cytotoxic T lymphocytes generated in human mixed-lymphocyte cultures from noncytotoxic precursors, *Cell. Immunol.*, 65, 230, 1981.
31. Strassman, G., Bach, F. H., and Zarling, J. M., Depletion of human NK cells with monoclonal antibodies allows the generation of cytotoxic T lymphocytes without NK-like cells in mixed cultures, *J. Immunol.*, 130, 1556, 1983.
31a. D'Amore, D. J., Shau, H., and Golub, S. H., unpublished data.
32. Golub, S. H., Golightly, M. G., and Zielske, J. V., NK-like cytotoxicity of human lymphocytes cultured in media containing fetal bovine serum, *Int. J. Cancer*, 24, 273, 1979.
33. Ortaldo, J. R., Bonnard, G. D., and Herberman, R. B., Cytotoxic reactivity of human lymphocytes cultured in vitro, *J. Immunol.*, 119, 1351, 1977.
34. Golightly, M. G., D'Amore, P. J., and Golub, S. H., Studies on cytotoxicity generated in human mixed lymphocyte cultures. III. Natural killer-like cytotoxicity mediated by human lymphocytes with receptors for IgM, *Cell. Immunol.*, 70, 219, 1982.
35. Abo, T. and Balch, C. M., Characterization of HNK-1+ (Leu-7) human lymphocytes. II. Distinguishing phenotypic and functional properties of natural killer cells from activated NK-like cells, *J. Immunol.*, 129, 1758, 1982.
36. Torten, M., Sidell, N., and Golub, S. H., Interleukin-2 and stimulator lymphoblastoid cells will induce human thymocytes to bind and kill K562 targets, *J. Exp. Med.*, 156, 1545, 1982.
37. Bolhuis, R. and Schellekens, H., Induction of natural killer cell activity and allocytotoxicity in human peripheral blood lymphocytes after mixed lymphocyte culture, *Scand. J. Immunol.*, 13, 401, 1981.
38. Jondal, M. and Merrill, J. E., Distribution of IgG and IgM receptors on human peripheral natural killer cells measured on the level of the single effector cell, *Eur. J. Immunol.*, 11, 531, 1981.
39. Merrill, J. E., Ullberg, M., and Jondal, M., Influence of IgG and IgM receptor triggering on human natural killer cell cytotoxicity measured on the level of the single effector cell, *Eur. J. Immunol.*, 11, 536, 1981.
40. Poros, A. and Klein, E., Cultivation with K562 leads to blastogenesis and increased cytotoxicity with changed properties of the active cells when compared to fresh lymphocytes, *Cell. Immunol.*, 41, 240, 1978.
41. Poros, A. and Klein, E., Distinction of anti-K562 and anti-allocytotoxicity in in vitro stimulated populations of human lymphocytes, *Cell Immunol.*, 46, 57, 1979.
42. Ausiello, C., Hokland, P., and Heron, I., Interferon-induced augmentation of cytotoxic killer cell generation in mixed lymphocyte cultures: analysis of the effector cell product, *Scand. J. Immunol.*, 13, 263, 1981.
43. Zarling, J. M. and Kung, P. C., Monoclonal antibodies which distinguish between human NK cells and cytotoxic T lymphocytes, *Nature*, 288, 394, 1980.
44. Zarling, J. M. and Bach, F. H., Stimulation of lymphocytes with allogeneic normal cells and autologous lymphoblastoid cell lines: distinction between NK-like cells and cytotoxic T lymphocytes by monoclonal antibodies, in *NK Cells and Other Natural Effector Cells*, Herberman, R. B., Ed., Academic Press, New York, 1982, 791.
45. Zarling, J. M., Bach, F. H., and Kung, P. C., Sensitization of lymphocytes against pooled allogeneic cells. II. Characterization of effector cells cytotoxic for autologous lymphoblastoid cell lines, *J. Immunol.*, 126, 375, 1981.
46. Takasugi, M., Mickey, M. R., and Terasaki, P. I., Reactivity of lymphocytes from normal persons on cultured tumor cells, *Cancer Res.*, 33, 2898, 1973.
47. Bolhuis, R. L. and Schellekens, H., Natural killer and mixed lymphocyte culture-activated AK cell-mediated lysis: induction of susceptibility to NK (like) lysis of target cells by phytohemagglutinin. *Hum. Lymphocyte Different.*, 1, 251, 1981.
48. Klein, E., Natural and activated cytotoxic T lymphocytes, *Immunol. Today*, 1(6), 4, 1980.

49. D'Amore, P. J., Golightly, M. G., and Golub, S. H., Heterogeneity of MLC-generated NK-like cells, in *NK Cells and Other Natural Effector Cells,* Herberman, R. B. Ed., Academic Press, New York, 1982, 785.
50. Zarling, J. M., Dierckins, M. S., Sevenich, E. A., and Clouse, K. A., Stimulation with autologous lymphoblastoid cell lines: lysis of Epstein-Barr virus-positive and -negative cell lines by two phenotypically distinguishable effector cell populations, *J. Immunol.,* 127, 2118, 1981.
51. Pawelec, G. P., Hadam, M. R., Schneider, E. M., and Wernet, P., Clonally restricted natural killer-like cytotoxicity displayed by cloned human T cell lines, *J. Immunol.,* 129, 2271, 1981.
52. Trinchieri, G., Santoli, D., Granato, D., and Perussia, B., Antagonistic effects of interferons on the cytotoxicity mediated by natural killer cells, *Fed. Proc., Fed. Am. Soc. Exp. Biol.,* 40, 2705, 1981.
53. Perussia, B., Manguni, L., Engers, H., and Trinchieri, G., Functional studies of Fc receptor-bearing human lymphocytes: effect of treatment with proteolytic enzymes, *J. Immunol.,* 123, 681, 1979.
54. Zarling, J. M., Eskra, L., Borden, E., Horoszewicz, J., and Carter, J. M., Activation of human natural killer cells cytotoxic for human leukemia cells by purified interferon, *J. Immunol.,* 123, 63, 1979.
55. Targan, S. and Dorey, F., Interferon activation of "Pre-Spontaneous Killer" (PRE-SK) cells and alteration in kinetics of lysis of both "PRE-SK" and active SK cells, *J. Immunol.,* 124, 2157, 1980.
56. Landegren, V., Ramstedt, R., Axberg, I., Orn, A., and Wigzell, H., Cyclosporin A permits the distinction between specific T and NK activity generated in a human MLC, *Int. J. Cancer,* 28, 725, 1981.
57. Ausiello, C., Hokland, P., and Heron, I., Interferon-induced augmentation of cytotoxic killer cell generation in mixed lymphocyte cultures: analysis of the effector cell product, *Scand. J. Immunol.,* 13, 263, 1981.
58. Argov, S. and Klein, E., Generation of lytic potential in mixed cultures and its modification by IFN-α, in *NK Cells and Other Natural Effector Cells,* Herberman, R. B. Ed., Academic Press, New York, 1982, 799.
59. Whisler, R., Bakenhaster, K., and Opremcak, E., Autologous mechanisms generating natural killer activity within human peripheral lymphocytes depleted of NK target-binding cells, *Cell. Immunol.,* 66, 342, 1982.
60. D'Amore, P. J. and Golub, S. H., Suppression of human NK cytotoxicity by an MLC-generated cell population, *J. Immunol.,* 134, 272, 1985.
61. D'Amore, P. J. and Golub, S. H., Suppression of NK cytotoxicity by HNK-1+ lymphocytes, in *Natural Killer Activity and Its Regulation,* Hoshino, T., Koren, H. S., and Uchida, A., Eds., Excerpta Medica, Tokyo, 1984, 258.

Chapter 13

LGL LYMPHOPROLIFERATIVE DISEASES IN MAN AND EXPERIMENTAL ANIMALS: THE CHARACTERISTICS OF THESE CELLS AND THEIR POTENTIAL EXPERIMENTAL USES

Craig W. Reynolds and Jerrold M. Ward

TABLE OF CONTENTS

I. INTRODUCTION

Although the existence of natural killer (NK) activity has been known for about 10 years, it was not until very recently that the characteristics of the effector cells were clearly defined. The cell responsible for most, if not all, NK and antibody-dependent cell-mediated cytotoxicity (ADCC) in the human, [1-3] rat, [3,4] and mouse[5,6] has recently been shown to be the large granular lymphocyte (LGL). The ability to isolate LGL on discontinuous Percoll density gradients, first reported by Timonen et al.,[7] has provided an extremely useful and productive tool for examining the morphological characteristics and functions of these cells. A summary of the general features of LGL from the mouse, rat, and human can be found in Table 1. Additional details regarding the features of LGL can be found elsewhere in this volume. In general, LGL are a distinct population of lymphocytes with an eccentric kidney-shaped nucleus and prominent azurophilic granules in the cytoplasm. Although the lineage of these cells is still not clear, rat and mouse LGL arise from bone marrow precursors and their differentiation does not require the presence of the thymus.[8,9] These results, along with the absence of cytoplasmic peroxidase, surface immunoglobulins, and the inability to phagocytose or adhere to plastic and glass clearly separates these cells from mature T cells, B cells, macrophages, and granulocytes.

In addition to helping establish the morphological characteristics of NK cells, the isolation of LGL has also led to a further definition regarding the function of these cells. It had been suggested that NK cells may play an important role in the first line of defense against some viral,[10-12] mycoplasma,[13] and parasitic infections,[14-16] as well as being a major means of immunosurveillance against the development of primary tumors and their metastases.[17-20] The isolation or culture of highly enriched effector cells for in vitro studies and in vivo transfer experiments has provided direct support for many of these theories.[21,22] In addition, recent experiments have suggested that LGL may play a critical role in controlling the proliferation and homeostasis of normal bone marrow populations.[21,23] Furthermore, experiments using highly purified populations of LGL have indicated that these cells can produce a variety of cytokines, thereby providing a basis for interacting with other leukocytes in the immune response.[24-26]

Although the isolation of highly purified LGL has been very useful in analyzing the morphological characteristics and function of NK cells, there is a practical limitation to the number of LGL which one can isolate from peripheral blood or spleen. This limitation has meant that many of the crucial detailed experiments requiring large numbers of cytotoxic effector cells have gone undone. Recently, two methods have become available for obtaining larger numbers of cytotoxic cells: (1) in vitro culture of LGL in IL-2-containing media and (2) spontaneously occurring LGL tumors. In both cases, large numbers of cytotoxic cells can be obtained for use in those experiments which require abundant starting material. These experiments include the isolation of LGL-produced lymphokines, cytoplasmic granules, cell membrane receptors, and enzymatic pathways required for regulation.

The present manuscript reviews the morphological, histochemical, antigenic, and functional nature of spontaneous human and rat LGL tumors. In addition, we will discuss some of the recent experiments which have suggested that these tumor cells may be extremely useful in addressing a number of questions regarding the recognition and mechanism of NK cell cytotoxicity.

Table 1
COMPARISON OF THE CHARACTERISTICS OF MOUSE, RAT, AND HUMAN LGL

Characteristic	Mouse	Rat	Human
Size	Medium (8—10 μm)	Large (10—14 μm)	Large (12—15 μm)
Adherence	–	–	–
Phagocytosis	–	–	–
E rosette			
4°C	NA	NA	50%
29° or 37°C	NA	NA	–
$Fc_\gamma R$	+	+	+
$Fc_\mu R$	–	–	–
sIg	–	–	–
Ia	–	20%	20%
Asialo GM_1	+	+	+
Other cell membrane Ags	Low Thy 1 (50%) Ly 5; M1/70	W3/13, OX-8 RT-7	OKT10; some OKT8 (25%) OKT11 (50%); OKM1 (75%)
ANAE	NT	Weak +	Weak +
ANBE	NT	–	–
Nonspecific esterase	–	–	–
AP	NT	+	+
Peroxidase	–	–	–
β-Glucuronidase	NT	+	+
TdT	NT	–	–

Note: NA = not applicable; NT = not tested.

II. HUMAN T_γ-LYMPHOPROLIFERATIVE DISEASE (T_γ-LPD)

Since the discovery that human NK and ADCC activities are highly associated with LGL, there have been a number of reports of human LPD with LGL-like characteristics. Although some difficulties occur in the interpretation and classification of these cases,[27] it is clear that many of these LPD are LGL in origin. The diseases in which the abnormal cells most closely resemble LGL are the chronic T_γ-LPD. This classification includes both a lymphocytosis of nonmalignant cells as well as those malignant cases comprising the chronic T_γ-lymphocytic leukemias (T_γ-CLL). In addition to these T_γ-LPD cases, there have recently been described a few cases of CLL which the authors have designated as LGL in origin. Since it is virtually impossible to distinguish these cases from the previously described T_γ-LPD, this review will designate all of these cases as T_γ-LPD and consider each one as a potential example of human LGL LPD.

Since 1980, over 30 cases of T_γ-LPD have been reported. This relatively small number of cases makes it difficult to draw accurate conclusions regarding the etiology or prognosis of patients with this disorder; however, a number of general cellular or clinical characteristics can be assigned to this disorder. These characteristics occur in >50% of the cases of T_γ-LPD studied, and in general are quite similar to the features of normal human LGL. A summary of these characteristics can be found in Table 2.

Morphologically, the cells from a majority of patients which comprise the human T_γ-LPD are granular lymphocytes,[28,41] which form E rosettes,[28,29,32,34,35,37,39-60] are $Fc_\gamma R$-positive,[28-32,34,35,39-43,45-53,55-60] and $Fc_\mu R$- and complement receptor-negative.[28-33,36,37,39,41,43,44,47,48,50,53,55-60,61] Histochemically these lymphocytes are positive for acid phosphatase (AP),[28,30,31,35,37,39,48-50,52,55,56,60] β-glucuronidase,[28,31,35,37,39,50] and periodic acid Schiff (PAS);[35,41,59] and negative for nonspecific esterase[39,41,50,52,60] and peroxidase

Table 2
COMPARISON OF NORMAL HUMAN LGL TO CHRONIC T_γ-LPD CELLS

Characteristic	LGL	T_γ-LPD
Cell morphology		
Cytoplasmic granules	+	+
Kidney-shaped nucleus	+	+
PTA	+	Some
Cell surface receptors		
E rosette (4°C)	Most	+
$Fc_\gamma R$	+	+
$Fc_\mu R$	−	−
C_3R	−	−
Histochemistry		
AP	+	+
ANAE	Weak	Weak
ANBE	−	−
Nonspecific esterase	−	−
β-Glucuronidase	+	+
Peroxidase	−	−
TdT	−	−
Cell surface antigens		
T_3 (pan T)	−	Most
T_4 (helper/inducer)	−	−
T_6	−	−
T_8 (suppressor/cytotoxic)	Some	Most
T_{10}	+	Some
T_{11}	+	+
M_1	Most	Most
Ia	Some	Some
sIg	−	−
Asialo GM_1	+	−
Other		
Adherent	−	NT
Erythrophagocytic	Ab-coated RBC	Some

Note: + = >50% of cases tested were positive; − = <10% of cases tested were positive; NT = not tested.

(PER).[32,40,60] These cells generally have little or no terminal deoxynucleotidyl transferase (TdT)[31,35,49,50,52,53] or adenosine deaminase activity,[62] but do contain relatively high amounts of 5′-nucleotidase and purine nucleoside phosphorylase.[62] These results demonstrate that the morphological and enzymatic profile of cells from T_γ-LPD are very similar to the pattern previously shown for normal human LGL (Table 2).

Recent studies using monoclonal antibodies (MoAb) have demonstrated that the cells comprising most T_γ-LPD express the T3, T8, and T11 antigens.[30-32,35,36,39-43,45,46,48,49,51,54,55,62] The majority of cells from T_γ-LPD have also been shown to be negative for sIg, T4, T6, and T10.[30-32,35,36,39-43,45,46,48,49,51,54-56,62] The expression of Ia,[30-32,35,36,39-43,45,46,50,56,59,62] M1,[39,40,45,46-48,51,55,62] and the HNK-1[39-41,48] markers are less consistent. In the only case reported, T_γ-CLL cells from one patient lacked detectable asialo-GM_1 expression.[48] With the exception of T3, these results demonstrate a pattern of cell surface antigens on the cells from the majority of patients with T_γ-LPD which are very similar to normal LGL.[63-65] Recently, increases in T3 and decreased T10 expression have also been seen with in vitro cultures of normal human LGL,[66] and suggest that the expression of these two antigens in LGL or LGL tumor cells may reflect changes in these cells upon enhanced cell proliferation.

The general phenotype of cells from patients with T_γ-LPD is similar to that of the T_γ-suppressor/cytotoxic cells. These data suggest that from a morphologic and histochemical perspective, chronic T_γ-LPD disorders represent a fairly uniform pattern of diseases. Since these characteristics are also very similar to the previous results using normal human LGL, we conclude that both normal LGL and cells from patients with T_γ-LPD represent a morphologically and histochemically homogeneous population of cells with some degree of heterogeneity in the expression of various cell surface antigens.

Clinically, T_γ-LPD cases are generally characterized as having elevated white blood count and absolute lymphocyte counts with variable levels of lymphocytic infiltration in the bone marrow (Table 3). Of the 29 cases in the literature, the median age at the time of T_γ-LPD diagnosis was 58 in males (range 41 to 83) and 61 in females (range 19 to 70). Interestingly, there have been 21 cases reported in males and only 8 cases in females. The reason for this sex difference is not clear but this is analogous to the previous observation that spontaneous LGL leukemias in rats occur slightly more frequently in males (see Section III, below). Additional clinical characteristics which occur in >50% of the cases of T_γ-LPD include recurrent skin lesions.[29,30,34-36,46,62] anemia,[28,35,41,42,46-49,53,59,67-70] neutropenia,[28-31,34,36,41-43,45,54,59] splenomegaly,[28-30,34,35,41,43,45,48,49,55,59,62,67] and hepatomegaly[28,34,39,45,46,48,49,59,67] with little or no lymphadenopathy.

Although anemia occurs in >50% of the patients with T_γ-LPD, the mechanism(s) by which this anemia occurs is not very clear. Red cell phagocytosis, although not a common finding, has been shown to occur with both normal T_γ-cells using antibody-coated erythrocytes,[71] and with some tumor cells from a small number of patients with T_γ-LPD.[59,67] In contrast, Coombs' tests for the detection of autoantibody to red cells have generally proven negative, suggesting that the anemia is not antibody-mediated.[41] One interesting mechanism for the development of anemia during T_γ-LPD may be the active suppression of erythrocyte generation. Although the bone marrow usually is infiltrated by large numbers of lymphocytes during T_γ-LPD, this bone marrow involvement is probably not sufficient to explain the development of severe anemia.[47,53,67,69,70,72] Several investigators have now suggested that the T_γ-lymphocytes can play a dramatic role in the suppression of both erythroid colony-forming units (CFU_E) and erythroid burst-forming units, (BFU_E), in vitro.[35,47,68,73] The production of large numbers of T_γ-cells in vivo could lead to an appreciable decrease in the total number of red cells produced. Furthermore, this type of red cell inhibition may not be restricted only to patients with T_γ-LPD. Recent studies also suggest that some patients with aplastic anemia also have T cells in the blood or bone marrow which suppress stem cell proliferation.[74-76]

Another characteristic which is present in the majority of patients with T_γ-LPD is the development of severe neutropenia. As with the development of anemia, the mechanism(s) behind this neutropenia is not clear but could reflect either the decreased production of granulocytes or an increase in the rate of their removal. Recent results suggest that LGL, or T_γ-cells in general, can inhibit the development of macrophage-granulocyte colony forming units (CFU_C) in vitro (see Chapter 4). Some patients with T_γ-LPD have normal levels of bone marrow CFU_C,[43,53] others have depressed numbers of CFU_C;[47] however, removal of T_γ-lymphocytes or tumor cells from the bone marrow does not affect the number of CFU_C observed, suggesting that in most cases, the depression in CFU_C is not due to an active suppression by tumor cells infiltrating the bone marrow. The production of antineutrophil antibodies also seems to be quite rare in cases of T_γ-LPD.[30,34,36,43,54] Therefore, at present, the role of these various mechanism(s) in the development of neutropenia in patients with T_γ-LPD remains a mystery.

Although the cellular characteristics and clinical symptoms suggest that many of the cases of T_γ-LPD could represent a proliferation of LGL, it is virtually impossible to

Table 3
FUNCTION AND CLINICAL FEATURES OF CHRONIC HUMAN T_γ-LPD AND RAT NK-TUMORS

Clinical feature/function	Human chronic T_γ-LPD	Rat NK tumors
Function		
NK activity	High[a]	High
ADCC	High	High
Suppressor activity	Some	NT
Mitogen proliferation	−	−
Clinical features		
Splenomegaly	+	+
Hepatomegaly	+	+
Anemia	+	+
Neutropenia	+	+
Skin lesions	+	−
Lymphadenopathy	−	+
Sex predominance	Male	Male
Malignant course	Chronic	Acute

Note: NT = not tested; + = >50% of the cases studied are positive; − = <10% of the cases studied are positive.

[a] Some cases have NK or ADCC, some have both.

distinguish on a morphological basis between a thymic-dependent T_γ-cell and the thymic-independent LGL. Although some functions of these two types of normal cells appear to be quite different,[109-77] the results from functional studies with cells from patients with T_γ-LPD suggest that the functional separation of T_γ-LDP of T_γ-cell vs. LGL origin may be very difficult. The lymphocytes from some patients have demonstrated either suppressor activity alone,[42,46,54] ADCC,[29,30,46,49,62] or NK activity[48] alone. However, many patients have cells with both suppressor activity and ADCC,[31,40,45,50,51,53] or both NK and ADCC.[34,39-41,46,55,58,59,62] It is likely that these results may reflect: (1) the accumulation of more than one functionally active cell population during the T_γ-LPD, (2) the possibility that LGL or suppressor T cells may express expanded functions during times of abnormal proliferation, or (3) merely the function of contaminating normal non-T_γ-lymphocytosis cells in the assay. At present, it is not clear which of these explanations may account for the variation in functions seen with T_γ-LPD cells; however, it is clear that cells from many of these patients can express suppressor and/or cytotoxic effector functions. The further analysis of a larger number of T_γ-tumors for other characteristics could allow for the separation of functionally and morphologically different T_γ-cell leukemias from LGL leukemias.

It should be emphasized, however, that not all chronic T cell LPD share a large number of characteristics with LGL.[78,79] Because the number of reported cases is still very small, it would be premature to speculate on the percentage of cases of chronic T LPD which may be LGL in origin; however, the results reviewed in this paper do suggest that at least some of the previously diagnosed chronic T cell LPD may have come from cells in the LGL lineage. This distinction between T cell and LGL tumors, first made by Pandolfi et al.,[32] may be an important distinction to make since the response of LGL and T cell tumors to standard therapies might be quite different. At present, however, additional information regarding the ontogeny, morphology, and function of LGL and T_γ-cells will be needed to clearly separate malignant cells of these lineages.

Table 4
COMPARISON OF MORPHOLOGICAL CHARACTERISTICS OF NORMAL RAT LGL AND LGL (RNK) TUMORS

Characteristics	LGL	RNK tumors
Cell morphology		
Cytoplasmic granules	+	+
Kidney-shaped nucleus	+	+
Large size (area)	75 μm^2	80 μm^2
Histochemistry		
AP	+	+
Alkaline phosphatase	NT	−
Nonspecific esterase	−	−
Chloroacetate esterase	NT	−
β-Glucuronidase	+	+
Peroxidase	−	−
Lysozyme	−	−
γ-Glutamyl transpeptidase	NT	−
Cell surface antigens		
Leukocyte common (L-C)	100%	6/10[a]
W3/13 (Pan T)	85%	7/7
W3/25 (helper/inducer T)	−	0/10
OX-8 (suppressor/cytotoxic T)	75%	8/10
Thy 1.1	−	8/10
Ia	20%	4/9
sIg	−	0/10
Asialo GM_1	80%	7/7
BC-84 (RT-7)	60%	6/10

Note: NT = not tested.

[a] Number positive/number tested.

III. SPONTANEOUS RAT LGL LEUKEMIAS

Probably the best studied example of an LGL LPD is the spontaneous leukemias in aged Fischer (F344) rats. This mononuclear cell leumemia was first described in 1969[80] and later shown to have the morphology, histochemistry, cell surface antigens, and functional activity of rat LGL.[81-85] A comparison between normal rat LGL and cells from these spontaneous mononuclear cell leukemias can be found in Table 4. Since the spontaneous leukemias in F344 rats share many characteristics with rat NK cells, we have termed these leukemias rat NK (RNK) tumors and feel confident that they represent the neoplastic transformation of cells within the LGL lineage. The mechanism behind the selective development of LGL leukemias in these ras is not yet clear, but may reflect the susceptibility of LGL or LGL precursors to transformation by an oncogenic retrovirus.[86]

These RNK tumors are rarely detected before 18 months of age, with an average appearance time at 22 months of age, with the duration of disease rarely lasting more than 6 weeks.[80] The reported incidence of this leukemia is 10 to 25% in conventional animals[80,87,88] but is higher in germ-free animals (26 to 36%).[89] The organs involved in this disease include the spleen, liver, blood, lymph nodes, and bone marrow.[81,85,87] Many of the clinical and laboratory signs are very similar to the previously described characteristics for human T_γ-LPD (Table 3). These include splenomegaly, hepatomegaly, icterus; elevated bilirubin, aminotransferase and serum alkaline phosphatase levels; reduced serum albumin levels, and anemia.[80,81,90] As in human T_γ-LPD, this anemia seems to be due to a combination of factors including erythrophagocytosis by the RNK tumor cells[81,90] and an infiltration of the bone marrow by leukemia cells.[81,87] As in human T_γ-LPD, Coombs' tests have generally been negative,[80] suggesting that the production of antibodies against red cells does not contribute to the development of this anemia. The major causes of death in these animals seem to be pulmonary infections, lung congestion, and liver failure.[87]

Early reports described this LPD as a mononuclear cell leukemia, with prominent azurophilic granules in the cytoplasm, and with a nucleus frequently having the appearance of a large lymphocyte.[80,87,91] These early studies suggested that the granules were acid phosphastase-positive, with the cytoplasm negative for peroxidase and nonspecific esterase. Our recent results confirm these reports and also show that the RNK leukemias are β-glucuronidase-positive and lysozyme-negative.[81] In addition, we have extensively studied the cell surface antigens and cytotoxic function of these tumor cells.[82] These results, summarized in Table 4, demonstrate that both normal LGL and the RNK leukemias are morphologically identifiable as large lymphocytes with azurophilic granules in the cytoplasm. Both populations are found to express the receptor for the Fc portion of IgG ($Fc_\gamma R$), the NK-associated asialo GM_1 antigen, and the majority of LGL and LGL tumor cells express the T cell-associated antigens recognized by the BC-84, W3/13, and OX-8 MoAb. In contrast, neither the LGL nor the RNK tumor cells express the W3/25 phenotype found on the helper/inducer subset of T lymphocytes. In addition, both normal rat LGL and the RNK leukemias have been shown to be weakly Ia-positive and sIg-negative. These results suggest that, as in the human, both LGL and the LGL leukemias most closely resemble the phenotype of the subpopulation of T cells that include cytotoxic/suppressor cells, expressing both the Fc_γ-R and the OX-8 antigens.[92,93]

An interesting difference between the rat LGL leukemias and normal LGL is the detection of the Thy 1.1 antigen on most LGL tumors.[82] The expression of this antigen, previously shown to be a marker on early lymphocyte precursors in the bone marrow,[94] probably reflects the relatively immature state of the transformed LGL. In addition, this antigenic difference separates RNK tumor cells from normal LGL and suggests that those cells in the spleens of tumor-bearing animals are not merely the accumulation of normal LGL. Further evidence for the malignant nature of the RNK cells has come from studies in F_1 recipients. These studies clearly demonstrate that the accumulation of large numbers of LGL in the spleen are the result of tumor cell proliferation, since these cells do not share the hosts' F_1 alloantigens.[82]

Ultrastructurally, RNK leukemia cells have irregular or kidney-shaped nuclei, with cytoplasmic granules which appear as lysosomes in association with Golgi vesicles. A few leukemia cells have been shown to contain crystals within the granules although, as with normal rat LGL, no virus or parallel tubular arrays (PTA) could be found.[81] With the exception of an absence of PTAs, these results are quite similar to the ultrastructural characteristics found on normal human LGL and on cells from patients with T_γ-LPD.[39,71,95,96]

As in human T_γ-LPD, some, but not all, of the spontaneous LGL leukemias of F344 rats have been found to have high NK and/or ADCC activity.[81,82] Both 4- and 18-hr assays have been used when testing these RNK lines for NK activity since some tumor cells kill at a much slower rate than previously shown for normal LGL.[8] In these assays a rather wide range of activity has been seen when tumor cells were tested for cytotoxicity against NK-susceptible target cells. The analysis of primary tumors indicated that tumors could be categorized into those with high, intermediate, and low or undetectable NK activity. Following transplantation, however, the functional activity of some tumors has been found to change.[82] Some tumor lines have increased activity, some

Table 5
CHARACTERISTICS OF CYTOPLASMIC GRANULES ISOLATED FROM RAT LGL TUMORS[98,99]

Purified granule preparations contain the lysosomal enzymes α-L-fucose, AP, α-hexaminadase, and β-glucuronidase

The cytolytic activity from purified granule preparations are
- Dependent on Ca^{+2} or Sr^{+2} for activity
- Active against a wide variety of both normal and neoplastic target cells
- Effective at equivalent E/T ratios of 0.2—0.2:1 (0.1—1 μg/mℓ protein)
- Temperature-dependent
- Augmented by exogenous proteins (FCS, BSA, etc.)
- Inhibited by phosphorylated sugars and amino acids, or rabbit antisera against the granules
- Not affected by protease inhibitors or nonphosphorylated sugars

Similar granule preparations from rat liver cells, mast cells, peripheral blood T cells are *not* cytolytically active; preparations from normal rat or human peripheral blood LGL *are* active

decreased, and the cytotoxicity of some lines does not change. Although there has frequently been a change in the levels of cytotoxicity following transplantation, little or no shift in the cytotoxic specificity in the RNK-tumor lines has been detected. The results demonstrate that most of the RNK lines efficiently kill the NK-sensitive targets YAC-1 and G_1-TC, but have little or no cytotoxic activity against the NK-resistant targets (C58NT)D and P815. In addition, some lines demonstrate appreciable levels of ADCC activity when tested against antibody-coated P815. These results demonstrate a pattern of specificity which is very similar to that seen with normal rat LGL.[4,97] The fact that some lines have NK but no ADCC activity may suggest that separate populations of LGL can mediate these two functions. However, it is clear that a number of RNK-tumor lines have both activities, suggesting that either more than one effector cell is present in these tumor cell lines or that a single LGL is capable of killing both NK-sensitive and antibody-coated targets. Interestingly, as yet, no rat tumors have been found which have ADCC activity in the absence of NK.

These results demonstrate a remarkable similarity between the spontaneous LGL tumors which appear in aged F344 rats and the majority of T_γ-LPD cases. These morphological, functional, and clinical similarities suggest that the RNK tumor lines may serve as an excellent experimental model for further examining the ontogeny, function, and response to treatment of LGL tumors.

IV. POTENTIAL EXPERIMENTAL USES OF LGL LEUKEMIA CELLS

Although the isolation of highly purified normal LGL has been very useful in analyzing the morphological and functional characteristics of NK cells, the limitation in the number of LGL which can easily be obtained has limited the scope of projects which can be carried out with these cells. However, the use of functionally active LGL leukemia cells can be extremely useful in overcoming this difficulty in obtaining enough highly enriched effector cells for analysis. In particular, the LGL leukemias are an excellent source of cells for those projects which involve the isolation and characterization of subcellular or secretory products which may be present in very small amounts in each cell. One example of this type of application is the recent studies by Henkart et al.[98] and Millard et al.[99] who have demonstrated that the LGL leukemias from the rat can be a very useful source of cells for the isolation, purification, and characterization of LGL cytoplasmic granules. A summary of the characteristics and functional activity of these granules is presented in Table 5. It should be emphasized that the amount of granule material required to do these detailed studies clearly could not have been obtained from normal LGL. These granule preparations have been found to contain a number of lysosomal enzymes (α-L-fucose, acid phosphatase, α-hexaminadase, and β-glucuronidase) but no detectable amounts of those enzymes that are normally associated with plasma membranes (5′-nucleotidase), mitochondria (succinic dehydrogenase), or soluble cytoplasm (lactate dehydrogenase). Under the electron microscope these granule preparations are relatively pure but do contain a variety of granules with different shapes, sizes, and staining densities. In the presence of calcium, purified granules are highly cytotoxic to a wide variety of cells. Red cells are completely lysed at 0.1 to 1 μg/mℓ of granule protein, corresponding to an equivalent effector to target cell ratio of 0.02 to 0.2:1 based on the yield of granules per LGL tumor cell. Most nucleated targets are also lysed but require concentration of granules 100-fold greater than red cells. In contrast, no cytolytic activity is found associated with other cellular fractions of LGL tumor homogenates. Purified rat liver lysosomes or cytoplasmic granule preparations from several other lymphoid cell populations contain 100 to 10,000 less cytolytic activity on a per protein basis. These results further support the hypothesis that some component(s) of the LGL cytoplasmic granules is an integral part of the mechanism of NK and ADCC tumor cell lysis. Further studies along this line should help us understand the molecular nature of NK cell lysis.

The use of LGL leukemias should also be quite useful in examining a number of questions related to the structure and function of intracellular and cell-surface LGL components. For example, the large number of available cells would allow for the analysis of intracellular RNA or protein changes associated with interferon (IFN) activation or prostaglandin inhibition of cytotoxicity. Cell surface studies designed to isolate and characterize a number of surface membrane structures could be carried out with the large amount of material available from LGL tumor cells. The studies might include experiments to analyze the cell surface receptors for IFN, target cell receptor(s), and additional structures required for NK cell activation and granule release.

In addition to the analysis of cellular components, LGL tumor cells could be quite useful in examining the synthesis and excretion of cytokines by LGL.[24-26] Recently, cells from several patients with T_γ-LPD were found to produce significant amounts of immune IFN ($_\gamma$-IFN).[31,48] This spontaneous production of $_\gamma$-IFN serves as an additional similarity to normal LGL[24] and could be further studied in more detail by using tumor cells which produce this molecule. Wright and Bonavida[100] have also recently shown that rat LGL tumor cells produce very high amounts of a soluble NK cytotoxic factor (NKCF) during short-term culture with NK target cells. The requirements for NKCF production are very similar to that for normal LGL; however, the large number of tumor cells which can be stimulated to produce this factor should allow for a more detailed analysis of the cellular mechanisms which are responsible for the production and release of NKCF. Furthermore, the large amounts of factor which can be generated using these LGL tumor lines should provide an excellent source for the purification and physiochemical characterization of the NKCF molecule.

The ability to clone and culture LGL tumor cells might also be quite useful in examining the clonal nature of both target cell specificity and lymphokine production. Since this pattern of cytotoxic specificities also exists for the RNK tumor cell lines,[82] these differences might be examined at a clonal level and further details regarding the mechanism(s) of this specificity addressed. In particular, one could investigate whether the cytotoxic specificities seen with these LGL tumor lines is due to a lack of target cell recognition molecules, or the production of cytotoxic molecules with inherent specificities for selected target cells, as has been proposed for the NKCF molecule.[101]

Some observations with the rat LGL leukemias may also provide some insight into the lineage of LGL. Moloney et al. first reported that low-dose irradiation (450 R) given at 4 months of age dramatically reduced the incidence of this tumor in W/Fu rats.[80] They later extended these results to F344 animals and demonstrated that 240 R significantly reduced the incidence of leukemia below that of unirradiated controls.[102] These authors have also shown that splenectomy at 1 to 2 months of age reduced the incidence of leukemia from approximately 20 to <4%.[103] These results suggest that the source of progenitors for this leukemia may be a highly radiosensitive cell which resides in the spleen. The results are consistent with the spleen being a rich source of normal LGL and would support the hypothesis that this organ may serve as a primary site for LGL differentiation and/or maturation.[104]

It therefore seems clear that the LGL leukemias from both man and experimental animals may provide important reagents for examining a number of detailed questions regarding the cellular structure, mechanism of action, specificity, and molecular nature of regulating LGL function. However, the use of these cells should not affect the importance of further studies on effector cells from normal animals. Instead, the use of LGL leukemias should be considered as complementary to these studies of normal NK and ADCC effector cells, and employed primarily for those studies which require large numbers of cells which could not be practically or economically obtained from normal animals. This approach should lead to the development and refinement of new ideas and hypotheses which can be subsequently tested in cells from normal animals.

REFERENCES

1. Timonen, T., Ranki, A., Saksela, E., and Häyry, P., Human natural cell-mediated cytotoxicity against fetal fibroblasts. III. Morphological and functional characterization of the effector cells, *Cell. Immunol.*, 48, 121, 1979.
2. Timonen, T., Ortaldo, J. R., and Herberman, R. B., Characteristics of human large granular lymphocytes and relationship to natural killer and K cells, *J. Exp. Med.*, 153, 569, 1981.
3. Timonen, T., Reynolds, C. W., Ortaldo, J. R., and Herberman, R. B., Isolation of human and rat natural killer cells, *J. Immunol. Methods*, 51, 269, 1982.
4. Reynolds, C. W., Timonen, T., and Herberman, R. B., Natural killer (NK) cell activity in the rat. I. Isolation and characterization of the effector cells, *J. Immunol.*, 127, 282, 1981.
5. Luini, W., Boraschi, D., Alberti, S., Aleotti, A., and Tagliabue, A., Morphological characterization of a cell population responsible for natural killer activity, *Immunology*, 43, 663, 1981.
6. Kumagai, K., Itoh, K., Suzuki, R., Hinuma, S., and Saitoh, F., Studies of murine large granular lymphocytes. I. Identification as effector cells in NK and K cytotoxicity, *J. Immunol.*, 129, 388, 1982.
7. Timonen, T., Saksela, E., Ranki, A., and Häyry, P., Fractionation, morphological, and functional characterization of effector cells responsible for human natural killer activity against cell-line targets, *Cell. Immunol.*, 48, 133, 1979.
8. Reynolds, C. W., Timonen, T., Holden, H. T., Hansen, C. T., and Herberman, R. B., Natural killer cells activity in the rat. Analysis of effector cell morphology and effect of interferon on natural killer cell function in the athymic (nude) rat, *Eur. J. Immunol.*, 12, 577, 1982.
9. Itoh, K., Suzuki, R., Umezu, Y., Hanaumi, K., and Kumugai, K., Studies on murine large granular lymphocytes. II. Tissue, strain and age distribution of LGL and LAL, *J. Immunol.*, 129, 395, 1982.
10. Santoli, D., Trinchieri, G., and Leifn, F. S., Cell-mediated cytotoxicity against virus-infected target cells in humans. I. Characterization of the effector lymphocytes, *J. Immunol.*, 121, 526, 1978.
11. Welsh, R. M., Jr., Zinkernagel, R. M., and Hallenbeck, L. A., Cytotoxic cells induced during lymphocytic choriomeningitis virus infection of mice. II. Specificities of the natural killer cells, *J. Immunol.*, 122, 475, 1979.
12. Lopez, C., Kirkpatrick, D., and Fitzgerald, P., The role of NK (HSV-1) effector cells in resistance to Herpesvirus infections in man, in *NK Cells and Other Natural Effector Cells*, Herberman, R. B., Ed., Academic Press, New York, 1982, 1445.
13. Brooks, C. G., Rees, R. C., and Leach, R. H., High nonspecific reactivity of normal lymphocytes against mycoplasma-infected target cells in cytotoxicity assays, *Eur. J. Immunol.*, 9, 159, 1979.
14. Trischmann, T., Tanowitz, H., Wittner, M., and Bloom, B. R., *Trypanosoma cruzi:* role of the immune response in the natural resistance of inbred strains of mice, *Exp. Parisitol.*, 45, 160, 1978.

15. Attallah, A. M., Lewis, F. A., Urritia-Shaw, A., Folks, T,. and Yeatman, T. J., Natural killer cells (NK) and antibody-dependent cell-mediated cytotoxicity (ADCC) components of *Schistosoma mansoni* infection, *Ant. Arch. Allergy Appl. Immunol.,* 63, 351, 1980.
16. Hatcher, F. M. and Kuhn, R. E., Natural killer (NK) cell activity against extracellular forms of *Trypanosoma cruzi,* in *NK Cells and Other Natural Effector Cells,* Herberman, R. B., Ed., Academic Press, New York, 1982, 1091.
17. Haller, O., Hansson, M., Kiessling, R., and Wigzell, H., Role of nonconventional natural killer cells in resistance against syngeneic tumor cells in vivo, *Nature (London),* 270, 609, 1977.
18. Hanna, N. and Fidler, I., Role of natural killer cells in the destruction of circulating tumor emboli, *J. Natl. Cancer Inst.,* 65, 801, 1980.
19. Riccardi, C., Santoni, T., Barlozzari, T., Puccetti, P., and Herberman, R. B., In vivo natural reactivity of mice against tumor cells, *Int. J. Cancer,* 25, 475, 1980.
20. Gorelik, E., Wiltrout, R. H., Okumura, K., Habu, S., and Herberman, R. B., Role of NK cells in the control of metastatic spread and growth of tumor cells in mice, *Int. J. Cancer,* 30, 107, 1982.
21. Warner, J. and Dennert, T., Effects of a cloned cell line with NK activity on bone marrow transplants, tumour development and metastasis in vivo, *Nature,* 300, 31, 1982.
22. Barlozzari, T., Reynolds, C. W., and Herberman, R. B., In vivo role of natural killer cells: involvement of large granular lymphocytes in the clearance of tumor cells in anti-asialo GM_1-treated rats, *J. Immunol.,* 131, 1024, 1983.
23. Hansson, M., Beran, M., Andersson, B., and Kiessling, R., Inhibition of in vitro granulopoiesis by autologous allogeneic human NK cells *J. Immunol.,* 129, 126, 1982.
24. Djeu, J. Y., Stocks, N., Zoon, K., Stanton, G. J., Timonen, T., and Herberman, R. B., Positive self regulation of cytotoxicity in human natural killer cells by production of interferon upon exposure to influenza and herpes virus, *J. Exp. Med.,* 156, 1222, 1982.
25. Domzig, W. and Stadler, B. M., The relation between human natural killer cells and interleukin 2, in *NK Cells and Other Natural Effector Cells,* Herberman, R. B., Ed., Academic Press, New York, 1982, 409.
26. Kasahara, T., Djeu, J. Y., Dougherty, S. F., and Oppenheim, J. J., Capacity of human granular lymphocytes (LGL) to produce multiple lymphokines: interleukin 2, interferon, and colony stimulating factor, *J. Immunol.,* 131(5), 2379, 1985.
27. Scala, G., Allavena, P., Djeu, J. Y., Kasahara, T., Ortaldo, J. R., Herberman, R. B., and Oppenheim, J. B., Human large granular lymphocytes (LGL) are potent producer of interleukin 1, *Nature,* 309(5963), 56, 1984.
28. McKenna, R. W., Parkin, J., Kersey, J. H., Gail-Peczalska, K. J., Peterson, L., and Brunning, R. D., Chronic lymphoproliferative disorder with unusual clinical, morphologic, ultrastructural and membrane surface marker characteristics, *Am. J. Med.,* 62, 588, 1977.
29. Bom-Van Noorloos, A. A., Pegels, H. G., van Oers, R. H. J., Silerbusch, J., Feltkamp-Vroom, T. M., Goudsmit, R., Zijlemaker, W. P., von dem Borne, A. E. G., and Melief, C. J. M., Proliferation of T_γ cells with killer-cell activity in two patients with neutropenia and recurrent infections, *N. Engl. J. Med.,* 302, 933, 1980.
30. Aisenberg, A. C., Wilkes, B. M., Harris, N. L., Ault, K. A., and Carey, R. W., Chronic T-cell lymphocytosis with neutropenia: report of a case studied with monoclonal antibody, *Blood,* 58, 818, 1981.
31. Hooks, J. J., Haynes, B. F., Detrich-Hooks, B., Diehl, L. F., Gerrard, T. L., and Fauci, A. S., Gamma (immune) interferon production by leukocytes from a patient with a T_G cell proliferation disease, *Blood,* 59, 198, 1982.
32. Pandolfi, F., Quinti, I., DeRossi, G., Frielingsdorf, A., Tonietti, G., Pasqualetti, D., and Aiuti, F., A population of sheep rosetting cells lacking T- and monocyte-specific antigens, as detected by monoclonal antibodies, *Clin. Immunol. Immunopathol.,* 22, 331, 1982.
33. Pandolfi, F., DeRossi, G., Semenzato, G., Quinti, I., Ranucci, A., DeSanctis, G., Lopez, M., Gasparotto, G., and Aiuti, F., Immunologic evaluation of T chronic lymphocytic leukemia cells: correlation among phenotype, functional activities, and morphology, *Blood,* 59, 688, 1982.
34. Pross, H. F., Pater, J., Dwosh, I., Giles, A., Gallinger, L. A., Rubin, P., Corbett, W. E. N., Galbraith, P., and Baines, M. G., Studies of human natural killer cells. III. Neutropenia associated with unusual characteristics of antibody-dependent and natural killer cell-mediated cytotoxicity, *J. Clin. Immunol.,* 2, 126, 1982.
35. Hocking, W. G., Singh, R., Schroff, R., and Golde, D. W., Cell mediated inhibition of erythropoiesis and megablastic anemia in T-cell chronic lymphocytic leukemia, *Cancer,* 51, 631, 1983.
36. Starkebaum, G., Martin, P. J., Singer, J. W., Lum, L. G., Price, T. H., Kadin, M. E., Raskind, W. H., and Fialkow, P. J., Chronic lymphocytosis with neutropenia: evidence for a novel abnormal T-cell population associated with antibody-mediated neutrophil destruction, *Clin. Immunol. Immunopathol.,* 27, 110, 1983.

37. Gallart, T., Anegón, I., Woessner, S., de la Fuente, R., Florensa, L., Sans-Sabafrén, C., and Vives, J., Clinically benign adult T-cell chronic lymphocytosis with unusual phenotype, *Lancet,* 769, 1983.
38. Stein, P., Peiper, S., Butler, D., Melvin, S., Williams, D., and Stass, S., Granular acute lymphoblastic leukemia, *Am. J. Clin. Pathol.,* 79, 126, 1983.
39. Ferrarini, M., Romagnani, S., Montesaro, E., Zicca, A., DePrete, G. F., Nocera, A., Maggi, E., Leprini, A., and Grossi, C. E., A lymphoproliferative disorder of the large granular lymphocytes with natural killer activity, *J. Clin. Immunol.,* 3, 30, 1983.
40. Pandolfi, F., Semenzanto, G., DeRossi, G., Quinti, I., Guglielmi, C., Pezzutto, A., Lopez, M., Tonietti, G., Fontana, L., Abo, T., and Aiuti, F., HNK-1 monoclonal antibody (Leu-7) in the identification of abnormal expansions of large granular lymphocytes, *Clin. Exp. Immunol.,* 529, 641, 1983.
41. Palulke, M., Eisneberg, L., Kaplan, J., Hussain, M., Kithier, K., Tabaczka, P., Mirchandani, I., and Tenenbaum, D., Natural killer and suppressor T-cell chronic lymphocytic leukemia, *Blood,* 62, 627, 1983.
42. Callard, R. E., Smith, C. M., Worman, C., Linch, D., Cawley, J. C., and Beverley, P. C. L., Unusual phenotype and function of an expanded subpopulation of T cells in patients with haemopoietic disorders, *Clin. Exp. Immunol.,* 43, 497, 1981.
43. Linch, D. C., Cawley, J. C., Worman, C. P., Galvin, M. C., Roberts, B. E., Callard, R. E., and Beverley, P. C. L., Abnormalities of T-cell subsets in patients with neutropenia and an excess of lymphocytes in the bone marrow, *Br. J. Haematol.,* 48, 137, 1981.
44. Gupta, S. and Fernandes, G., Natural killer and antibody-dependent cytotoxicity by T leukaemic blasts from acute lymphoblastic leukaemia, *Scand. J. Immunol.,* 16, 477, 1982.
45. Pandolfi, F., Semenzato, G., DeRossi, G., Strong, D. M., Quinti, I., Pezzutto, A., Mandelli, F., and Aiuti, F., Heterogeneity of T-CLL defined by monoclonal antibodies in nine patients, *Clin. Immunol. Immunopathol.,* 24, 330, 1982.
46. Rumke, H. C., Miedema, F., ten Berge, I. J. M., Terpstra, F., van der Reijden, J. H., van de Griend, R. J., de Briun, H. G., von dem Borne, A. E. G. K., Smit, J. W., Zeijlemaker, W. P., and Melief, C. J. M., Functional properties of T cells in patients with chronic T_γ lymphocytosis and chronic T cell neoplasia, *J. Immunol.,* 129, 419, 1982.
47. Linch, D. C., Cawley, J. C., MacDonald, S. M., Masters, G., Roberts, B. E., Antonis, A. H., Waters, A. K., Sieff, C., and Lydyard, P. M., Acquired pure red-cell aplasia associated with an increase of T cells bearing receptors for the Fc of IgG, *Acta Haematol.,* 65, 270, 1981.
48. Itoh, K., Tsuchikawa, K., Awataguchi, T., Shiiba, K., and Kumagai, K., A case of chronic lymphocytic leukemia with properties characteristic of natural killer cells, *Blood,* 61, 940, 1983.
49. Siegal, F. P., Rambotti, P., Siegal, M., Lopez, C., Smith, M., Davies, T. F., Osband, M., and Estren, S., Helper cell function of leukemic Leu-2a$^+$, histamine receptor$^+$, T_γ lymphocytes, *J. Immunol.,* 129, 1775, 1982.
50. Pandolfi, F., Strong, D. M., Slease, R. B., Smith, M. L., Ortaldo, J. R., and Herberman, R. B., Characterization of a suppressor T-cell chronic lymphocytic leukemia with ADCC but not NK activity, *Blood,* 56, 653, 1980.
51. Beverley, P. C. L., Linch, D. C., Callard, R. E., Worman, C. P., and Cawley, J. C., Cytopenia and T cell proliferation, *J. Clin. Immunol.,* 2, 1355, 1982.
52. Costello, C., Catovsky, D., O'Brien, M., Morilla, R., and Varadi, S., Chronic T-cell leukemias. I. Morphology, cytochemistry and ultrastructure, *Leukemia Res.,* 4, 463, 1980.
53. Nagasawa, T., Abe, T., and Nakagawa, T., Pure red cell aplasia and hypogammaglobulinemia associated with T_γ-cell chronic lymphocytic leukemia, *Blood,* 57, 1025, 1981.
54. Delforge, A., Bron, D., and Stryckmans, P., Neutropenia associated with excess of T cell lymphocytes, *Br. J. Haematol.,* 49, 488, 1981.
55. Riethmüller, G., Lohmeyer, J., Rieber, E. P., Feucht, H., Schlimok, G., and Thiel, E., Unique combination of surface markers on human NK cells: a phenotypic compromise at last, in *NK Cells and Other Natural Effector Cells,* Herberman, R. B., Ed., Academic Press, New York, 1982, 53.
56. Thiel, E., Stünkel, K., Rieber, E. P., Rodt, H., Thierfelder, S., Feucht, H., Meier, C. R., Goldstein, G., Kung, P. C., and Schlimok, G., Chronic lymphocytic leukemia of T_G-type with NK- and ADCC activity: demonstration of T-lymphocytic and monocyte antigens, *Immunobiology,* 159, 141, 1981.
57. Thiel, E., Schlimok, G., Stünkel, K., Rieber, E. P., Huhn, D., and Feucht, H., Chronic lymphocytic leukemia of T_G-type with NK- and ADCC-activity: demonstration of T-lymphocytic and monocytic antigens, in *Mechanisms of Lymphocyte Activation,* Resch, K. and Kirchner, H., Eds., Elsevier, Amsterdam, 1981, 294.
58. Schlimok, G., Thiel, E., Rieber, E. P., Huhn, D., Feucht, H., Lohmeyer, J., and Riethmüller, G., Chronic leukemia with a hybrid surface phenotype (T lymphocyte/myelomonocytic): leukemic cells displaying natural killer activity and antibody-dependent cellular cytotoxicity, *Blood,* 59, 1157, 1982.

59. Schlimok, G., Thiel, E., Rieber, E. P., Huhn, D., Feucht, H., Renner, D., and Riethmüller, G., Proliferation of T_γ-lymphocytes in two patients: clinical features and functional properties of the proliferating cells, *Klin. Wochenschr.*, 60, 133, 1982.
60. Huhn, D., Thiel, E., Rodt, H., Schlimok, G., Theml, H., and Rieber, P., Subtypes of T-cell chronic lymphocytic leukemia, *Cancer*, 51, 1434, 1983.
61. Kai, S., Hamano, T., Fujita, S., Nakamuta, K., Hara, H., and Nagai, K., Suppression of mitogen- and alloantigen-induced proliferation by chronic lymphocytic leukemia cells of T-cell origin, *Clin. Immunol. Immunopathol.*, 17, 427, 1980.
62. van de Griend, R. J., van der Reijden, J. H., Bolhuis, R. L. H., Melief, C. J. M., van dem Borne, A. E. G., and Roos, D., Analysis of lymphoproliferative diseases by use of enzyme parameters: a useful addition to monoclonal antibodies for subclassification, *Blood*, 62, 669, 1983.
63. Ortaldo, J. R., Sharrow, S. O., Timonen, T., and Herberman, R. B., Determination of surface antigens on highly purified human NK cells by flow cytometry with monoclonal antibodies, *J. Immunol.*, 127, 2401, 1981.
64. Lohmeyer, J., Rieber, P., Feucht, H., Johnson, J., Hadam, and Riethmüller, G., A subset of human natural killer cells isolated and characterized by monoclonal antibodies, *Eur. J. Immunol.*, 11, 997, 1981.
65. Lohmeyer, J., Reiber, E. P., Feucht, H., and Riethmüller, G., Heterogeneity of human natural killer cells (NK) revealed by monoclonal antibodies, *Immunobiology*, 159, 138, 1981.
66. Timonen, R., Ortaldo, J. R., Vose, B. M., Henkart, M., Alvarez, J., and Herberman, R. B., Cultures of human natural killer cells (large granular lymphocytes) and T cells in the presence of interleukin-2-containing conditioned medium, *J. Reticuloendothel. Soc.*, 33, 67, 1983.
67. Hoffman, R., Kopel, S., Hsu, S. D., Dainiak, N., and Zanjani, E. D., T cell chronic lymphocytic leukemia: presence in bone marrow and peripheral blood of cells that suppress erythropoiesis in vitro, *Blood*, 52, 255, 1978.
68. Mangan, K. F., Chikkappa, G., Scharfman, W. B., and Desforges, J. F., Evidence for reduced erythroid burst (BFU-E) promoting functions of T lymphocytes in the pure red cell aplasia of chronic lymphocytic leukemia, *Exp. Haematol. (Copenhagan)*, 9, 489, 1981.
69. Mangan, K. F., Chikkappa, G., Bieler, L. Z., and Scharfman, W. B., The role of T lymphocytes bearing Fc receptors for IgM or IgG in the pathogenesis of pure red cell aplasia in a patient with chronic lymphocytic leukemia, in *Experimental Hematology Today*, Baum, S. J., Ledney, G. D., and Khan, A., Eds., S. Karger, Basel, 1981, 161.
70. Mangan, K. F., Chikkappa, G., and Farley, P. C., T gamma (T_γ) cells suppress growth of erythroid colony-forming units in vitro in the pure red cell aplasia of B-cell chronic lymphocytic leukemia, *J. Clin. Invest.*, 70, 1148, 1982.
71. Grossi, C. E., Webb, S. R., Zicca, A., Lydyard, P. M., Moretta, L., Mingari, M. C., and Cooper, M. D., Morphological and histochemical analysis of two human T-cell subpopulations bearing receptors for IgM or IgG, *J. Exp. Med.*, 147, 1405, 1978.
72. Dainiak, N., Kulkarni, V., Howard, D., Kalmanti, M., Dewey, M. C., and Hoffman, R., Mechanism of abnormal erythropoiesis in malignancy, *Cancer*, 51, 1101, 1983.
73. Torok-Storb, B., Martin, P. J., and Hansen, J. A., Regulation of in vitro erythropoiesis by normal T cells: evidence for two T cell subsets with opposing function, *Blood*, 58, 171, 1981.
74. Górski, A., Rowińska, D., Skopinska, E., and Orlowski, T., Circulating suppressor cells in aplastic anemia, *Vox. Sang.*, 36, 356, 1979.
75. Amore, M., Abdou, N. L., Robinson, M. G., and Abdou, N. I., Aplastic anemia associated with bone marrow suppressor T-cell hyperactivity: successful treatment with antithymocyte globulin, *Am. J. Hematol.*, 5, 25, 1978.
76. Ascensão, J., Kagan, W., Moore, M., Pahwa, R., Hansen, J., and Good, R., Aplastic anaemia: evidence for an immunological mechanism, *Lancet*, 669, 1976.
77. Moretta, L., Moretta, A., Canonica, G. W., Bacigalupo, A., Mingari, M. C., and Cerottini, J. C., Receptors for immunoglobulins on resting and activated human T cells, *Immunol. Rev.*, 56, 141, 1981.
78. Insel, R. A., Melewicz, F. M., LaVia, M. F., and Balch, C. M., Morphology, surface markers, and in vitro responses of a human leukemic T cell, *Clin. Immunol. Immunopathol.*, 4, 382, 1975.
79. Uchiyama, T., Sagawa, K., Takatsuki, K., and Uchino, H., Effect of adult T-cell leukemia cells on pokeweed mitogen-induced normal B-cell differentiation, *Clin. Immunol. Immunopathol.*, 10, 24, 1978.
80. Moloney, W. C., Boschetti, A. E., and King, V. P., Observations on leukemia in Wistar Furth rats, *Cancer Res.*, 29, 938, 1969.
81. Ward, J. M. and Reynolds, C. W., Large granular lymphocyte leukemia, a heterogenous lymphocytic leukemia in F344 rats, *Am. J. Pathol.*, 111, 1, 1983.

82. Reynolds, C. W., Bere, E. W., Jr., and Ward, J. M., Natural killer activity in the rat. IV. Characterization of transplantable large granular lymphocyte (LGL) leukemias in the F344 rat, *J. Immunmol.*, 132, 534, 1984.
83. Reynolds, C. W., Ward, J. M., Denn, A. C., III, and Bere, E. W., Characterization of large granular lymphocyte (LGL) tumors in the rat, in *B and T Cell tumors,* Vitetta, E. S., Ed., Academic Press, New York, 1982, 51.
84. Reynolds, C. W., Ward, J. M., Denn, A. C., III, and Bere, E. W., Jr., Identification and characterization of large granular lymphocyte (LGL) leukemias in F344 rats, in *NK Cells and Other Natural Effector Cells,* Herberman, R. B. Ed., Academic Press, New York, 1982, 1161.
85. Reynolds, C. W., Denn, A. C., III, Bere, E. W., and Ward, J. M., Characterization of large granular lymphocyte (LGL) tumors in the F344 rat, *Immunobiology,* 163, 409, 1982.
86. Fish, D. C., Djurickovic, D. B., and Huebner, R. J., Conversion of two lethal rat tumors to protective vaccines, submitted.
87. Davey, F. R. and Moloney, W. C., Postmortem observations on Fischer rats with leukemia and other disorders, *Lab. Invest.*, 23, 327, 1970.
88. Goodman, D. G., Ward, J. M., Squire, R. A., Chu, K. C., and Linhart, M. S., Neoplastic and nonneoplastic lesions in aging F344 rats, *Toxicol. Appl. Pharmacol.*, 48, 237, 1979.
89. Sachsteder, M. R., Occurrence of spontaneous tumors in the germfree F344 rat, *J. Natl. Cancer Inst.*, 57, 1371, 1976.
90. Kusewitt, D. F., Hahn, F. F., and Pickrell, J. A., Hematologic and serum chemical characteristics of mononuclear leukemia in Fischer 344 rats, *Lab. Anim. Sci.*, 32, 275, 1982.
91. Moloney, W. C., Boschetti, A. E., and King, V. P., Spontaneous leukemia in Fischer rats, *Cancer Res.*, 30, 41, 1970.
92. Cantrell, D. A., Robins, R. A., Brooks, C. G., and Baldwin, R. W., Phenotype of rat natural killer cells defined by monoclonal antibodies marking rat lymphocyte subsets, *Immunology,* 45, 97, 1982.
93. Reynolds, C. W., Sharrow, S. O., Ortaldo, J. R., and Herberman, R. B., Natural killer (NK) activity in the rat. II. Analysis of surface antigens on LGL by flow cytometry, *J. Immunol.*, 127, 2204, 1981.
94. Goldschneider, I., Metcalf, D., Battyl, F., and Mandel, T., Analysis of rat hemopoietic cells on the fluorescence-activated cell sorter. I. Isolation of pluripotent hemopoietic stem cells and granulocyte-macrophage progenitor cells, *J. Exp. Med.*, 152, 419, 1980.
95. Grossi, C. E., Cadoni, A., Zicca, A., Leprini, A., and Ferrarini, M., Large granular lymphocytes in human peripheral blood: ultrastructural and cytochemical characterization of the granules, *Blood,* 59, 277, 1982.
96. Payne, C. M. and Glasser, L., Evaluation of surface markers on normal human lymphocytes containing parallel tubular arrays: a quantitative ultrastructural study, *Blood,* 57, 567, 1981.
97. Reynolds, C. W. and Herberman, R. B., In vivo augmentation of rat natural killer (NK) cell activity, *J. Immunol.*, 126, 1581, 1981.
98. Henkart, P., Millard, P., Reynolds, C., and Henkart, M., Purification of cytoplasmic granules from rat NK tumors, *Immunobiology,* 163, 404, 1982.
99. Millard, P. J., Henkart, M. P., Reynolds, C. W., and Henkart, P. A., Purification and properties of cytoplasmic granules from cytotoxic rat LGL tumors, *J. Immunol.*, 132, 3197, 1984.
100. Wright, S. and Bonavida, B., personal communication.
101. Wright, S. and Bonavida, B., Selective lysis of NK-sensitive target cells by a soluble mediator released from murine spleen cells and human peripheral blood lymphocytes, *J. Immunol.*, 126, 1516, 1981.
102. Hellman, S., Moloney, W. C., and Meissner, W. A., Paradoxical effect of irradiation on tumor incidence in the rat: implications for radiation therapy, *Cancer Res.*, 42, 433, 1982.
103. Moloney, W. C. and King, V. P., Reduction of leukemia incidence following splenectomy in the rat, *Cancer Res.*, 33, 573, 1973.
104. Levy, E. M., Kumar, V., and Bennett, M., Natural killer activity and suppressor cells in irradiated mice repopulated with a mixture of cells from normal and ^{89}Sr-treated donors, *J. Immunol.*, 127, 1428, 1981.

INDEX

A

B

C

D

E

F

G

H

I

K

L

M

N

O

T

V

X

Y

Shepherd College Library
QR 185.8.K54I46 1986 rusc
Immunobiology of natural killer cells /
3 4550 200103955 9

QR
185.8
.K54
I46
1986
v.1

0172308

DATE DUE

MAR 18 1997
MY 15 '98